Percutaneous Nephrolithotomy

Guohua Zeng • Kemal Sarica
Editors

Percutaneous Nephrolithotomy

Springer

Editors
Guohua Zeng
Department of Urology
and Guangdong Key Laboratory
of Urology
The First Affiliated Hospital of
Guangzhou Medical University
Guangzhou, Guangdong
China

Kemal Sarica
Department of Urology
Biruni University Medical School
Istanbul
Turkey

ISBN 978-981-15-0574-4 ISBN 978-981-15-0575-1 (eBook)
https://doi.org/10.1007/978-981-15-0575-1

This Springer imprint is published by the registered company Springer Nature Singapore Pte Ltd.
The registered company address is: 152 Beach Road, #21-01/04 Gateway East, Singapore 189721, Singapore

Foreword

It is refreshing to find a book that is totally devoted to percutaneous stone extraction. I am delighted with the dramatic changes that have occurred in the field over the past 40 years, and this book will bring the reader up to date. It covers all aspects of percutaneous stone extraction starting with the early days of endourology to the present time.

There are invariably different approaches in treating stones that vary in size and consistency as well as stone location. It is important that the competent endourologist is not only aware of these techniques but also is facile with them. For example, one may prefer to have a patient in the prone position for renal access. However, if the patient has stones in an upper calyx and additional stones in an adjacent upper calyx, a different approach may be preferable. In such a situation, one can use a two-team approach with simultaneous ureteroscopy and stone extraction ureteroscopically or alternatively grasp the stone ureteroscopically and pass it to the endourologist who has the nephroscope in the kidney.

When I started doing percutaneous procedures, I elected to dilate the tract to 30 French in order to extract a 1 cm stone. The downsizing of instruments diminishes the morbidity of the procedure, and hopefully further reduction in the size of instruments will continue.

I congratulate the editors in their selection of authors for the various chapters. They are all knowledgeable and highly respected endourologists and undoubtedly the reader will benefit from their extensive experience.

This book is a "must" for both the young and more experienced endourologists, as the guidance it provides will certainly benefit their patients.

Hempstead, NY, USA — Arthur D. Smith

Preface

Percutaneous nephrolithotomy (PCNL) was originally introduced back at 1976 by Fernström and Johansson. Since then, it has gradually evolved to be one of the main endourologic treatment options. Over the past four decades, tremendous changes have occurred in the PCNL technique. Miniaturization of the working instruments, improvement of patient positioning, safer and more accurate tract creation techniques, new imaging modalities, evolvement of intracorporeal lithotripters, and incorporation of flexible instruments for efficient collecting system screening have allowed the continuous reshaping of this field.

Given such advances, there is a need for a "textbook" that brings together all aspects of PCNL techniques. The goal of this book is to provide the most recent clinical information on PCNL techniques and innovative materials. For that purpose, we have been fortunate to be able to recruit experts and opinion leaders around the world to outline their techniques clearly and concisely. We are deeply grateful to the authors for contributing their enlightening, informative chapters. This book could never have appeared without the exceptional cooperation of all concerned.

The book begins with some historical data, which will support the reader in understanding the evolution of the instruments and techniques. The renal anatomy, armamentariums, operating room setup, and anesthesia-related PCNL are then described and presented in illustrations. The book continues with the description of the new developments in the PCNL techniques (mini-Perc, micro-PCNL, UMP, SMP, ECIRS). The next chapters are dedicated to the PCNL in special situations and pediatric cases. Finally, there are entire sections on patient's follow-up and training in PCNL. Each chapter is supported by a shortlist of up-to-date references that provide a basis for further reading if needed. Selected figures illustrate key concepts.

We believe that this is the most comprehensive reference book on PCNL techniques currently available. In a work of this nature, there is bound to be some overlap between some of the chapters. However, this only enhances the information provided rather than being repetitive. We truly hope this book offers real support for every practitioner in general, and every urologist in particular.

Guangzhou, China — Guohua Zeng
Istanbul, Turkey — Kemal Sarica

Contents

1 **History of PNL** 1
Peter Alken

2 **Anatomy for PNL** 13
Wen Zhong

3 **Armamentariums Related to Percutaneous Nephrolithotripsy (PCNL)** 23
Athanasios Dellis and Athanasios Papatsoris

4 **Operating Room Setup for PCNL** 31
Victoria Jahrreiss and Mehmet Özsoy

5 **Preoperative Assessment and Patient Preparation for PCNL Surgery** 37
Simon K. S. Choong and Gautam Kumar

6 **Positioning During PNL** 43
András Hoznek

7 **Anesthesia** 53
Wenqi Wu

8 **Principles of a Perfect Puncture for Percutaneous Nephrolithotomy** 69
David B. Bayne and Thomas L. Chi

9 **Tract Dilation During PNL** 79
Thomas Knoll

10 **Intracorporeal Lithotripsy During PCNL** 83
Xiaofeng Gao, Ziyu Fang, Hao Dong, Fei Xie, Chaoyue Lu, and Zeyu Wang

11 **Tubeless PCNL** 93
Julian Veser and Christian Seitz

12 **Complications Related with PCNL and Their Management** 103
Iliya Saltirov and Kremena Petkova

13 Microperc 113
Stefano Paolo Zanetti, Matteo Fontana, and Emanuele Montanari

14 Ultra-Mini PCNL (UMP) 127
Janak D. Desai

15 Super-Mini-PCNL (SMP) 131
Guohua Zeng and Wei Zhu

16 Minimal-Invasive PCNL (Mini-PCNL) 137
Sven Lahme

17 ECIRS (Endoscopic Combined IntraRenal Surgery): From Background Actor to Main Character of the Endourological Treatment of Urolithiasis 151
Cesare Marco Scoffone and Cecilia Maria Cracco

18 PCNL in Special Situations 161
Diego M. Carrion, Ramón Cansino, Cristina Ballesteros Ruiz, Juan Gómez Rivas, Juan A. Mainez Rodríguez, Jose R. Pérez-Carral, and Luis Martínez-Piñeiro

19 Percutaneous Nephrolithotomy in Children (Pediatric PNL) 179
Rasim Guzel and Kemal Sarica

20 Natural History of Residual Stone Fragments Following PCNL 187
Mohammad A. Alomar and Alaa A. Mokhtar

21 Training in Percutaneous Nephrolithotomy 195
Abdullatif Aydın, Ahmed Al-Jabir, Brandon Smith, and Kamran Ahmed

History of PNL

1

Peter Alken

1.1 Introduction

A general belief is that the past is well known just as the future is unpredictable. If the past is presented as history its facts are inevitably transformed into personal views. The view of the historian will depend on the integrity of his data mining, which is bound to be incomplete. Easy access to ancient archives of medical journals is difficult and practically limited to what is electronically accessible in the English language; early and very early reports probably remain dormant in old textbooks in many countries. Many of these known or unknown historical reports have one thing in common: they did not stimulate a breakthrough into a new era. As English has become the prevailing scientific language, articles written in other languages are lost because they cannot be read and understood by the scientific community. Consequently facts and procedures are unintentionally reinvented or described as new and the past becomes "unpredictable". History is a personal story and reading publications on the same topic offers confusing if not conflicting views [1–5].

History is not a bus that everybody jumped on at the same time to go in the same direction.

P. Alken (✉)
Department of Urology, University Clinic Mannheim, Mannheim, Germany
e-mail: peter.alken@medma.uni-heidelberg.de

1.2 Nephrostomy

Operative nephrostomy as done until the 1970s was a relatively simple surgical procedure from a mere technical point of view, but the necessary dissection and exposure of the kidney could be difficult to perform in the acute or the chronic situation. Despite being a kind of least-invasive surgical approach reserved as a last resort measure in the acute critically sick patient, it was accompanied by substantial risks and a frequently complicated postoperative course [6]. Offered to patients with a complicated chronic situation like recurrently failed urinary diversion, operative nephrostomy was a palliative, permanently disabling procedure.

Percutaneous nephrolithotomy is an operative procedure with several consecutive steps. Access can be established in different positions and by different techniques using fluoroscopy, sonography or both. Tract dilation may be achieved by a variety of instruments or is omitted with the one-step technique. Tract size and instrument type are a matter of choice just as the technique of stone disintegration. The type of postprocedural drainage depends on the perfection of the individual procedure. The two common core processes of PNL are establishment of access by a

G. Zeng, K. Sarica (eds.), *Percutaneous Nephrolithotomy*,
https://doi.org/10.1007/978-981-15-0575-1_1

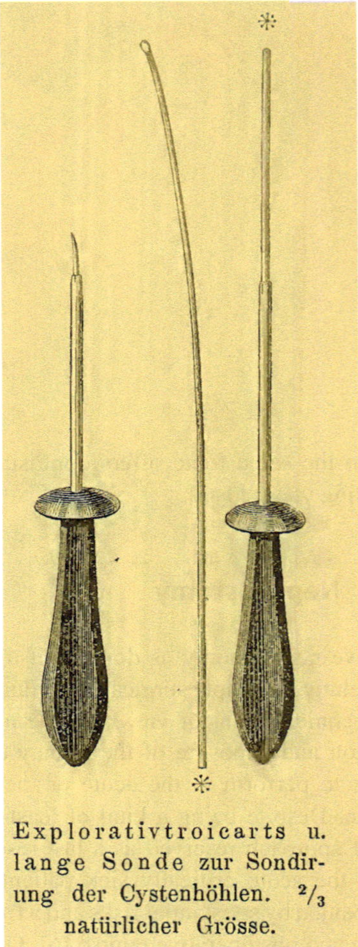

Fig. 1.1 Straight trocar for percutaneous puncture of the kidney by Simon 1876 [7]

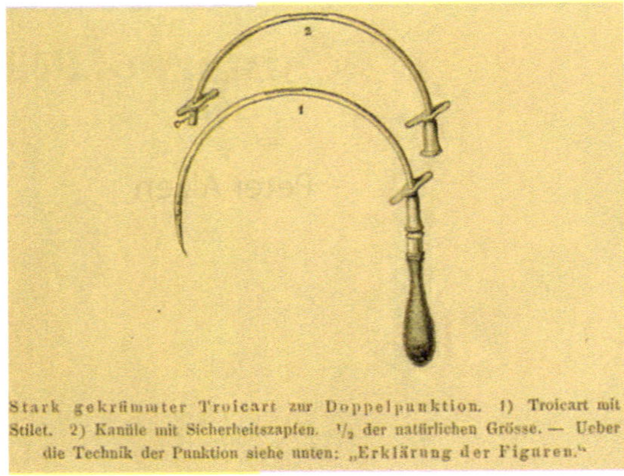

Fig. 1.2 Curved trocar for percutaneous puncture of the kidney by Simon 1876 [7]

non-operative procedure and endoscopy of the renal collecting system.

Nonsurgical percutaneous procedures to the kidney, the renal collecting system, or the perirenal space for different indications are not exclusively recent. Simon who performed the first successful nephrectomy describes in his textbook from 1871 in the chapter about hydro- and pyonephrosis the trocar puncture of the kidney (Figs. 1.1 and 1.2) with or without leaving a cannula. He refers to other cases described in the German, French and English literature [7].

Also in modern times percutaneous drainage of the kidney was an outgrowth of renal punctures originally done to establish proper diagnosis in silent kidneys or cases of renal displacement due to unknown space-occupying lesions [8]. These procedures were done with injection of a contrast dye to differentiate cysts from solid tumors; in case of hydronephrotic kidneys, this could be used to perform antegrade pyelography as described by Casey and Goodwin: "Our use of this technique was an accidental discovery during needle biopsy of a "nonfunctioning" kidney in August 1953" [9]. In their publication, they refer to earlier or simultaneous work [10–12]. Typically, these authors punctured the collecting system, drained a little bit of urine or pus, depending on the case and, subsequently, submitted the patient to operative nephrostomy. Goodwin and his colleagues described in the same year percutaneous pyelostomy as the logical next step after percutaneous pyelography [13].

This procedure did not get widespread acceptance. A simple explanation might be the fact that Goodwin and his colleagues were exceptionally, radiologically active urologists. In 1950 they had published a paper on translumbar aortography [14] mentioning the "unfailing cooperation" of a radiologist but not listing the latter as co-author. Different from this group, most urologists at that time obviously had no such direct access to fluoroscopy and X-ray equipment and preferred keeping the patients requiring drainage of obstructed kidneys in the urologist's hands instead of referring them to a radiologist. This strict typical American division of urologists' and radiologists' tasks has continued through the years up to today and explains procedural differences between America and other countries. In 2002 Segura commented on this problem [15]:

> *Goodwin used plain x-ray films to confirm placement of his trocars and tubes. Fluoroscopy was much less commonly available than today and, when available, it was securely in the hands of radiology … it seems clear that it was the widespread availability of fluoroscopy that was the key to the popularity that percutaneous nephrostomy tube placement enjoys today. I believe that had there existed something like an "endourology table" in those days, we, and not radiology, would be putting these tubes in today, and we would have been doing it for 50 years and not just 25.*

The question who should establish percutaneous access to the kidney is handled differently in different countries, and there is considerable conflicting literature on this topic.

It is only in the late 1960s and early 1970s that percutaneous nephrostomy became popular in various countries. In 1977 Barbaric and Wood [16] reviewed the 121 cases described in the literature up to that time, of which a third was treated because of obstructing calculous disease. All these stone patients were submitted to open stone surgery after temporary percutaneous drainage despite the fact that reports on endoscopy through operatively established tracts were known. These single series of percutaneous nephrostomy were usually small and authored by radiologists. In 1978 the total number of cases published was >500 with a very low major complication rate of 4% [17]. Already at that time approximately 20% of the cases were done in supine position. But it took another 10 years until this position was suggested again for percutaneous stone removal [18].

As radiologists were the primary intervening physicians for PNL in many countries, percutaneous nephrostomies were done without a preceding ureteral catheterization and retrograde pyelography [17, 19]. Also in our series, even after taking over access establishment from radiologists to urologists, we did not use preliminary retrograde pyelography and the patient was kept in a prone position during the whole procedure.

1.2.1 Ultrasound-Assisted Nephrostomy

Pedersen was the first to use sonography and fluoroscopy to guide and control the puncture [20].

In our experience, adopting the technique of sonographically controlled puncture on an x-ray table in 1978 was the step to become independent of the radiologist and take the whole procedure into urological hands [21, 22].

1.3 Tract Dilation, Tract Size, Timing

Tract dilation was initially a several-days-to-weeks-session procedure done with whatever available, plastic tubes, catheters of different material, or hollow metallic Hegar cervical dilators (Fig. 1.3).

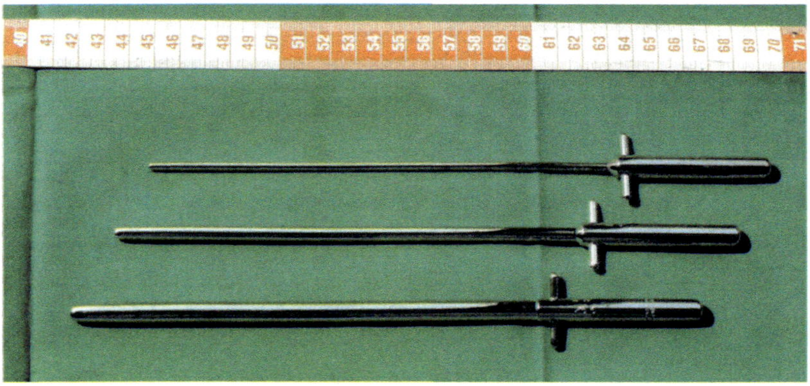

Fig. 1.3 Hollow cervical Hegar dilators used for nephrostomy tract dilation

All techniques using malleable conical dilators and plastic sheaths are outgrowths of angiographic radiological procedures originally introduced by Seldinger in 1953 [23].

The principle is "the catheter being introduced on a flexible leader through the puncture hole after withdrawal of the puncture needle" [23]. Radiologists introduced these procedures into PNL. The material was available by companies serving radiologists.

Tract size was a matter of stone size regarded as appropriate for removal and the equipment available for stone disintegration. Those who had no technique to disintegrate stones used large diameter tracts to expand the indication. Establishment of access, tract dilation, and stone removal was initially done [24] and is still done in many places as a several-days-, several- or separate-steps procedure especially if the urologist-surgeon does not establish the access. Fernström, a radiologist, primarily used Couvelaire catheters up to 24 F [25] and later on tapered plastic dilators rarely up to 32 F [26]. In 1982 the radiologist Rusnak et al. described the use of polyurethane dilators gradually enlarging to 30 F to allow the introduction of large catheters for the removal of stones up to 1 cm in diameter. A 34 F sleeve that remained in place after removal of the dilator is known today as the Amplatz sheath [27]. The largest tract size reported in 1982 was 50 F [28].

Clayman et al. introduced balloon dilation of the tract [29]. This balloon dilator was also primarily in radiological use for angioplasties [30].

The principle of the metallic telescope dilators developed in 1980 was to allow for a safe one-session procedure. They were the first purposely designed instruments for PNL (Fig. 1.4) [31, 32].

During the dilation, a straight puncture path was maintained; the tract was continuously tamponaded to reduce bleeding; the sheaths of the 18, 21 and 26 F nephroscopes were advanced like one of the dilators. No additional sheaths of larger size like a 34 F Amplatz sheath were used as the 26 F was the actual sheath of the continuous flow nephroscope [33].

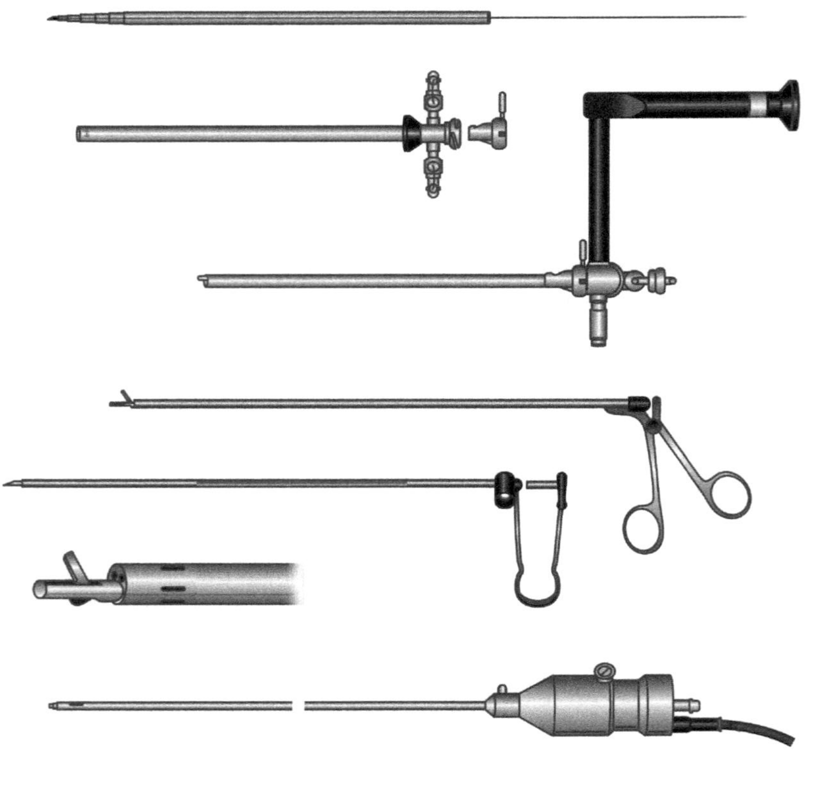

Fig. 1.4 Instruments for PNL (telescope dilators, sheath, nephroscope, graspers, ultrasound disintegrator)

The dilators were initially produced by Karl Storz in 1980 and later on by Wolf [34] and Olympus [35] to realize the same principles with their instruments.

Small size tracts are nowadays popular. In China, Wu et al. did Mini-PNL with a 12.5 F ureteroscope for staghorn stones since 1988 [36]. An 11/13 F sheath and a 7.7 F pediatric cystoscope were used by Jackman et al. in their "mini-perc" series in 1998. Somehow their procedure also included one-step dilation [37]. A similar procedure in pediatric PNL was published by Helal et al. [38]. Single-step dilation has become even more popular [39] and goes perfectly well with smaller tracts [40].

1.3.1 Timing

All first-day urological Matadors—the Mainz (Alken), the Freiburg (Korth), the Vienna (Marberger), the Mayo (Segura), the Minnesota (Smith) and the London (Wickham) groups—of modern PNL started with puncture, dilation, endoscopy done in several sessions. Changing to a one session PNL was not easy: We failed in a third of our first 90 one-session patients [32], Clayman et al. in 69% [41] and Wickham et al. in 5 of 10 patients [42].

1.4 Stone Removal

Percutaneous procedures were initially done endoscopically because fluoroscopy was not available; Chester D. Allen from Memphis, Tennessee reported in 1935 on a successive dilation of a 14 F operatively established nephrostomy tract within a few days to 24 F to pass a 24 F cystoscope for stone removal [43]. Rupel and Brown are usually given credit to have done this first [44]. Only 10 more well-documented similar cases were published between 1941 and 1980 [45].

The switch to radiological control came with Fernström's publication [25]. Stimulated by reports on percutaneous extraction of missed biliary stones, the radiologist Fernström extracted kidney stones under radiological control through percutaneously established tracts since 1974 and published in 1976 three cases together with the urologist Johansson [25]. They dilated the tract to 22–32 F during several weeks, later on days, and removed the stones with Dormia baskets or Randall forceps. Extractable stone size was limited by tract size, but in some cases the stones broke during removal attempts and fragments were extracted thereafter. By 1982 they had successful treated 34 patients with percutaneous tracts and 5 with operative nephrostomies with a mean stone size of 1 cm [26]. Until the first world congress on percutaneous renal surgery, their successful case number had increased to 63 patients. They never had proceeded to endoscopic procedures and Fernström consequently concluded that 2 cm represents the upper limit for stone extraction. These were exceptional cases and the mean diameter in their series was 1 cm [46]. However, at that time endoscopically controlled PNL had already begun.

Urologists had the patients but radiologists had the necessary x-ray equipment and experience with percutaneous techniques. Therefore, to establish access for PNL was initially a radiologically controlled procedure and still is a shared business in many countries. This is frequently demonstrated by the authorship of publications.

The first five cases published by Smith et al. in 1978 and 1979 [47, 48] were treated under radiological control by chemolysis in four and/or extraction in two cases. But the authors knew and quoted the publications by Rupel and Brown [44] and Bissada [49] who had done endoscopy.

In 1982 the Minnesota team—with six radiologists and three urologists involved—regarded "the introduction of large tubes into the kidney as key to successful percutaneous extraction of urinary calculi." The 25 patients were treated preferably, by extraction through 34 and 50 F tracts [28].

Extraction was the predominant form of treatment in their subsequent publications on 100/126 patients in 1984 [41, 50]. This group initially focused on mechanical tools for stone removal [51, 52]. In a few cases, they used electrohydraulic lithotripsy, which was popular at that time for the treatment of bladder stones. Also Smith in his own series of the first 100 patients done since 1982 preferred to dilate the tract to 34 French, and remove stones up to 1.5 cm intact sometimes even together with the sheath [53]. The London Group also temporarily favored it because of an unacceptable but exceptionally high complication rate with ultrasound lithotripsy [54].

Electrohydraulic lithotripsy, having been applied in operatively established tracts first in 1969 [55], is a disintegration technique with highest risk to tissue and instruments and is used today only very rarely [56].

Two German groups independently worked on ultrasound lithotripsy together with Storz [57, 58] and Wolf, respectively [59]. In 1976 two cases of ultrasound disintegration through operatively established tracts were independently performed [60, 61]. Our series of PNL was based on the positive in-house experience with the Storz ultrasound lithotripter [61] and initially also on the skills of our radiologist [6, 62, 63]. We—the radiologist Günther, the urologists Hutschenreiter and the author—never relied on stone extraction or chemolysis alone but on combined endoscopy and ultrasound lithotripsy from the very start [45, 64–66]. With the development of purposely built instruments the numbers of PNL steadily increased until PNL had replaced 50% of our surgical procedures for stones (Figs. 1.5 and 1.6).

Marberger [67] and Segura [68] used the Wolf equipment and published their first series in 1982.

As they had a reliable disintegration technique, they did not need large tracts and had

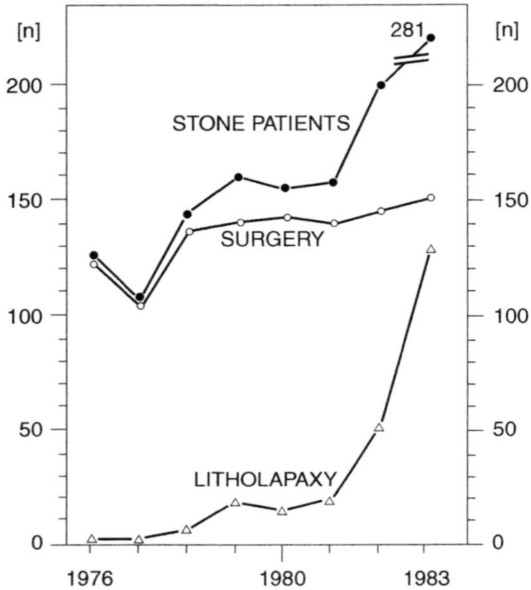

Fig. 1.5 Frequency of stone therapy at the Department of Urology, Mainz University, Germany 1976–1983 (litholapaxy = PNL)

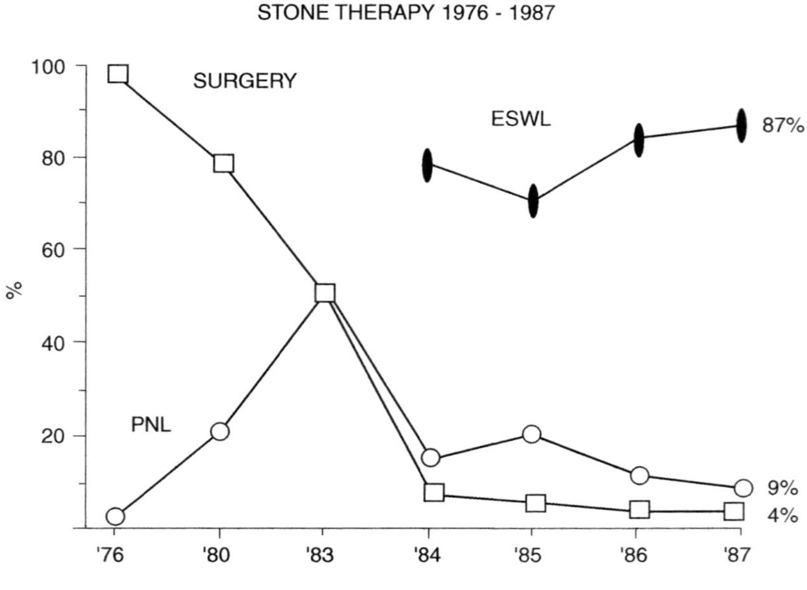

Fig. 1.6 Frequency of stone therapy at the Department of Urology, Mainz University, Germany 1976–1987

adopted our technique with 24 F continuous flow nephroscopes.

Wickham had seen PNL during his visits to our department in Mainz and the author's presentation about our technique "Percutaneous stone removal from the kidney" at the fourth annual meeting of the European Intra-Renal Surgery Society in Bern in 1979. In that year he started his series [69] without ultrasound lithotripsy [70]. He seems to have been unhappy after his first 36 cases [70] and with the first 50 patients [71] using the ultrasonic lithotripter in 9: "The necessity for ultrasonic lithotripsy greatly prolonged the operative time … The Wolf lithotripter was cumbersome, slow and unpleasantly noisy." His experience was in contrast to ours and that of Marberger [67] and Segura [68]. Ultrasound lithotripsy has been developed further and is still the preferred method to treat large stones [56].

1.5 Exit Strategy

In the old days when matured tracts were used, it was not necessary to leave a nephrostomy tube after stone extraction and an uneventful procedure because the tract would still be open for a few hours in case of postoperative problems and would close by itself.

With the one session approach the postoperative outcome is less predictable. Bellman et al. were the first to report on a large series with a planned no-nephrostomy strategy and a positive outcome [72]. Initially the "no-nephrostomy" strategy was leaving a double-J-stent instead of a nephrostomy and leaving nothing is the "no-tube" solution.

1.6 The Effects of ESWL and URS

The fact that we got very early, in December 1983, the fourth ESWL machine in Germany led to a steep decrease of the PNL numbers. Our PNL procedures were reduced to approximately 10% of all stone cases referred to us (Fig. 1.6). At the same time the combined use of PNL and ESWL for branched stones or stone extensions not easily accessible with the rigid nephroscope became routine in our hands. This allowed us to dispense with multiple tracts or flexible nephroscopy. By 1985 we had done 408 cases of percutaneous nephrolithotomy (PNL), 1002 cases of ESWL and 84 cases of ureterorenoscopy (URS) [73]. Similar reductions in PNL numbers to approximately 10% happened wherever ESWL was installed, in April 1985 in the Mayo Clinic [74] or in 1984 in London where John Wickham was working [75].

Presently URS replaces ESWL worldwide but PNL seems to maintain its position with the advent of mini-PNL techniques, laser lithotripsy and no-nephrostomy or no-tube solutions.

It is surprising to see that voting for URS or PNL at stone conferences favors the latter probably because of the ease demonstrated in life surgery sessions, the short OR-time, the comparably low cost and durability of equipment and the fact that PNL can be successfully applied regardless of the stone size and location.

1.7 A Personal Hit List

History iteself is objectively not existing. It is always the personal, subjective view of the person who selectively collects and presents the data:

- Fernström and Johansson publishing percutaneous access to radiologically controlled percutaneous renal stone extraction [25]
- Kurth et al. removing a staghorn stone with ultrasound lithotripsy [61]
- Our—Rolf Günther, Gerd Hutschenreiter and the author—decision in 1976 to develop unlimited endoscopically controlled percutaneous renal stone removal
- The hostile attacks of some senior academic German urologist upon my first presentation of 21 cases at the German urological convention in 1979 [65]
- Arthur Smith enthusiastically giving me his "Endo-Urology" flyer (Fig. 1.7) at the 75th AUA meeting in San Francisco in May 1980 after my presentation of our 34 cases of PNL.

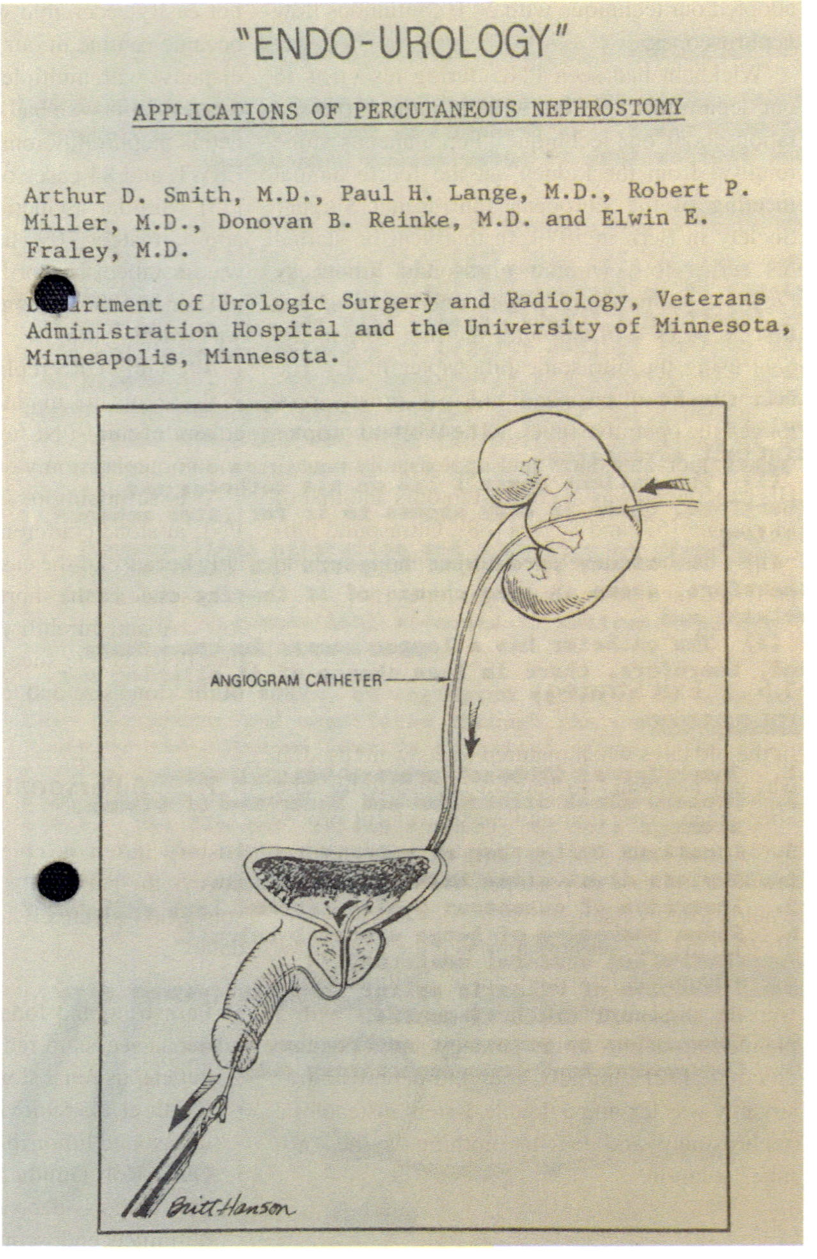
"ENDO-UROLOGY"

APPLICATIONS OF PERCUTANEOUS NEPHROSTOMY

Arthur D. Smith, M.D., Paul H. Lange, M.D., Robert P. Miller, M.D., Donovan B. Reinke, M.D. and Elwin E. Fraley, M.D.

Department of Urologic Surgery and Radiology, Veterans Administration Hospital and the University of Minnesota, Minneapolis, Minnesota.

Fig. 1.7 The 1980 "Endo-Urology" flyer of Arthur Smith

- A letter from W. W. Scott the then editor of the *Journal of Urology*: In 1980, he commented on our manuscript submission [66] which was based on my presentation at the AUA meeting in May 1980. We had concluded:
- "Percutaneous stone manipulation as a deliberate alternative to open surgery has to compete with the techniques for operative stone removal established over the past 100 years. Its specific place among the various techniques of stone therapy will be defined on the basis of further experience."
- He wanted us to change this paragraph and his comment was: "The Journal of Urology is not

a Medicine Man's paper." We were of course keen on the publication; so the new text was:

- "Most of the instruments in current use are primarily designed for the treatment of bladder stones. Further improvement of intrarenal stone manipulation is expected when instruments especially designed for the purpose of percutaneous manipulation are available." We changed the text [66] but not our ideas.
- John Wickham's decision to organize the First World Congress in Percutaneous Renal Surgery in London in 1983 [76].
- The book published in 1984 by the Minnesota group, Ralph Clayman and Wilfrido Castaneda-Zuniga; this was a real PNL cookery book covering every aspect of PNL at that time [77].
- The impressive series of Segura et al.: till the end of June 1984 they had treated 1000 patients [78].
- When I learned in 1994 that the German Urologist Heinrich von Rohr (1911–1978) had developed instruments for percutaneous endoscopic procedures and had designed an x-ray apparatus to guide a puncture needle to the right place in the kidney (Figs. 1.8 and 1.9). He had published studies on cadavers and animals in the East German *Zeitschrift für Urologie und Nephrologie* in 1958 [4, 79]. At that time this periodical was probably only read in East Germany and traditional thinking hampered his innovation. We do not know why von Rohr never proceeded to clinical studies. But sometimes the right thoughts need the right time to become reality.
- To see the continuously growing, extensive, worldwide dissemination of endoscopically controlled PNL, e.g. in India or in China when visiting Mahesh Desai in the Muljibhai Patel Urological Hospital at Nadiad, India [80] or Guohua Zeng in the Guangzhou Institute of Urology at Guangzhou, China [81].
- To learn that our 1981 publication [66] was included in the centennial supplement issue of the *Journal of Urology* in 2017 [82].

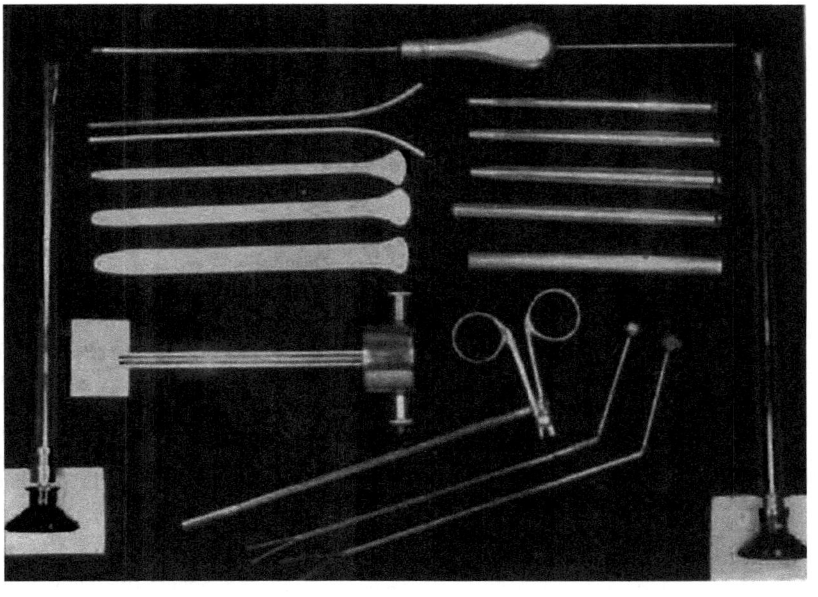

Fig. 1.8 Instruments for PNL designed by H. von Rohr [79]

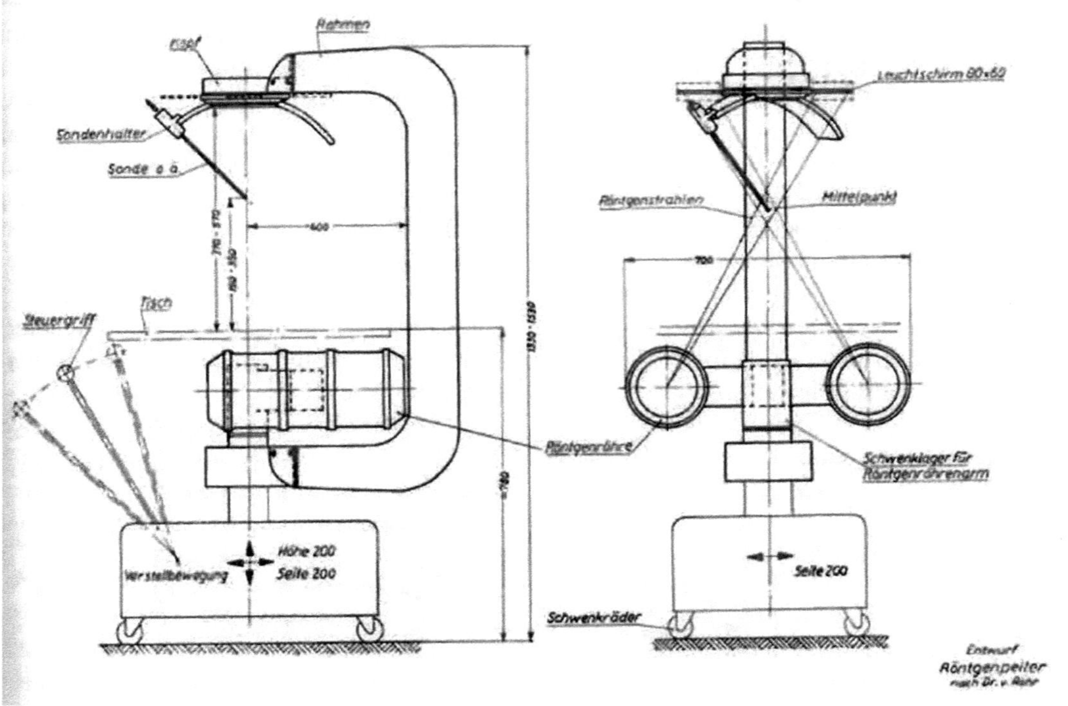

Fig. 1.9 X-ray localization and needle guide apparatus for percutaneous puncture of the renal collecting system designed by H. von Rohr [79]

References

1. Wickham JE. Treatment of urinary tract stones. BMJ. 1993;307(6916):1414–7.
2. Smith AD. A personal perspective on the origins of endourology and the endourological society. J Endourol. 2002;16(10):705–8.
3. Dasgupta P, Rose FK, Wickham JE. Percutaneous renal surgery: a pioneering perspective. J Endourol. 2006;20(3):167–9.
4. Alken P. The early history of percutaneous nephrolithotomy (PNL). In: Scoffone CM, Hoznek A, Cracco CM, editors. Supine percutaneous nephrolithotomy and ECIRS. Paris: Springer; 2014.
5. Patel SR, Nakada SY. The modern history and evolution of percutaneous nephrolithotomy. J Endourol. 2015;29(2):153–7.
6. Günther R, Alken P, Altwein JE. Percutaneous nephropyelostomy using a fine-needle puncture set. Radiology. 1979;132(1):228–30.
7. Simon G. Chirurgie der Nieren. Enke Erlangen. 1871. https://archive.org/details/chirurgiedernier00simo. Accessed 21 June 2019.
8. Lindblom K. Percutaneous puncture of renal cysts and tumors. Acta Radiol. 1946;27(1):66–72.
9. Casey WC, Goodwin WE. Percutaneous antegrade pyelography and hydronephrosis. J Urol. 1955;74(1):164–73.
10. Kapandji EM. Ponction de Bassinet et Radiomanometrie Meato-uretreo-pyelocalicielle. Rev C Par. 1949;68:270–90, (Abstracted in. Internat. Abstr. Surg. 1950 June; 90: 577–578
11. Weens HS, Florence TJJ. The diagnosis of hydronephrosis by percutaneous renal puncture. Urology. 1954;72(4):589–95.
12. Wickbom I. Pyelography after direct puncture of the renal pelvis. Acta Radiol. 1954;41(6):505–12.
13. Goodwin WE, Casey WC, Woolf W. Percutaneous trocar (needle) nephrostomy in hydronephrosis. JAMA. 1955;157:891–4.
14. Goodwin WE, Scardino PL, Scott WW. Translumbar aortic puncture and retrograde catheterization of the aorta in aortography and renal arteriography. Ann Surg. 1950;132(5):944–58.
15. Segura JW. Editorial comment. J Urol. 2002;167:829.
16. Barbaric ZL, Wood BP. Emergency percutaneous nephropyelostomy: experience with 34 patients and review of the literature. Am J Roentgenol. 1977;128(3):453–8.
17. Stables DP, Ginsberg NJ, Johnson ML. Percutaneous nephrostomy: a series and review of the literature. Am J Roentgenol. 1978;130(1):75–82.

18. Valdivia Uría JG, Lachares Santamaría E, Villarroya Rodríguez S, Taberner Llop J, Abril Baquero G, Aranda Lassa JM. Percutaneous nephrolithectomy: simplified technic (preliminary report). Arch Esp Urol. 1987;40(3):177–80.
19. LeRoy AJ, May GR, Bender CE, Williams HJ Jr, McGough PF, Segura JW, Patterson DE. Percutaneous nephrostomy for stone removal. Radiology. 1984;151(3):607–12.
20. Pedersen JF. Percutaneous nephrostomy guided by ultrasound. J Urol. 1974;112(2):157–9.
21. Hutschenreiter G, Alken P, Klippel KF. Percutaneous nephrostomy under ultrasound guidance. Urologe A. 1979;18(3):157–63.
22. Thüroff JW, Hutschenreiter G. Fallbericht: Perkutane Nephrostomie und instrumentelle Steinentfernung in Lokalanästhesie. Urol Int. 1980;35:375–80.
23. Seldinger SI. Catheter replacement of the needle in percutaneous arteriography: a new technique. Acta Radiol. 1953;39(5):368–76.
24. LeRoy AJ, May GR, Segura JW, Patterson DE, McGough PF. Rapid dilatation of percutaneous nephrostomy tracks. Am J Roentgenol. 1984;142(2):355–7.
25. Fernström I, Johannsson B. Percutaneous pyelolithotomy: a new extraction technique. Scand J Urol Nephrol. 1976;10:257–9.
26. Fernström I, Johansson B. Percutaneous extraction or renal calculi. Front Eur Radiol. 1982;1:1–24.
27. Rusnak B, Castaneda-Zuniga W, Kotula F, Herrera M, Amplatz K. An improved dilator system for percutaneous nephrostomies. Radiology. 1982;144(1):174.
28. Castaneda-Zuniga WR, Clayman R, Smith A, Rusnak B, Herrera M, Amplatz K. Nephrostolithotomy: percutaneous techniques for urinary calculus removal. Am J Roentgenol. 1982;139(4):721–6.
29. Clayman RV, Castaneda-Zuniga WR, Hunter DW, Miller RP, Lange PH, Amplatz K. Rapid balloon dilatation of the nephrostomy track for nephrostolithotomy. Radiology. 1983;147(3):884–5.
30. Olbert F, Hanecka L. Transluminale Gefässdilatation mit einem modifizierten Dilatationskatheter. Wien Klin Wochenschr. 1977;89:281–4.
31. Alken P. Teleskopbougierset zur perkutanen Nephrostomie. Aktuelle Urol. 1981;12:216–9.
32. Alken P, Gunther R, Thüroff J. Percutaneous nephrolithotomy—a routine procedure? BJU Special Suppl. 1983:1–5.
33. Alken P. The telescope dilators. World J Urol. 1985;3:7–10.
34. Marberger M, Stackl W, Hruby W, Kroiss A. Late sequelae of ultrasonic lithotripsy of renal calculi. J Urol. 1985;133(2):170–3.
35. Korth K. Percutaneous kidney surgery. Puncture and dilatation in the hands of the surgeon. Urologe A. 1986;25(6):315–21.
36. Wu KJ, et al. Secondary minimally invasive PCNL followed by nephrostomy for staghorn stones. Acad J Guangzhou Med Coll. 1993;2:13–6.
37. Jackman SV, Docimo SG, Cadeddu JA, Bishoff JT, Kavoussi LR, Jarrett TW. The "mini-perc" technique: a less invasive alternative to percutaneous nephrolithotomy. World J Urol. 1998;16(6):371–4.
38. Helal M, Black T, Lockhart J, Figueroa TE. The Hickman peel-away sheath: alternative for pediatric percutaneous nephrolithotomy. J Endourol. 1997;11(3):171–2.
39. Frattini A, Barbieri A, Salsi P, Sebastio N, Ferretti S, Bergamaschi E, Cortellini P. One shot: a novel method to dilate the nephrostomy access for percutaneous lithotripsy. J Endourol. 2001;15(9):919–23.
40. Alken P. Dilation of the nephrostomy tract. In: Smith A, Preminger G, Kavoussi L, Badlani G, editors. Smith's textbook of endourology. 4th ed. Hoboken: Wiley; 2019.
41. Clayman RV, Surya V, Miller RP, Castaneda-Zuniga WR, Smith AD, Hunter DH, Amplatz K, Lange PH. Percutaneous nephrolithotomy: extraction of renal and ureteral calculi from 100 patients. J Urol. 1984;131(5):868–71.
42. Wickham JEA, Miller RA, Kellett MJ. Percutaneous nephrolithotomy results and cost effectiveness. BJU Special Suppl. 1983:103–106.
43. Allen CD. Notes on nephrostomy drainage. Urol Cut Rev. 1935;39:389–93.
44. Rupel E, Brown R. Nephroscopy with removal of stone following nephrostomy for obstructive calculous anuria. J Urol. 1941;46:177–82.
45. Alken P. Percutaneous ultrasonic destruction of renal calculi. Urol Clin North Am. 1982;9(1):145–51.
46. Fernström I. Percutaneous extraction of renal calculi: technique and results. BJU Special Suppl. 1983:25–26.
47. Smith AD, Lange PH, Reinke DB, Miller RP. Extraction of ureteral calculi from patients with ileal loops: a new technique. J Urol. 1978;120:623–5.
48. Smith AD, Reinke DB, Miller RP, Lange PH. Percutaneous nephrostomy in the management of ureteral and renal calculi. Radiology. 1979;133:49–54.
49. Bissada NK, Meacham KR, Redman JF. Nephrostoscopy with removal of renal pelvic calculi. J Urol. 1974;112(4):414–6.
50. Clayman RV. Techniques in percutaneous removal of renal calculi. Mechanical extraction and electrohydraulic lithotripsy. Urology. 1984;23(5):11–9.
51. Smith AD, Clayman RV, Castaneda-Zuniga WR. Use of Mauermeyer stone punch via percutaneous nephrostomy. J Urol. 1982;128(6):1285–6.
52. Clayman RV, Surya V, Castaneda-Zuniga WR, Miller RP, Lange PH. Percutaneous nephrolithotomy with Mazzariello-Caprini forceps. J Urol. 1983;129(6):1213–5.
53. Lee WJ, Loh G, Smith AD, White E, Greenspan B, Vernace FM, Pochaczevsky R. Percutaneous extraction of renal stones: experience in 100 patients. Am J Roentgenol. 1985;144(3):457–62.
54. Miller RA, Payne SR, Wickham JE. Electrohydraulic nephrolithotripsy: a preferable alternative to ultrasound. Br J Urol. 1984;56(6):589–93.
55. Sachse H. Erfahrungen mit der Elektrolithotripsie. Verh Deutsche Ges Urol 1970;23:171–173.

56. Alken P. Intracorporeal lithotripsy. Urolithiasis. 2018;46(1):19–29.
57. Lutzeyer W, Pohlman R, Terhorst B, Cichos M. Die Zerstörung von Harnsteinen durch Ultraschall. I. Experimentelle Untersuchungen. Urol Int. 1970;25:47–63.
58. Terhorst B, Lutzeyer W, Cichos M, Pohlman R. Destruction of urinary calculi by ultrasound. II. Ultrasound lithotripsy of bladder calculi. Urol Int. 1972;27(6):458–69.
59. Gasteyer KH. A new method of bladder calculi fragmentation: ultrasonic lithotripsy. Urologe. 1971;10(1):30–2.
60. Rathert P, Stumpf U, Pohlman R, Lutzeyer W. Ultraschall-Lithotripsie von Ureter- und Nierensteinen: experimentelle und erst klinische Untersuchungen. Verh Deutsche Ges Urol 1976;28:365–367.
61. Kurth KH, Hohenfellner R, Altwein JE. Ultrasound litholapaxy of a staghorn calculus. J Urol. 1977;117:242–3.
62. Günther R, Altwein JE, Georgi M. Fine needle puncture for antegrade pyelography and percutaneous nephropyelostomy. Rofo. 1977;127(5):439–42.
63. Günther R, Alken P, Altwein JE. Percutaneous nephro-pyelostomy applications and results. Rofo. 1978;128(6):720–6.
64. Alken P, Kurth KH, Günter R. Die perkutane Instrumentation bei Nierensteinen. In: Gasser G, Vahlensieck W, editors. Fortschritte der Urologie und Nephrologie. Darmstadt: Steinkopf Verlag; 1977. p. 393–7.
65. Alken P, Altwein J. Die perkutane Nephrolitholapaxie. Verh Deutsche Ges Urol. 1979;36:109–12.
66. Alken P, Hutschenreiter G, Günter R, Marberger M. Percutaneous stone manipulation. J Urol. 1981;125:463–6.
67. Marberger M, Stackl W, Hruby W. Percutaneous litholapaxy of renal calculi with ultrasound. Eur Urol. 1982;8(4):236–42.
68. Segura JW, Patterson DE, LeRoy AJ, McGough PF, Barrett DM. Percutaneous removal of kidney stones. Preliminary report. Mayo Clin Proc. 1982;57(10):615–9.
69. Wickham JE, Kellett MJ. Percutaneous nephrolithotomy. Br J Urol. 1981;53(4):297–9.
70. Wickham JE, Kellet MJ. Percutaneous nephrolithotomy. Br Med J (Clin Res Ed). 1981;283(6306):1571–2.
71. Wickham JE, Kellett MJ, Miller RA. Elective percutaneous nephrolithotomy in 50 patients: an analysis of the technique, results and complications. J Urol. 1983;129(5):904–6.
72. Bellman GC, Davidoff R, Candela J, Gerspach J, Kurtz S, Stout L. Tubeless percutaneous renal surgery. J Urol. 1997;157(5):1578–82.
73. Alken P, Hardeman S, Wilbert D, Thüroff JW, Jacobi GH. Extracorporeal shock wave lithotripsy (ESWL): alternatives and adjuvant procedures. World J Urol. 1985;3(1):48–52.
74. Leroy AJ, Segura JW, Williams HJ Jr, Patterson DE. Percutaneous renal calculus removal in an extracorporeal shock wave lithotripsy practice. J Urol. 1987;138(4):703–6.
75. Webb DR, McNicholas TA, Whitfield HN, Wickham JE. Extracorporeal shockwave lithotripsy, endourology and open surgery: the management and follow-up of 200 patients with urinary calculi. Ann R Coll Surg Engl. 1985;67(6):337–40.
76. Wickham JAE, Miller R, editors. Percutaneous renal surgery. BJU Special Suppl. 1983.
77. Clayman R, Castaneda-Zuniga W, editors. Techniques in endourology: a guide to the percutaneous removal of renal and ureteral calculi. Chicago: Year Book Medical Publishers; 1984.
78. Segura JW, Patterson DE, LeRoy AJ, Williams HJ Jr, Barrett DM, Benson RC Jr, May GR, Bender CE. Percutaneous removal of kidney stones: review of 1000 cases. J Urol. 1985;134(6):1077–81.
79. von Rohr H. Die (endoskopische) Pyeloskopie: Neues Verfahren der Nierenheckendiagnostik und Grundlage der vereinfachten Entfernung von Nierenbeckensteinen: Ein Arbeitsbericht. Z Urol Nephrol. 1958;12:697–712.
80. Desai M, Grover R, Manohar T, Ganpule A. Simultaneous bilateral percutaneous nephrolithotomy: a single-center experience. J Endourol. 2007;21(5):508–14.
81. Zeng G, Mai Z, Zhao Z, Li X, Zhong W, Yuan J, Wu K, Wu W. Treatment of upper urinary calculi with Chinese minimally invasive percutaneous nephrolithotomy: a single-center experience with 12,482 consecutive patients over 20 years. Urolithiasis. 2013;41(3):225–9. https://doi.org/10.1007/s00240-013-0561-z.
82. Alken P, Hutschenreiter G, Günther R, Marberger M. Percutaneous stone manipulation. J Urol. 2017;197(2S):S154–7.

Anatomy for PNL

2

Wen Zhong

Percutaneous nephrolithotomy (PNL) involves percutaneous puncture into the target calyx, establishment of access, intraluminal lithotripsy, and insertion of nephrostomy tube and/or JJ stent. As an invasive procedure, a thorough understanding of the target organ anatomy is definitely necessary, to increase the success rate of the operation and also decrease complications. Typically, since stones are scattered over the renal collecting system, and the kidney is hidden in the retroperitoneum, a successful PNL should make a precise puncture into the target calyx, avoid perirenal viscera and interlobar artery injury, and get into different calyxes to remove the stones [1]. Since all these procedures are not carried out in open operation manner, several potential injuries are hard to avoid. Thus, the anatomy of kidney, perirenal viscera, renal collecting system, and renal vessels is significant in the guidance of PNL.

2.1 Kidney

2.1.1 General Anatomy

Kidneys are a pair of vital, broad bean-shaped organs. The lateral edge of the kidney is bulged, with a flat back and a convex front. The central depression area is called hilum, where the vessels, nerves, lymphatics, and ureter extend out. The kidney is 10–12 cm in length, 4–6 cm in width, and 3–4 cm in thickness, weighing 100–120 g. The size of the kidney varies, and the ratio of the size of the kidney to the body weight in newborns is about three times than that in adults.

The right kidney is little lower than the left kidney because of the location of liver. The upper edge of the right kidney is on the level of the 12th rib thoracic vertebra, and the lower edge is on the level of the third lumbar vertebra, while the upper edge of the left kidney is on the level of the 11th rib thoracic vertebra, and the lower edge is on the level of the second lumbar vertebra. The right kidney hilum is on the level of the second lumbar vertebra, while the left kidney hilum is on the level of the first lumbar vertebra. The location of kidneys also varies; the kidney in lean people is relatively lower, while it is higher in obese people.

Both the kidneys lie on the posterior abdominal wall, against the psoas major muscles, the longitudinal axis striding across the psoas major muscles. Moreover, since the psoas major muscles have a shape of a cone, the kidneys are also dorsal and inclined on the longitudinal axis. Therefore, the upper poles are more medial and more posterior than the lower poles. The lateral borders of both the kidneys are posterior positioned. Hence, the puncture from the upper pole is more prone to be close to the spine, while the

W. Zhong (✉)
Department of Urology and Guangdong Key Laboratory of Urology, The First Affiliated Hospital of Guangzhou Medical University Guangzhou, Guangdong, China

G. Zeng, K. Sarica (eds.), *Percutaneous Nephrolithotomy*,
https://doi.org/10.1007/978-981-15-0575-1_2

puncture from the lower pole is more prone to be away from the spine and deeper than the puncture from the upper pole.

2.1.2 Perirenal Covering

The surface of kidney is enclosed in a continuous covering of fibrous tissue called renal capsule. Each kidney within its capsule is surrounded by a mass of adipose tissue lying between the peritoneum and the posterior abdominal wall and called the perirenal fat (Fig. 2.1). The perirenal fat is enclosed by the renal fascia (so-called fibrous renal fascia of Gerota or, in this book, Gerota's fascia). The renal fascia is enclosed anteriorly and posteriorly by another layer of adipose tissue, which varies in thickness, called pararenal fat.

The renal fascia comprises a posterior layer (a well-defined and strong structure) and an anterior layer, which is a more delicate structure that tends to adhere to the peritoneum. The anterior and posterior layers of the renal Gerota's fascia subdivide the retroperitoneal space in three potential compartments (Fig. 2.1): (1) the posterior pararenal space, which contains only fat; (2) the intermediate perirenal space, which contains the suprarenal glands, kidneys, and proximal ureters, together with the perirenal fat; and (3) the anterior pararenal space, which extends across the mid-line from one side of the abdomen to the other. This space contains the ascending and descending colon, the duodenal loop, and the pancreas.

During normal PNL procedures, the nephroscope is inserted into the renal collecting system

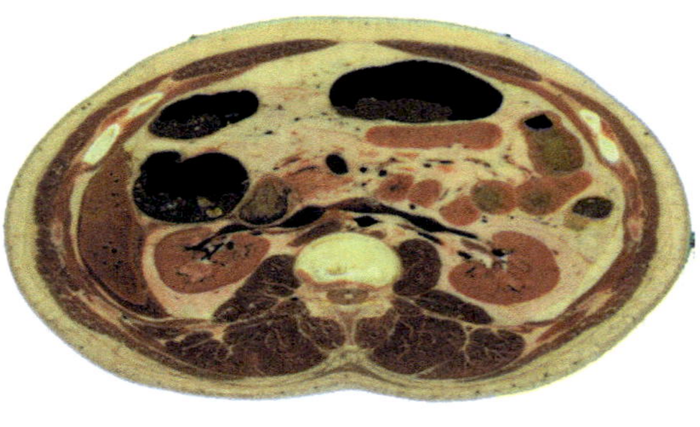

Fig. 2.1 Perirenal covering and potential compartments

which inspects the renal collecting system, but when the percutaneous tract is lost or the percutaneous access fails to enter the renal collecting system, the perirenal viscera organs are noted. The loose perirenal fat looks like cobweb or cloud cluster. Sometimes, the pink renal capsule is also found. Since kidney moves up and down with breathing, once the percutaneous tract is lost, it is difficult to find the original access into the renal collecting system. Retrograde injection of the methylene blue is helpful to trace the previous tract, which does not work every time. If the tract cannot be found in a short period of time, the irrigation would bring much more difficulty in the later puncture, since the irrigation would push the kidney far away to a deeper position. Thus, another puncture is required when the tract is lost and cannot be found in a short time.

2.1.3 Relationship Between Kidney and the Diaphragm, Pleural Cavity, and Ribs [2]

Both the kidneys lie below the diaphragm, which is almost symmetrical on both the sides. On the lower side, the liver and spleen lie on the right and left side, respectively. While on the upper area, pleura and ribs cover the upper pole and mostly middle pole of the kidney, respectively. Due to the position of the liver, the right kidney is lower than the left kidney. The posterior surface of the right kidney is crossed by the 12th rib, and the left kidney is crossed by the 11th and 12th ribs.

The posterior surface of the diaphragm is attached to the extremities of the 11th and 12th ribs, and the posterior aspect of the diaphragm arches as a dome above the superior pole of both the kidneys on each side. Therefore, most of the intercostal punctures into the upper pole traverse the diaphragm, but almost without any symptoms, while referring pain in shoulder in few cases. Regardless of the degree of respiration, middle or full expiration, the puncture between the 10th and 11th ribs has a risk of injury to the lung, but there is no report of lung injury during PNL. Intercostal puncture between the tenth and 11th ribs, even sometimes, subcostal puncture, would pass the pleural cavity. Because of the negative pressure in the pleural cavity during the inspiratory phase, gas or irrigation would be sucked into the pleural cavity during PNL, especially when torque the nephroscope and sheath, hydropneumothorax would be noted. However, most of the time, the tract passage through the pleural cavity will not bring hydropneumothorax, because the diaphragm would stop the leakage. Anyway, supracostal puncture should be done cautiously, especially when puncture from the tenth intercostal space.

In the course of PNL, we must pay attention to body surface positioning, which is helpful in the selection of percutaneous puncture points. Some patients may have received rib excision or truncation during previous open operation. Misjudgment of rib position might lead to the supracostal puncture site being above the tenth intercostal space, and cause pleural injury, in serious cases, hemothorax or pneumothorax.

Intercostal vessels often travel along the lower edge of the ribs. In order to avoid injury to intercostal vessels, any intercostal puncture should be performed below half of the intercostal space. While using sharp knife for incision on skin and subcutaneous tissue, attention should be paid to the direction of incision; it should go along the axis of intercostal space, so as to avoid longitudinal incision which would cause intercostal artery injury.

2.1.4 Relationship Between Kidney and the Liver and Spleen [2]

Below the diaphragm and above the kidney hilum, the liver and spleen lie on the right and left sides, respectively (Fig. 2.2). The liver and spleen lie exactly posterolaterally on each side. When hepatosplenomegaly is noted or sometimes when liver and spleen have deviation toward the midaxis, the lateral margin of the kidney would be covered by the liver or spleen. Preoperative CT scan is required to identify the relationship between kidney and perirenal organs. Intraoperative real-time ultrasonography guidance could guide the puncture and help avoid liver or spleen injury during PNL. Percutaneous puncture should be close to the inner side, rather than the outboard.

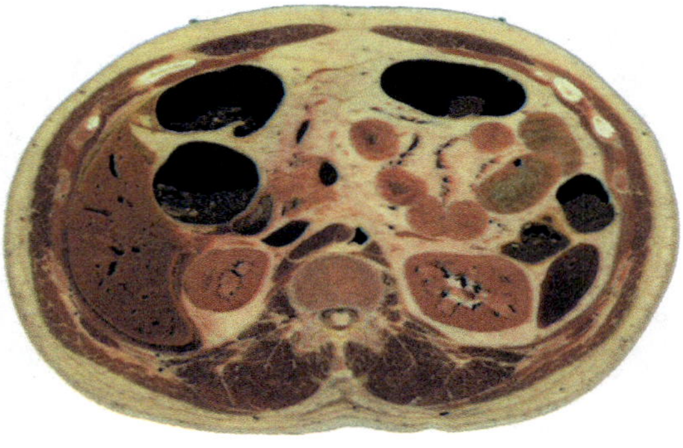

Fig. 2.2 Relationship between kidney and the liver and spleen

Very few liver and spleen injuries has been reported so far, but this complication is always worrisome, especially the spleen injury in PNL always causes severe bleeding, which leads to splenectomy. Liver injury in PNL is relatively not as urgently as spleen injury, because bleeding from liver vein would stop when nephrostomy tube is inserted, except when a large hepatic vein is injured.

2.1.5 Relationship Between Kidney and the Colons [3]

The ascending colon dips down from the ileocecal valve to the right colic flexure (hepatic flexure), where it passes into the transverse colon. The hepatic colic flexure (hepatic angle) lies anteriorly to the inferior portion of the right kidney. The descending colon extends inferiorly from the left colic flexure (splenic flexure) to the level of the iliac crest. The left colic flexure lies anterolateral to the left kidney.

It is important to consider the position of the retroperitoneal ascending and descending colons. It has been occasionally noted in routine abdominal CT scan that the retroperitoneal colon lies in a posterolateral or even a postrenal position. In these cases, there is a great risk of colon injury during PNL. The retrorenal colon is much more frequently noted in elder female, thin patients, at the left side, lower pole of kidney, and also a puncture into ante-

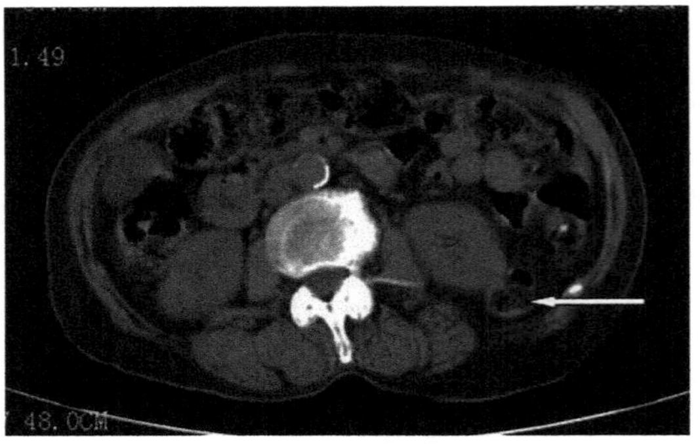

Fig. 2.3 Retrorenal colon

rior calyx (Fig. 2.3). Much more attention should be paid to these cases when puncture is made under fluoroscopy guidance. In some urologists'personal experience with colon injury during PNL, it has been stated that there is no special resistance when the needle puncture into colon, but the dilation into colon is different, since the colon serosa has high toughness and the colon would move away, thus obvious resistance would be noted.

2.2 Renal Collecting System

2.2.1 Pelviocalyceal System

The renal parenchyma basically consists of two kinds of tissues: the cortical and the medullar tissues. On a longitudinal section, from the lateral to the medial, there is successively the capsule, cortical tissue, medullar tissue, and renal calyx and renal pelvis.

The cortical tissue consists of glomerulus, which contains proximal and distal convoluted tubules. The renal pyramids comprise the loops of Henle and collecting ducts. These ducts join the papillary ducts, open at the papillary surface, where always the center of the fornix, and then drain into minor calyx and into renal pelvis at last. The renal papilla is at the apex of a pyramid-shaped medullar tissue. The layer of the cortical tissue between adjacent pyramids is named renal columns, where the interlobular artery passes through.

A minor calyx is defined as the calix that drains the papilla directly. The number of minor calyces varies, ranging from 5 to 14. The minor calyces may drain straightly into an infundibulum or join to form major calyces, which subsequently drains into an infundibulum. Finally, the infundibula drain into the renal pelvis [4].

The anatomy shape of renal collecting system varies extremely, even the left kidney and right kidney in one person is not symmetrical. Thus, there is no fixed pattern for the puncture in PNL procedures. When performing PNL, attention must be paid to the anatomical diversity of the renal collecting system, because the structure of the renal collecting system would directly affect the operating. Generally, the slender calyx seriously affects the operation using endoscopy, while the wide and shallow calyx is relatively easy to look over. However, the general consensus of renal collecting system should be well known.

In Smith's textbook of Endourology, Sampio analyzed three-dimensional polyester resin corrosion endocasts of the pelviocalyceal system [5]. According to the endocasts, the pelviocalyceal system is divided into two major groups A and B . Group A (62.2%) comprises pelviocalyceal systems that present two major calyceal groups (superior and inferior) as a primary division of the renal pelvis and a midzone calyceal drainage dependent on these two major groups. Group B (37.8%) comprises pelviocalyceal systems that present the kidney midzone (hilar) calyceal drainage independent of both the superior and the inferior calyceal groups.

Since the kidney looks like a bean, the middle pole is much more thick and solid than the upper and the lower poles. Regarding the calyceal drainage at different poles of the kidney, 98.6% of the upper poles are drained by a calyx; for the lower pole, 57.9% are drained by two calyces in pairs and 42.1% are drained by a single calyx; the middle pole is mostly composed of multiple pairs of anterior and posterior calyces. From this point of view, the calyces in the middle pole are much more complex, the parallel calyces, the anterior and posterior calyces, which would cause difficulty for puncture manipulation. Thus, the well understanding of the pelvio-calyceal systems was crucial to guide the puncture and manipulation during the PNL procedure.

2.2.2 Urography and Significance

A thorough understanding of the spatial anatomy of the pelvis and calyx is of great importance for PNL. However, it is difficult for the urologists to imagine the actual three-dimensional structure, since the excretory urography (IVU) or retrograde urography can only demonstrate the two-dimensional planar image. The anatomical background could help urologists to conceive a three-dimensional image of the renal collecting system, even though when observing a two-dimensional image (Fig. 2.4). Three-dimensional CT reconstruction is a powerful and significant tool to reconstruct the three-dimensional image of the renal collecting system and stones but had the limitation of high cost and radiation. In Smith's textbook of Endourology, Sampio analyzed three-dimensional polyester resin corrosion endocasts of the pelviocalyceal system. By comparing the urography and three-dimensional cast of the renal collecting system, we can have a preliminary impression of the three-dimensional structure of the renal collecting system.

Since the calyces stretch with different angle, length, and width, the projection on two-dimensional plain film varies. The renal stones and contrast in renal collecting system demonstrate different structures. Some calyces are arranged in parallel with others. Some calyces have the projection of a sealed ring with a transparent area in the middle. Some calyces overlap almost completely, and since the calyces are irregular, there would be some local area that shows dense shadow [6].

In several cases, perpendicular minor calyces go directly into the renal pelvis or into a major calyx (Fig. 2.5). The minor calyces almost perpendicular to the surface of the collecting system, thus in the projection, has been demonstrated as a black circle, which overlaps with the background. The residual stones in these perpendicular minor calyces are always posterior; hence, the anterior calyces are much easier to detect in PNL. Most of time, the puncture goes from the posterior calyx, thus for the residual stones in the perpendicular minor calyces, another puncture directly to the target calyx is required. It has to be noticed that most of these calyces lie near the infundibulum or renal pelvis, and the puncture and tract dilation are at high risk of vascular injury, thus a very precise puncture would not cause severe bleeding in these cases.

For these overlapping calyces, overlapped either almost together or into a circle (Fig. 2.6), a thorough understanding of the hierarchical relationship of posterior and anterior calyces is crucial. Unfortunately, the plain film could only demonstrate a two-dimensional planar image. The preoperative CT scan can provide an accurate

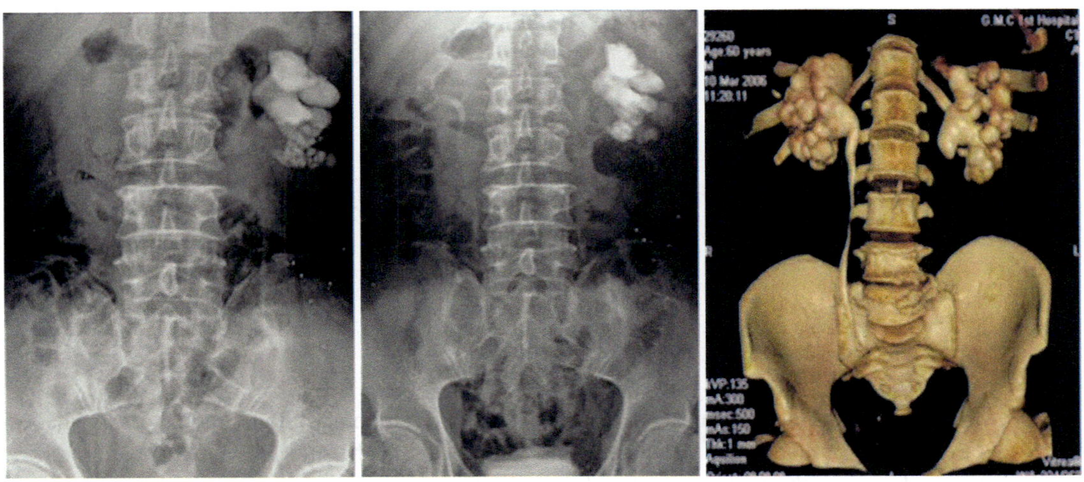

Fig. 2.4 The KUB, IVU, and 3D CT reconstruction of renal collecting system and stones

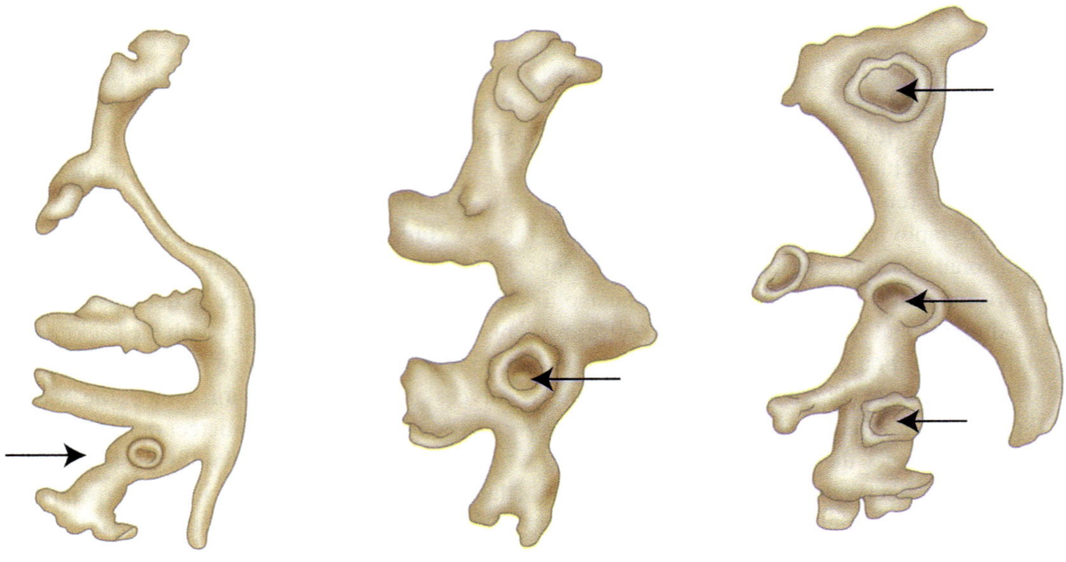

Fig. 2.5 Perpendicular minor calyces draining directly into the renal pelvis or into a major calyx

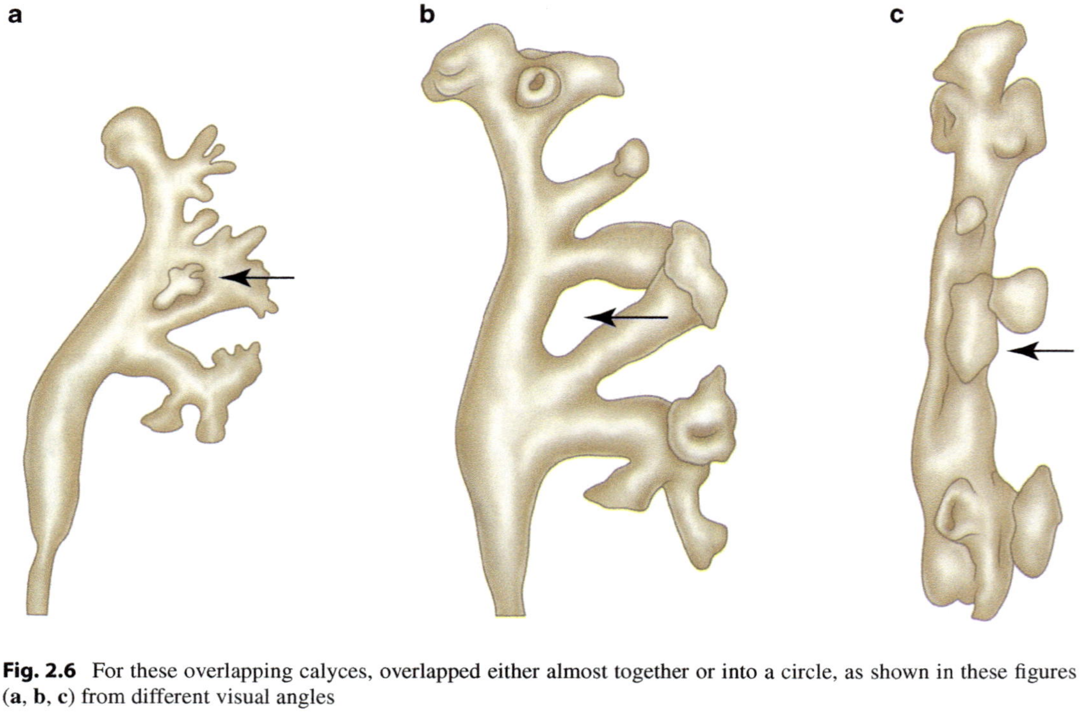

Fig. 2.6 For these overlapping calyces, overlapped either almost together or into a circle, as shown in these figures (**a**, **b**, **c**) from different visual angles

relationship of anterior and posterior calyx, but intraoperative CT guidance is unviable in PNL. Retrograde urography with contrast and air can also be performed to identify the posterior calyx. Even though the gradual deep–shallow relationship is helpful to identify the hierarchical relationship sometimes, a great deal of personal experience is required.

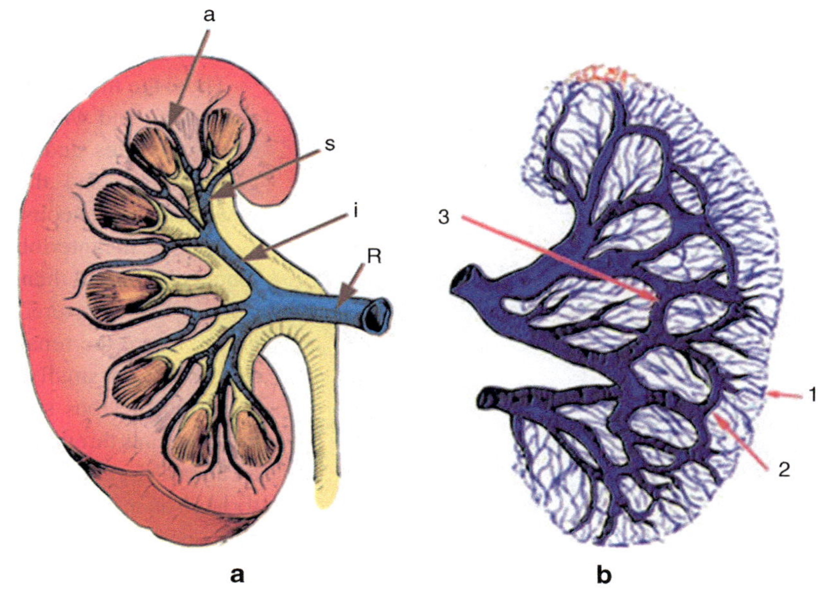

Fig. 2.7 A sketch from the anterior phase of the right kidney (**a**) showing four branches of the renal artery: *R* renal artery, *s* segmental artery, *I* interlobar (carotid) artery, and *a* arcuate artery. The right figure (**b**) shows three levels of arcuate veins

Since the percutaneous renal access to the renal collecting system through the posterior calyces could provide a better manipulation pattern in PNL with prone position, it is of great significance to identify which calyx is posterior calyx.

The angle of the posterior and anterior calyces with the horizontal plane is different. In most of time, anterior calyx stretches to a much more acute angle than posterior calyx. Thus, the projection of posterior calyx is prone to close to the renal pelvis, on the premise that the anterior and posterior calyces are in similar length. If the posterior calyx is much larger than the anterior calyx, the distal tip of projection of the posterior calyx is much more lateral rather than midway. However, the premise is not always working, and different angles and lengths destine that the hierarchical relationship of anterior and posterior calyx in projection is complex and hard to identify on plain film. Rotation of C-arm is helpful to identify the posterior calyx. When the bulb is rotated to 30°, the project direction is changed, the overlapped area is deviated, and then the posterior calyx would be displayed, since the top of posterior calyx would be highlighted in the 30° sagittal axis.

2.2.3 Intrarenal Vessels

Generally, the main renal artery divides into an anterior and a posterior branch after giving off the inferior suprarenal artery. The posterior branch (retropelvic artery) proceeds as the posterior segmental artery to supply the homonymous segment without further significant branching, whereas the anterior branch of the renal artery provides three or four segmental arteries [7].

The segmental arteries divide before entering the renal parenchyma into interlobar arteries (infundibular arteries), which progressed adjacent to the calyceal infundibula and the minor calyces, entering the renal columns between the renal pyramids (Fig. 2.7).

The interlobar arteries progress near the base of the pyramids, originating (usually by dichotomous division) the arcuate arteries (Fig. 2.8). The arcuate arteries give off the interlobular arteries, which reach to the periphery giving off the afferent arterioles of the glomeruli.

Unlike the renal artery, the renal vein is not segmental, but it has abundant circulatory anastomosis [8]. Cortical venules, also known as stellate veins, drain into the interlobular veins that form a series of arches. There are usually three longitudinal

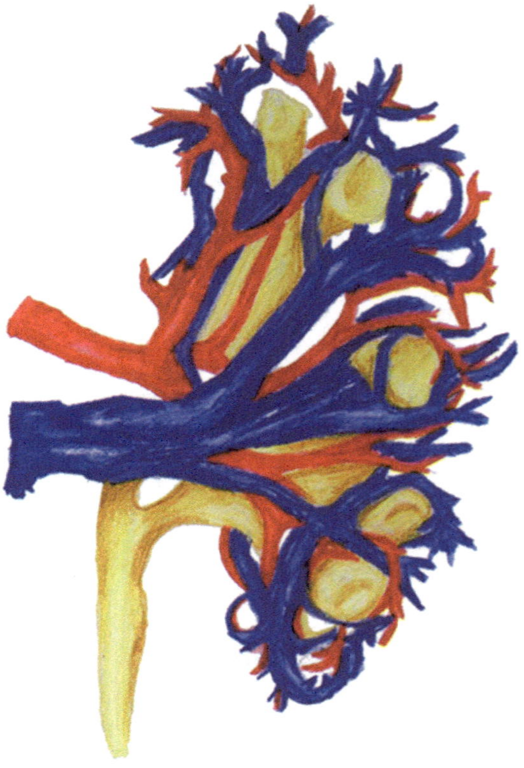

Fig. 2.8 Intrarenal vessels and the relationships between infundibulum and fornix

anastomotic arcuate systems in the renal parenchyma: between the stellate veins (more peripherally), between the arcuate veins (at the base of the pyramids), and between the interlobar (infundibular) veins (close to the renal sinus) (Fig. 2.7).

2.2.4 Anatomical Relationship Between Intrarenal Vessels and Renal Collecting System [9]

As shown in the previous text, the intrarenal vessels are hidden in the renal cortex and medulla, which constitute the periphery of the renal collecting system. The puncture into the desired calyx must travels through the parenchyma and has the risk of injury to renal vessels. Bleeding is one of the most frequently noted complications following PNL, thus an ideal puncture should be well designed and accurately performed without severe vessel injury.

Thus, the major artery is located near the kidney hilum, and when we move forward to interlobular arteries and arcuate arteries, the artery gets smaller, and the peripheral artery injury would be spontaneously solidified.

Exactly, the interlobular arteries travel through renal column and then extend as arcuate arteries. Thus, when punctured from the apical center of calyx, where the renal papilla originates, named as fornix, only small arcuate arteries are injured.

In the previous study, investigators compared the punctures through a calyceal infundibulum and a calyceal fornix. It has been noted that puncture through an infundibulum (in any region of the kidney) resulted in much more artery and vein injury. Puncture through the upper pole infundibulum is the most dangerous because this region is surrounded almost completely by large vessels. Infundibular arteries and veins course parallel to the anterior and posterior aspects of the upper pole infundibulum [7, 10]. The posterior aspect of the lower pole infundibulum is widely presumed by urologists and interventional radiologists to be free of arteries. It is considered, therefore, to be a safe region through which to gain access to the collecting system and to place a nephrostomy tube.

Large venous anastomoses are similar to collars around the calyceal infundibula (the so-called calyceal necks). A venous lesion usually heals spontaneously, but consequent hemorrhage may be cumbersome during the procedure.

Direct puncture into renal pelvis is also at high risk of bleeding, since large branches of renal artery and main branches of renal veins are all nearby the renal pelvis. The injury of these large vessel branches is fatal. On the other hand, the nephrostomy tube inserted directly into the renal pelvis is much more prone to fall off, and there are much more extravasations during the PNL procedure.

In conclusion, the high rate of vascular injury destined that the puncture from infundibulum is not feasible, while the puncture from the fornix is the ideal pathway to decrease bleeding in PNL.

References

1. Sampaio FJB. Renal anatomy: endourologic considerations. Urol Clin North Am. 2000;27(4):585–607.
2. Hopper KD, Yakes WF. The posterior intercostal approach for percutaneous renal procedures: risk of puncturing the lung, spleen, and liver as determined by CT. AJR Am J Roentgenol. 1990;154(1):115–7.
3. Hopper KD, Sherman JL, Luethke JM, et al. The retrorenal colon in the supine and prone patient. Radiology. 1987;162(2):443–6.
4. Sampaio FJB. Basic anatomic features of the kidney collecting system. Three-dimensional and radiologic study. In: Sampaio FJB, Uflacker R, editors. Renal anatomy applied to urology, endourology, and interventional radiology. New York: Thieme Medical Publishers; 1993. p. 7–15.
5. Sampaio FJB. Anatomic classification of the pelviocaliceal system. Urologic and radiologic implications. In: Sampaio FJB, Uflacker R, editors. Renal anatomy applied tourology, endourology, and interventional radiology. New York: Thieme Medical Publishers; 1993. p. 1–6.
6. Sampaio FJB, Mandarim-de-Lacerda CA. 3-dimensional and radiological pelviocaliceal anatomy for endourology. J Urol. 1988;140(6):1352–5.
7. Sampaio FJB. Relationships of intrarenal arteries and the kidney collecting system. Applied anatomic study. In: Sampaio FJB, Uflacker R, editors. Renal anatomy applied tourology, endourology, and interventional radiology. New York: Thieme Medical Publishers; 1993. p. 23–32.
8. Sampaio FJB, Aragio AHM. Anatomical relationship between the renal venous arrangement and the kidney collecting system. J Urol. 1990;144(5):1089–93.
9. Sampaio FJB. Renal collecting system anatomy: its possible role in the effectiveness of renal stone treatment. Curr Opin Urol. 2001;11(4):359–66.
10. Sampaio FJB. Intrarenal access by puncture. Three-dimensional study. In: Sampaio FJB, Uflacker R, editors. Renal anatomy applied to urology, endourology, and interventional radiology. New York: Thieme Medical Publishers; 1993. p. 68–76.

Armamentariums Related to Percutaneous Nephrolithotripsy (PCNL)

3

Athanasios Dellis and Athanasios Papatsoris

3.1 Nephroscopes

The choice of the nephroscope is of utmost importance. Although most of the scopes used are rigid ones, the nephroscope's choice depends absolutely on personal preference and availability [1].

3.1.1 Rigid Nephroscopes

Rigid nephroscopes have the advantage of superior optical quality due to the rod lens system, excellent irrigation and working channels. The optimal nephroscope should have a sufficient working length, a large working channel, a reduced outer diameter and a watertight entry site for instruments and accessories [1].

Practically, all nephroscope models have their optical and light cables and the irrigation lines located on the same side of the shaft. Most nephroscope models are designed with a continuous flow system, managed with an inflow and an outflow valve. However, when using a plastic Amplatz sheath, the outer shaft with the outflow valve loses its role; in fact, the irrigation fluid can flow out between the nephroscope and the Amplatz sheath. Although rigid nephroscopes have proven their efficacy and safety through years, they are characterized by limited maneuverability through long tracks (e.g. in cases of horseshoe kidneys) or around complex intrarenal anatomy due to the distance and the spatial location of calculi in the calyces [1, 2].

3.1.2 Flexible Nephroscope

A flexible cystoscope/nephroscope is essential during a contemporary single tract PCNL since it allows access in peripheral calyces that are not reachable with a rigid instrument (e.g. in staghorn stones). With the flexible scope the number of tracts can be minimized. However, through the working channel only flexible instruments can be utilized. For instance, stone fragmentation can be performed only with laser lithotripsy [2].

3.2 Renal Access

Safe and accurate percutaneous renal access is of utmost importance [3]. The best approach to the kidney is ideally achieved by a transpapillary

A. Dellis
University Department of Surgery, Aretaieion Hospital, Athens, Greece

University Department of Urology, Sismanoglio Hospital, Athens, Greece

A. Papatsoris (✉)
University Department of Urology, Sismanoglio Hospital, Athens, Greece

G. Zeng, K. Sarica (eds.), *Percutaneous Nephrolithotomy*,
https://doi.org/10.1007/978-981-15-0575-1_3

puncture with direct access to the renal pelvis [2, 3]. Identifying the ideal target calyx preoperatively as well as obtaining a three-dimensional knowledge of the kidney anatomy and stone burden is the hallmark of a state-of-the-art PCNL. The principal steps of PCNL are primarily puncture of the calyx, followed by tract dilation, stone fragmentation and proper pelvicalyceal system drainage. Standard methods for obtaining access include fluoroscopic and/or ultrasound guidance performed either by radiologists or solely urologists, regardless of the operator's experience [4].

Initially, under fluoroscopic guidance, a 5–7 F ureteric catheter should be inserted cystoscopically (either with a rigid or with a flexible cystoscope) into the renal pelvis or at about 1 cm above the obstructing stone [2].

Non-ionic contrast medium (diluted at 1:2–1:3 ratio in normal saline) sometimes with a few drops of methylene blue is injected for opacification of the collecting system and distend it so that the puncture would be more accurate [2, 5].

The ureteric catheter is fixed to a urethral catheter in order to prevent displacement and provide free access for contrast injection or guide wires insertion.

Equipment

- 5–7 F open-ended ureteric catheter with a Luer-lock fixed proximally
- Urethral (Foley) catheter 14–18 F
- Contrast medium diluted with 0.9% saline and if needed 0.2–0.5 mL of methylene blue in order to give a faint blue color to the mixture so as to be distinguished from urine or blood
- A two-part puncture needle: usually 18-G straight stiff puncture needle, with an oblique beveled tip, 2 cm longer than the Amplatz sheath
- Guide wires (Table 3.1): Preferably, hydrophilic guide wires 0.035–0.038 inch in diameter/150 cm in length, with a straight floppy tip. They are called "slippery" because they can easily slip out of the kidney or through the surgeon's or assistant's hands [5]. They are more expensive than standard polytetrafluoroethylene (PTFE) wires [5, 6]. They can easily find their way and coil in the pelvicalyceal system, by-pass ureteric or renal stones or advance through ureter in the urinary bladder. In rare conditions they can pass through the pelvicalyceal system or ureteric wall, causing a "false route" passage. In order to avoid the latter, we may use a "J-tip" wire, whose tip is a half-circle [5–7]. However, when there is resistance while advancing the hydrophilic wire through the needle there is a risk of striping its surface. Therefore, the hydrophilic wire should not be pushed in and out the wire when there is resistance

Table 3.1 Guide wire types

Type	Tip	Characteristics
Hydrophilic	Straight or "J"	Diameter: 0.035–0.038 inch Length: 150 cm
Super stiff	Straight	
PTFE	Straight or "J"	

3.2.1 Standard MiniPerc (Table 3.2)

- 12 F rigid nephroscope and 15 F sheath [8, 9]. MiniPerc is the term used for PCNL cases with tract size less than or equal to 18–20 F [10, 11].

3.2.2 Super MiniPerc

- Use of active irrigation and active suction.
- 7 F nephroscope and 8 F sheath. The telescope consists of a 3 F fibre-optic bundle [12].

3.2.3 Ultra MiniPerc

- 3.5 F miniature nephroscope and 11/13 F sheath [13].

3.2.4 Micro PCNL

- Micro-fiber optics of 2–3 F, all-seeing needle 4.8 F or 8 F micro-sheath. Drainage of collecting system is provided through a ureteral catheter inserted preoperatively [14].

Table 3.2 Conventional and miniaturized PCNL

	Conventional	Mini	Super mini	Ultra mini	Micro
Dilatation	Yes	Yes	Yes	Yes	No
Fragmentation	Ultrasound Pneumatic Combined Laser	Laser	Laser	Laser	Laser
Amplatz sheath	30 F	15 F (<18–20 F)	8 F	11 F/13 F	No
Nephrostomy	Mostly	Rare	No	No	No

3.3 Renal Tract Dilation

Tract dilation is the second crucial step for a successful PCNL procedure where costly disposables could be utilized. There are five standard tract dilation techniques for PCNL: Amplatz fascial dilation (AFD) [15], metal telescopic dilation of the Alken type (AT) [16, 17], balloon dilation (BD) [18], one-shot dilation (OSD) [19] and radially expanding single-step nephrostomy dilator (RESN) [20]. Each of the five types has its own advantages and disadvantages. In general, the choice depends on the availability and the surgeon experience and, therefore, there is no consensus regarding the best dilation technique [21]. For instance, there are no significant differences in stone-free and transfusion rates between OSD and AT while there are significant differences in tract dilatation fluoroscopy time and hemoglobin decrease between the OSD and AT groups. Significant differences in transfusion rates were found between the BD and AT groups while among patients without previous open renal surgery those who underwent BD exhibited a lower blood transfusion rate and a shorter surgical duration compared with those who underwent AFD. The OSD technique is safer and more efficient than the AT technique for tract dilation during PCNL, particularly, in patients with previous open renal surgery, resulting in a shorter tract dilatation fluoroscopy time and a lesser decrease in hemoglobin. The efficacy and safety of BD are better than AFD in patients without previous open renal surgery. As a result, the OSD technique should be considered for most patients who undergo PCNL therapy [21–23].

Equipment

1. Amplatz fascial dilators [15, 24]
   - Polyurethane, single use
   - 8F flexible polyurethane dilator sliding over the working guidewire and whenever it is possible descending into the ureter
   - The polyurethane dilator protects the guidewire and prevents kinking during progressive dilation
   - Stepwise tract dilation until the desired caliber is reached (usually up to 30–32 F)
   - Each dilator has to be removed before next insertion of the larger dilator and, therefore, in the time interval the tract may bleed
   - In cases of large hydronephrosis, the kidney can collapse between dilator exchanges
2. Alken-type telescopic dilators [16]
   - Metal, reusable and autoclavable
   - Prevent bleeding between each dilator insertion due to parenchymal tamponade
   - No hydronephrotic system deflation, no serial exchange
   - Particularly fit for patients with previous open renal surgery/scar tissue
3. Balloon dilator [18]
   - Olbert balloon catheter 8–10 mm in diameter and 4 cm long attached to an Amplatz gauge system, a racket and screw mechanism as well as a syringe
   - Single use
   - Balloon over the guide wire (through the fasciae and into the kidney) and inflated under fluoroscopy, usually up to 20 atm
   - Radial inflation, not shearing process
   - Kidney tamponade with inflation
   - Difficult to inflate in dense scar tissue

4. One-shot (single-stage) dilator [19]
   - A single 25 F or 30 F Amplatz dilator pulled in on the Alken guide or on the 8 F first polyurethane dilator of the Amplatz set
   - Single use
   - Dilator inserted over guidewire in a single rotating maneuver
   - Kidney tamponade during insertion
5. Radially expanding single-step dilator [20]
   - 8 F woven sleeve with an inner stylet
   - 30 F tapered fascial dilator
   - Amplatz-like working sheath
   - Significantly low axial forces transmitted in kidney
6. Amplatz sheath [5]
   - Firm Teflon or polyurethane tube
   - Not to be advanced blindly
   - Usually with diameter of 30 F
   - The hydrostatic pressure perioperatively is always less than 10 cm H_2O
   - Smaller Amplatz sheaths, those compatible with 22 F nephroscopes
   - Conventional Amplatz sheaths are inadequate for obese patients. Place a suture at the outer edge to avoid inward migration
   - "Peel away" sheath to facilitate nephrostomy tube placement in the end of procedure

3.4 Lithotripsy

Several fragmentation devices are available for clinical use. The three mostly used devices for intra-corporeal lithotripsy, include ultrasound, ballistic and laser lithotripters, or a combination of these energies.

3.4.1 Ultrasound Lithotripters

Contemporary ultrasonic lithotripters consist of a handpiece containing a piezoelectric crystal which is stimulated by electric energy and is activated by a pedal switch [25, 26]. The stone fragmentation is achieved by high-frequency vibration (23.000–27.000 Hz) [1, 5, 8]. The longitudinal vibration is transmitted to the stone with the help of a hollow probe, resulting in rapid fragmentation especially in cases of soft stones [27]. The handpiece has also a central channel on the same axis of the probe, allowing suction of the irrigation fluid and stone particles during all the fragmentation process as well by keeping the visual field clear in the unlikely event of bleeding [28]. Unfortunately, it may be obstructed by fine stone remnants or collapse the collecting system of the kidney, thus limiting vision intraoperatively. It is usually atraumatic to tissues and also helps to cool both probe and handpiece. It can remove large volumes of stone without needing to remove and re-insert the nephroscope; however, since it should be directly applied to the stone, the stone should be immobilized. For conventional PCNL, usually 10 F probes are used [1, 5, 8].

3.4.2 Pneumatic (Ballistic) Lithotripters

Pneumatic lithotripsy works similarly to a pneumatic jackhammer [29]. It functions with the use of compressed air that practically bursts against the head of the metal probe at a frequency up to 12 cycles per second [1, 5, 30]. Shots can be triggered by a foot pedal switch in a single- or a multiple-pulse mode setting. It is more effective in large and hard renal stones that should preferably be immobilized but the latter combined with the "jackhammer effect" may cause bleeding [31, 32].

A relatively novel handheld pneumatic lithotripter has been presented [1]. It is a cordless handheld device that is powered by a disposable, detachable compressed carbon dioxide (CO_2) cartridge [1, 5]. The shot is initiated by a hand-activated trigger rather than a foot pedal. When the CO_2 abruptly expands, its pressure projects the hammer against the firing pin, transmitting the kinetic energy to a metallic probe that should be held in contact with the stone. One significant advantage of this device is the minimal displacement at the tip of the probe, despite the high energy of the mechanical shock [33]. The amount of pressure transmitted to the stone is 31 bars, compared with the 3 bars of standard pneumatic lithotripters.

Large fragments are easily generated and can be quickly extracted. Because of progressive drop of the gas pressure inside the cartridge, the energy of the impulses simultaneously decreases. One cartridge provides approximately 70 shocks [1, 5].

3.4.3 Combined Pneumatic and Ultrasound Lithotripter

This device consists of a combined generator delivering simultaneously pneumatic ad ultrasonic energy. The two sources of energy are transmitted to a handpiece and triggered with a dual foot switch. The 3 F pneumatic probe, set to a 5 Hz frequency, is advanced through the hollow 10 F ultrasonic probe without protruding [1, 5]. The pneumatic shockwave produces gross fragmentation. The ultrasound completes the fragmentation and allows for aspiration of fine stone fragments. Suction is synchronized with ultrasound fragmentation [34–36].

3.4.4 Laser

The principle of laser fragmentation of the stones consists of the localized explosive boiling of water near the stone, resulting in a shockwave [37–39]. Lasers used for stone treatment should have a wavelength belonging to the infrared spectrum, such as erbium:YAG, holmium:YAG or CO_2.

The holmium:YAG laser is characterized by high water absorption and a penetration that does not exceed 0.4 mm with pulse duration varying between 150 and 1000 μs. Lasers are mostly used for miniaturized PCNL as presented above with fibers up to 500 um [1, 5].

3.5 Retrieval Equipment

3.5.1 Graspers

Alligator forceps have an active grasping mechanism, similar to surgical forceps, practically having a scissor handle that allows to open and close its jaws [40]. The jaws open in a "V" shape and, therefore, cannot grasp large fragments (bigger than 4 mm) since they are pushed away as the jaws close [41].

Triradiate forceps have a passive grasping mechanism with a U-shaped handle without joints or complex hinges [1, 5]. Stones are grasped by three-serrated jaws with a sharp claw at the tip [42, 43]. They can grasp larger stone fragments. However, since the jaws are sharp and thin and when widely spreading out they can easily perforate the collecting system and further tear it during closure. In practice, they are better used in dilated or larger than confined spaces. In order to avoid trauma to the collecting system the forceps could be slightly rotated before retrieval in order to check all three jaws.

3.5.2 Baskets

Tipless dismembered baskets are very useful, especially for large fragment extraction. Basket wires are of smaller caliber compared to metallic grasper jaws and, therefore, allow removal of larger stone fragments through the Amplatz sheath [43, 44].

3.5.3 Flashing out Fragments

In cases of fragments that can pass through the Amplatz sheath, a cut nasogastric tube (14–16 F) can be inserted through the sheath—if possible next to or behind the fragments. By repeatedly moving forward and backward in a "jerking" motion while saline is instilled under some pressure to create turbulence, the mechanical flushing out of stone fragments is achieved based on the "Bernoulli effect" [45].

3.6 Nephrostomy/Exit Strategies

Most urologists leave a 10–18 F nephrostomy/catheter in the kidney following PCNL in order to achieve *nephrostomy trifecta*: kidney drainage (primarily of urine, blood clots and small stone debris), hemostasis and healing and access of collecting system postoperatively (reentry, imaging or chemolysis). It is usually left open draining the kidney for first 24–48 h postoperatively [46, 47]. It is initially closed, left in place and re-opened if the patient experiences pain or fever or removed if the case is uneventful [48].

3.6.1 Loop Nephrostomy

The fine self-retaining (pig-tail-like) nephrostomy with an internal string attached in order to form a loop into collecting system can be easily removed by cutting the string. Care must be taken when a loop nephrostomy is inside the upper loop of a JJ stent [49]. In this case they can be tangled, and the JJ stent accidentally removed with nephrostomy removal [1, 5, 8].

3.6.2 Balloon Catheter

Simple or two-piece balloon catheters 12–18 F which are easily placed and removed [50]

3.6.3 Tubeless Nephrostomy

No nephrostomy/drainage is left while a JJ stent may be or may not be in situ. This is an advantage of miniaturized PCNL which is gaining popularity with novel laser technology [51].

3.6.3.1 Tubeless but Stented PCNL

In particular cases, where an alternative ureteral drainage is needed in order to prevent urine leakage through the percutaneous tract, a JJ stent is placed. Ureteral spasm or stenosis or UPJ edema revealed with difficult passage of the contrast medium down the ureter to the bladder small stone fragments in the ureter or cases with risk of clot formation, which are the most frequent criteria for JJ stent placement [1]. JJ stents used are either with a string attached that can be removed by the patient within a few days or without string that are usually left for longer periods (e.g. 3–6 weeks). Advantages of JJ stent placement are urine drainage facilitation leading to better percutaneous tract healing, dilation of the ureter in cases of spasm, edema or stenosis and ease of small stone fragment passage. Disadvantages of JJ stent placement are stent-related symptoms that need to be relieved with medication, cost increase and need for further endoscopic procedure to remove it [52–56].

3.6.3.2 Totally Tubeless (Unstented) PCNL

The totally tubeless PNL (tubeless and stentless with no postoperative drainage of the operated collecting system at all) is reserved for very selected cases with no bleeding, no residual stone fragments or other complicating elements [1].

References

1. Scoffone CM, Hoznek A, Rode J. Instruments and accessories for ECIRS. In: Scoffone CM, et al., editors. Supine percutaneous nephrolithotomy and ECIRS. Paris: Springer-Verlag; 2014.
2. Skolarikos A, Dellis A. Tips to puncture the kidney using the triangular technique. In: Rane A, et al., editors. Practical tips in urology. London: Springer-Verlag; 2016.
3. Fernstrom I, Johansson B. Percutaneous pyelolithotomy. A new extraction technique. Scand J Urol Nephrol. 1976;10:257–9.
4. Skolarikos A, Alivizatos G, Papatsoris A, et al. Ultrasound-guided percutaneous nephrostomy performed by urologists: 10-year experience. Urology. 2006;68(3):495–9.
5. Webb DR. Percutaneous renal surgery. A practical clinical handbook. Cham: Springer International Publishing; 2016.
6. Turna B, Nazli O, Demiryoguran S, et al. Percutaneous nephrolithotomy: variables that influence hemorrhage. Urology. 2007;69:603–7.
7. Michel MS, Trojan L, Rassweiler JJ. Complications in percutaneous nephrolithotomy. Eur Urol. 2007;51:899–906.
8. Autorino R, Liatsikos E, Porpiglia F. New technologies and techniques in minimally invasive urologic surgery. An ESUT collection. Torino: Edizioni Minerva Medica SpA; 2019.
9. Lahme S, Bichler KH, Stohmaier WL, et al. Minimally invasive PCNL in patients with renal pelvic and calyceal stones. Eur Urol. 2001;40:619–24.
10. Sabnis RB, Ganesamoni R, Scarpal R. Miniperc: what is its current status? Curr Opin Urol. 2012;22:129–33.

11. Li X, He Z, Wu K, et al. Chinese minimally invasive percutaneous nephrolithotomy: the Guangzhou experience. J Endourol. 2009;23:1693–7.
12. Zhao Z, Tuerxu A, Liu Y, et al. Super-mini PCNL (SMP): material, indications, technique, advantages and results. Arch Esp Urol. 2017;70:211–6.
13. Desai J, Solanki R. Ultra-mini percutaneous nephrolithotomy (UMP): one more armamentarium. BJU Int. 2013;112:1046–9.
14. Bader MJ, Gratzke C, Seitz M, et al. The "all-seeing needle": initial results of an optical puncture system confirm in access in percutaneous nephrolithotomy. Eur Urol. 2011;59:1054–9.
15. Segura JW, Patterson DE, Leroy AJ, et al. Percutaneous lithotripsy. J Urol. 1983;130:1051–4.
16. Alken P, Hutschenreiter G, Gunher R, et al. Percutaneous stone manipulation. J Urol. 1981;125:463–7.
17. Alken P. Telescopbougierset zur perkutanen Nephrostomie. Aktuel Urol. 1981;12:216–9.
18. Clayman RV, Castaneda-Zuniga WR, Hunter DW, et al. Rapid balloon dilatation of the nephrostomy track for nephrostolithotomy. Radiology. 1983;147:884–5.
19. Frattini A, Barbieri A, Salsi P, et al. One shot: a novel method to dilate the nephrostomy access for percutaneous lithotripsy. J Endourol. 2001;15:919–23.
20. Goharderakhshan RZ, Schwarz BF, Rudnick DM, et al. Radially expanding single-step nephrostomy tract dilator. Urology. 2001;58:693–8.
21. Dehong C, Liangren L, Huawei L, et al. A comparison among four tract dilation methods of percutaneous nephrolithotomy: a systematic review and meta-analysis. Urolithiasis. 2013;41(6):523–30.
22. Dellis AE, Skolarikos AA, Nastos K, et al. The impact of technique standardization on total operating and fluoroscopy times in simple endourological procedures: a prospective study. J Endourol. 2018;32(8):747–52.
23. Karagiannis A, Skolarikos A, Alexandrescu E, et al. Epidemiologic study of urolithiasis in seven countries of South-Eastern Europe: S.E.G.U.R. 1 study. Arch Ital Urol Androl. 2017;89(3):173–7.
24. Rusnak B, Castaneda-Zuniga W, Kotula F, et al. An improved dilator system for percutaneous nephrostomies. Radiology. 1982;144:174.
25. Mulvaney WP. Attempted disintegration of calculi by ultrasonic vibrations. J Urol. 1953;70:704–7.
26. Gasteyer KH. Eine neue Methode der Blasensteinzertrummerung: Die Ultraschall-Lithotripsie. Urologe. 1971;10:30–2.
27. Pietropaolo A, Proietti S, Geraghty R, et al. Trends of 'urolithiasis: interventions, simulation, and laser technology' over the last 16 years (2000-2015) as published in the literature (PubMed): a systematic review from European Section of Uro-technology (ESUT). World J Urol. 2017;35(11):1651–8.
28. Durutovic O, Dzamic Z, Milojevic B, et al. Pulsed versus continuous mode fluoroscopy during PCNL: safety and effectiveness comparison in a case series study. Urolithiasis. 2016;44(6):565–70.
29. Hemal AK, Goel A, Aron M, et al. Evaluation of fragmentation with single or multiple pulse setting of lithoclast for renal calculi during percutaneous nephrolithotripsy and its impact on clearance. Urol Int. 2003;70:265–8.
30. Teichman JM, Vassar GJ, Bishoff JT, et al. Holmium:YAG lithotripsy yields smaller fragments than lithoclast, pulsed dye laser or electrohydraulic lithotripsy. J Urol. 1998;159:17–23.
31. Bourdoumis A, Papatsoris A, Calleary JG, et al. The evolution of urolithiasis assessment and management in the new millennium. Panminerva Med. 2016;58(3):222–36.
32. Bourdoumis A, Stasinou T, Kachrilas S, et al. Thromboprophylaxis and bleeding diathesis in minimally invasive stone surgery. Nat Rev Urol. 2014;11(1):51–8.
33. Kachrilas S, Papatsoris A, Bach C, et al. The current role of percutaneous chemolysis in the management of urolithiasis: review and results. Urolithiasis. 2013;41(4):323–6.
34. Bach C, Goyal A, Kumar P, et al. The Barts 'flank-free' modified supine position for percutaneous nephrolithotomy. Urol Int. 2012;89(3):365–8.
35. Papatsoris AG, Shaikh T, Patel D, et al. Use of a virtual reality simulator to improve percutaneous renal access skills: a prospective study in urology trainees. Urol Int. 2012;89(2):185–90.
36. Kumar P, Bach C, Kachrilas S, et al. Supine percutaneous nephrolithotomy (PCNL): 'in vogue' but in which position? BJU Int. 2012;110(11 Pt C):E1018–21.
37. Hoffman N, Lukasewycz SJ, Canales B, et al. Percutaneous renal stone extraction: in vitro study of retrieval devices. J Urol. 2004;172:559–61.
38. Kachrilas S, Papatsoris A, Bach C, et al. Colon perforation during percutaneous renal surgery: a 10-year experience in a single endourology centre. Urol Res. 2012 Jun;40(3):263–8.
39. El-Husseiny T, Moraitis K, Maan Z, et al. Percutaneous endourologic procedures in high-risk patients in the lateral decubitus position under regional anesthesia. J Endourol. 2009;23(10):1603–6.
40. Skolarikos A, Papatsoris AG. Diagnosis and management of postpercutaneous nephrolithotomy residual stone fragments. J Endourol. 2009;23(10):1751–5.
41. Papatsoris A, Masood J, El-Husseiny T, et al. Improving patient positioning to reduce complications in prone percutaneous nephrolithotomy. J Endourol. 2009;23(5):831–2.
42. Papatsoris AG, Zaman F, Panah A, et al. Simultaneous anterograde and retrograde endourologic access: "the Barts technique". J Endourol. 2008;22(12):2665–6.
43. Papatsoris AG, Masood J, Saunders P. Supine valdivia and modified lithotomy position for simultaneous anterograde and retrograde endourological access. BJU Int. 2007;100(5):1192.
44. Bissas A, Dellis A, Bafaloukas N, et al. Percutaneous nephrolithotomy to remove a cartridge detonating cap mimicking a renal pelvic stone 12 years after renal trauma. J Endourol. 2005;19(6):719–21.

45. Panah A, Masood J, Zaman F, et al. A technique to flush out renal stone fragments during percutaneous nephrolithotomy. J Endourol. 2009;23(1):5–6.
46. Somani B, Dellis A, Liatsikos E, et al. Review on diagnosis and management of urolithiasis in pregnancy: an ESUT practical guide for urologists. World J Urol. 2017;35(11):1637–49.
47. Skolarikos A, Dellis A, Knoll T. Ureteropelvic obstruction and renal stones: etiology and treatment. Urolithiasis. 2015;43(1):5–12.
48. Paul EM, Marcovich R, Lee BR, et al. Choosing the ideal nephrostomy tube. BJU Int. 2003;92:672–7.
49. Srinivasan AK, Herati A, Okeke Z, et al. Renal drainage after percutaneous nephrolithotomy. J Endourol. 2009;23:1743–9.
50. Armitage JN, Irving SO, Burgess NA. Percutaneous nephrolithotomy in the United Kingdom: results of a prospective data registry. Eur Urol. 2012;61:1188–93.
51. Aldoukhi AH, Black KM, Shields J, Ghani KR. Ambulatory tubeless mini-percutaneous nephrolithotomy using Moses technology and dusting technique. Urology. 2019;124:306.
52. Papatsoris A, Dellis A, Daglas G, et al.; EAU Young Academic Urology Working Parties (Endourology). Management of JJ stent-related symptoms. Acta Chir Iugosl. 2014;61(1):73–4.
53. Dellis A, Joshi HB, Timoney AG, et al. Relief of stent related symptoms: review of engineering and pharmacological solutions. J Urol. 2010;184:1267–72.
54. Deliveliotis C, Chrisofos M, Gougousis E, et al. Is there a role for alpha1-blockers in treating double-J stent-related symptoms? Urology. 2006;67:35–9.
55. Dellis AE, Keeley FX Jr, Manolas V, et al. Role of a-blockers in the treatment of stent-related symptoms: a prospective randomized control study. Urology. 2014;83:56–61.
56. Dellis A, Papatsoris A, Keeley FX, et al. Tamsulosin, Solifenacin, and their combination for the treatment of stent-related symptoms: a randomized controlled study. J Endourol. 2017;31(1):100–9.

Operating Room Setup for PCNL

4

Victoria Jahrreiss and Mehmet Özsoy

To ensure ideal working conditions, a dedicated operating room (OR) setup for endourological procedures is essential. In order to enable efficiency and safety within the OR, strategic placement of the required equipment is crucial, allowing free movement of the equipment and the surgeon to view multiple screens at the same time [1].

In an ideal setting, PCNL should be performed in a lead-shielded endourology-dedicated operating room, which consists of a urology-specific endoscopy table with fluoroscopic capabilities and at least two monitors that receive fluoroscopic and endoscopic images.

In order to fit the large equipment required for endourologic procedures the recommended size for a fluoroscopy-compatible endoscopic operating room is around 50 m^2 with a ceiling height of at least 3 m and an additional 50–70 cm for an over ceiling space, containing cables for equipment booms, electrical wires, nitrous oxide, oxygen, compressed air, pipelines for air conditioning and a sterile air distributor. The sterile air distributer filters viruses, bacteria and dust and thus provides a hygienic, low-turbulence air supply for the operating room. A suspended metal ceiling with individually removable tiles enables easy maintenance of the infrastructures in the over ceiling space. Ideally at least two booms should be mounted to the ceiling, one for the anesthesiologist and one for the surgical team, supplying electrical sockets, pipelines and space to hold equipment. In order to provide radiation protection, the walls of a dedicated endourological OR can be either lead shielded or have a wall thickness equivalent to 2 mm of lead. The walls should be painted a light, washable color and have fixtures for a plasma screen, wall-mounted cameras, an X-ray film illuminator and drawers for endoscopic disposables. Materials for wall and floor surfaces need to be strong, slip resistant, impermeable and either seamless or have minimum joints. Recommended is laminated polyester or smooth paint for the walls and linoleum, jointless conductive tiles or similar materials for the flooring. Floor conductivity can range between minimum 1mΩ and a maximum of 10 mΩ. To provide proper drainage during endourological procedures, it is recommended for the OR to have a central drain outlet, centered underneath the operating table and the floors to have a slight tilt towards the central drain. The main OR gate should have a width of 1.5–2 m, facilitating movement of the larger appliances needed for endourological procedures. To minimize air currents, a sliding door is recommended. The operating suite should be equipped with a hydraulically operated OR table with large twin-wheel castors so that it

V. Jahrreiss · M. Özsoy (✉)
Department of Urology, Medical University of Vienna, Vienna, Austria
e-mail: mehmet.oezsoy@meduniwien.ac.at

G. Zeng, K. Sarica (eds.), *Percutaneous Nephrolithotomy*,
https://doi.org/10.1007/978-981-15-0575-1_4

can also be used for patient transportation to and from the operating suite. The table should have both battery and mains power supply. It should be divided into multiple segments: head plate, upper back plate, lower back plate, seat plate and leg plates, aiding the effortless placement of the patient in lithotomy position as well as supine and prone patient positioning. Additionally, the table needs to be rotatable in various axes with a stable base construction allowing the tilting of different body parts for optimal patient positioning. Furthermore, the OR table needs to be fluoroscopy compatible. For this purpose it is important for the tabletop to be padded with multiple layers of radiolucent foam and free of cross bars. During endourologic procedures different levels of lighting are required. Therefore, dimmable, freely movable lights are a necessity. Light-emitting diode lights provide adjustable light characteristics, a multicolor temperature facility and low heat generation at an unlimited lifespan. As in a general operating theater, overhead lights should provide shadowless lighting between 25,000 and 125,000 Lux with at least 15,000 Lux at the periphery and 50,000–100,000 Lux at the center. Color-corrected fluorescent lights produce smooth illumination and minimal glare. A separate sterilization room for the delicate endourological instruments should be set up close to the OR, enabling swift sterilization and, therefore, allowing multiple procedures to be performed in a day. Equipment should comprise of automated processing disinfection machines as well as units for manual cleaning and rinsing. If autoclavation of the endoscopic instruments is not possible, a unit for chemical sterilization and ethylene oxide needs to be set up.

For endourological procedures a number of appliances are necessary. In order to provide ideal working conditions, strategic placement of the equipment is essential as shown in Fig. 4.1. At least two monitors that receive fluoroscopic and endoscopic images are needed. The monitors should be placed in front of the surgeon ensuring an ergonomic working environment. Additionally, video monitoring ensures a more ergonomic procedure for the urologist and facilitates training for urologic residents. Moreover, it enables video or photo documentation that can be incorporated into the patient's electronic records.

A mobile C-arm is an essential appliance in an endourological operating room and should be placed on the opposite side of the surgeon for PCNL. The C-arm should supply graduated, balanced movement at all angles and produce a high-quality image, allowing the surgeon to make precise and quick assessments intraoperatively. It should also facilitate image processing, DICOM imaging and last image hold memory and provide a high resolution image to its display, ideally a TFT monitor, as well as to a hanging monitor [2].

Fluoroscopy (C-arm or table) is necessary to guide positioning of puncture needles, wires, dilators and catheters and to perform pyelography. Moreover, placement of the working shaft can be performed under fluoroscopic guidance over the working guidewire. Fluoroscopy can also identify radiopaque stones and help to assess success following stone defragmentation.

The surgeon should confirm that fluoroscopy is correctly positioned and can be easily manipulated prior to surgery. The surgeon should control fluoroscopy by activation of a foot pedal. An ultrasound device with an abdominal ultrasound probe should be placed in the vicinity of the surgeon and should be covered with a sterile draping in order to allow the surgeon to manipulate it during the procedure.

Everyone in the operating room should use lead aprons and thyroid shields for personal protection. Dosimetry badges are needed to record individual radiation exposure. Lead glasses are especially recommended for endoscopic surgeons due to their proximity to the radiation source and chronic exposure.

Before starting with PCNL, the operating room staff should confirm that all potential instruments and disposable equipment are available and ready for use. The surgeon should confirm that this equipment is correct for the chosen surgical modality.

The steps of the procedure should be anticipated and the operation table should be set up to ensure a smooth course of operation. In complex cases where access to the renal stone may be difficult, additional equipment

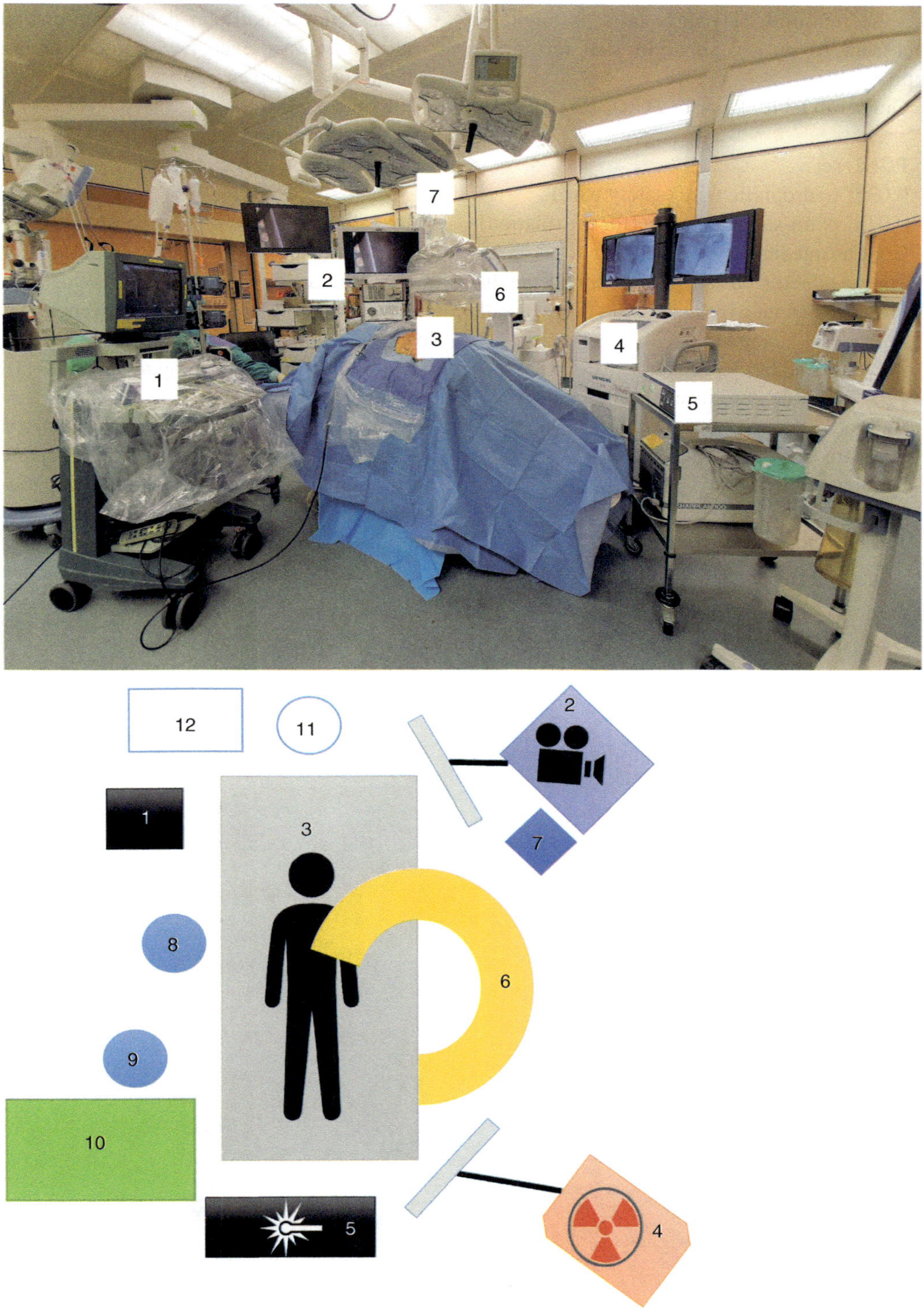

Fig. 4.1 OR floorplan PCNL setup. (1) Ultrasound, (2) Video tower, (3) OR table, (4) Fluoroscopy monitor, (5) Lithotripter, (6) C-arm, (7) Irrigation fluid (8) Surgeon, (9) Scrub nurse, (10) Scrub table, (11) Anesthesiologist, (12) Anesthesiology equipment

may be required. If access fails, it might be necessary to pursue an additional retrograde approach.

Our scrub table setup for PCNL (Fig. 4.2):

- PCNL set
- 0.035″ hydrophilic wire (safety wire)
- 0.035″ extra-stiff guidewire (for the dilation)
- Contrast media
- For the puncture, a two-part Trocar needle that provides enhanced visualization of the needle tip under ultrasound
- Polyethylene fascial dilator set (6–16 Fr)
- 11 Fr peelable introducer sheath
- Balloon dilator
- Amplatz working sheath
- Rigid nephroscope
- Rigid graspers
- 10 Fr nitinol tipless stone extractor
- Dual-action lithotripter device that combines ultrasonic wave energy with intermittent ballistic shockwave energy
- Flexible nephroscope
- 2.4 Fr nitinol basket
- 14–18 Fr Councill catheter

Irrigation under low pressure should be performed using an isotonic saline solution at body temperature as there is always a risk of absorption from pyelolymphatic or pyelovenous backflow or from ureteral or renal perforation. Irrigation bag should be hung at about 30–50 cm above patient's level.

Stone disintegration can be achieved with a variety of endoscopic lithotripters. While pneumatic and ultrasonic systems are most commonly used in standard PCNL, for miniaturized instruments the use of laser lithotripters has increased [3].

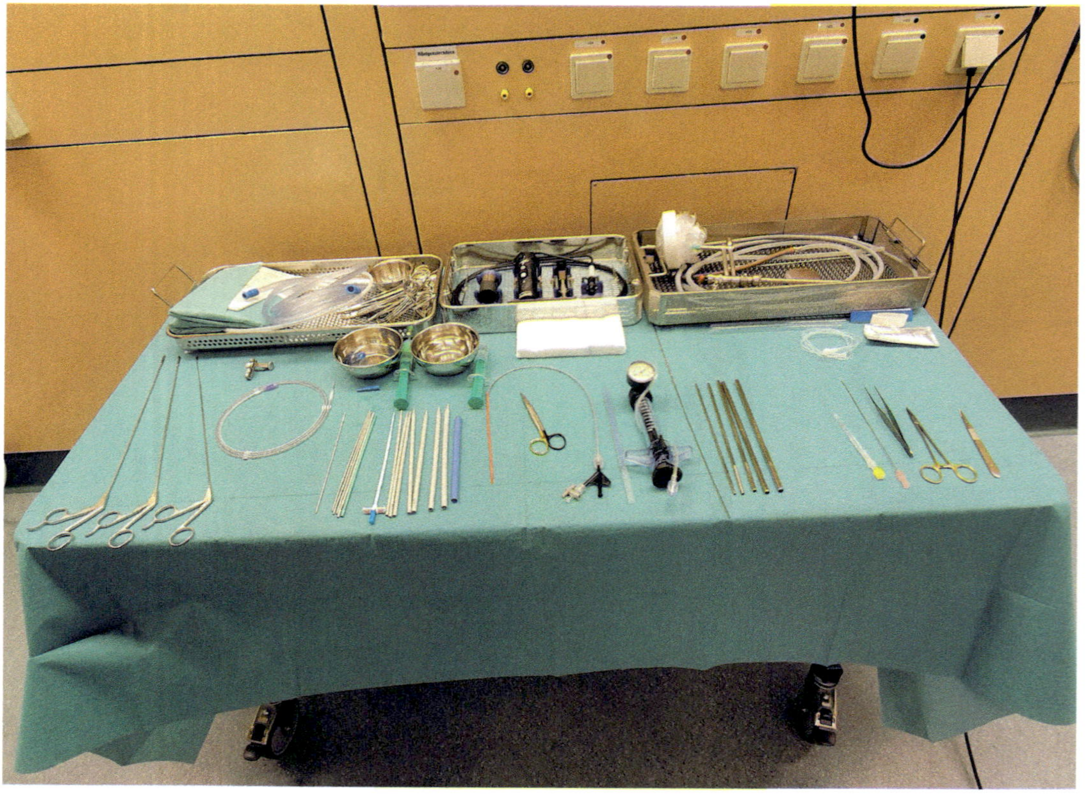

Fig. 4.2 A scrub table setup for PCNL

It is recommended to incorporate video cameras into the operating room: one directed to the top of the operating table, one giving an overview of the entire operating room and one covering the screens. Video recordings aid the surgical education of urologic residents and enable live surgery screenings for scientific meetings and workshops.

The requirements for a dedicated endourological operating room differ from those of a general OR. Endourological procedures demand modern technology as well as large appliances that have to be placed strategically. Thus, a well thought out setup for dedicated endourological operating suites is of great significance in order to enable optimal working conditions for the surgeon, minimize changeover times and facilitate surgical training for residents [2].

References

1. Reijnen M, Zeebregts CJ, Meijerink W. Future of operating rooms. Surg Technol Int. 2005;14:21–7.
2. Sabnis RB, Mishra S, Sharma R, Desai MR. Preoperative planning and designing of a fluoro-compatible endourology operating room. J Endourol. 2009;23(10):1579–85.
3. Ganesamoni R, Sabnis RB, Mishra S, Parekh N, Ganpule A, Vyas JB, et al. Prospective randomized controlled trial comparing laser lithotripsy with pneumatic lithotripsy in miniperc for renal calculi. J Endourol. 2013;27(12):1444–9.

5 Preoperative Assessment and Patient Preparation for PCNL Surgery

Simon K. S. Choong and Gautam Kumar

Prior to any type of surgery, including PCNL, patients undergo preoperative assessment. There are two main components to this and to patient preparation. The first is centered on the delivery of safe and appropriate surgery and anaesthesia. This is principally a safety check and communication process generally performed separately on the day of surgery by the surgeon and anaesthetist involved in the case. The second component is the concept of preoperative assessment to optimise patients in order to improve outcomes and reduce perioperative risk.

It is generally accepted that there is a need to assess the potential of benefit and of harm afforded by any surgical or anaesthetic procedural intervention and this information should be communicated to the patient. This should form the basis for the shared decision-making process, which will lead to the selection of appropriate intraoperative and postoperative care that considers the patient's personal preferences, expectations and values. The aim is to ensure the patient is fully informed and ready for surgery. This will involve a health check and possibly optimisation of their health and current therapies. It involves planning with the patient their admission to hospital and discharge after surgery. This will help prevent cancellations on the day of surgery and lead to an improved patient experience and outcome.

Preoperative assessment and preparation are a process. It involves primary care, anaesthesia, surgery and possibly other specialties. The general practitioner has a role to play by ensuring that patients are 'fit for referral' (for example with optimised blood pressure, diabetic management and medication) and by initiating the shared decision-making process. Development of strong links with primary care can facilitate this. Part of the process is an assessment to check it is safe to proceed with anaesthesia and surgery. It is also about both optimising and preparing the patient for anaesthesia and surgery. The anaesthetist plays a key role in co-ordinating this process with other medical specialties and healthcare professionals.

Shared decision making ideally should run throughout the whole patient journey; it is now viewed as an ethical imperative by the professional regulatory bodies, which expect clinicians to work in partnership with patients. The majority of patients want to be more involved than they currently are in making decisions about their own health, treatment, and healthcare, and there is compelling evidence that patients who are active participants in managing their health and healthcare have better outcomes than patients who are passive recipients of care. If the patient decides to

S. K. S. Choong (✉) · G. Kumar
Institute of Urology, University College London Hospitals, London, UK
e-mail: gautamkumar@doctors.org.uk

G. Zeng, K. Sarica (eds.), *Percutaneous Nephrolithotomy*,
https://doi.org/10.1007/978-981-15-0575-1_5

proceed, he or she should be as fit as possible for surgery and anaesthesia. Preoperative assessment and preparation allow risks to be clearly identified and mitigated or managed in a planned and consistent way.

5.1 Preoperative Assessment

Preoperative assessment largely comprises of the following steps:

- A patient interview and medical case notes review to establish current diagnoses, current medicines and past medical and anaesthetic history. This is primarily conducted by preassessment nursing staff with additional assessment by an anaesthetist if deemed necessary. All complex patients, as mentioned below, are assessed by a consultant anaesthetist, who decides upon the need for further investigations, decides if further optimization is needed and decides whether the patient needs postoperative critical care/high-dependency/intensive care management
- Examination, including airway assessment
- Review of results of relevant investigations (see below)
- The presence of any risk factors, including methicillin-resistant Staphylococcus aureus (MRSA) screening and risk of venous thromboembolism
- The need for further tests to give the patient more information about their individual risk

In addition to general risk factors and considerations for all patients undergoing anaesthesia (ischaemic heart disease, diabetes, etc.) the following are of specifically related to patients undergoing PCNL surgery:

- Spina bifida—The incidence of spina bifida (SB) is ~1:1000, and risk of stone disease is substantially raised in SB (up to 15% of all patients undergoing PCNL surgery have spina bifida, kyphoscoliosis or spinal cord injury.) (Fig. 5.1) PCNL in patients with SB is associated with multiple parameters of poor outcome. Patients with SB should be counselled about increased peri-operative risk and likelihood of stone recurrence.
- Raised BMI—Patients with an increase bodyweight (Fig. 5.2) prove a risk as many of them are operated on in the prone position, and hence there may be difficulty ventilating them and they possess an increased risk of pressure injury and nerve damage. Alternative treatment option by retrograde intrarenal surgery (RIRS) should be considered. There is also risk of injury to theatre staff who have to prone

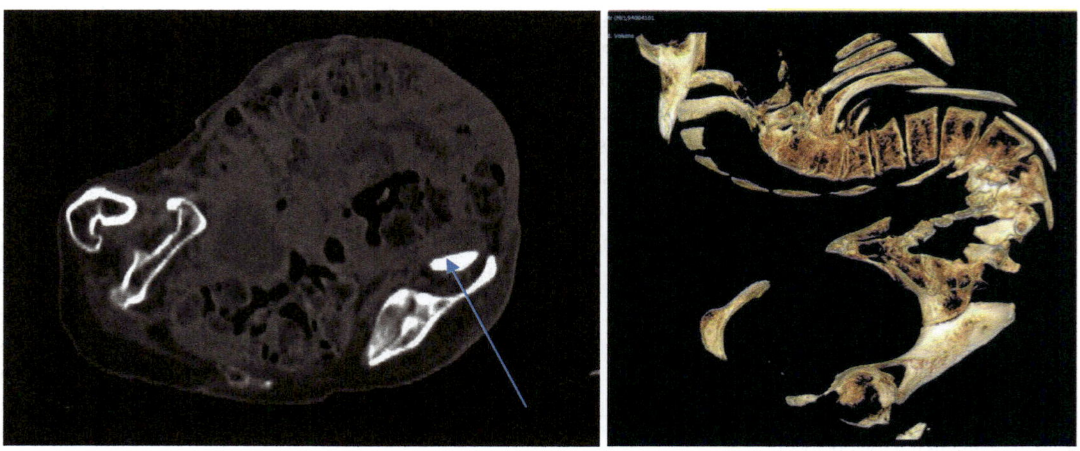

Fig. 5.1 CT scan of patient with spina bifida with severe kyphoscoliosis. Blue arrow shows kidney with stone

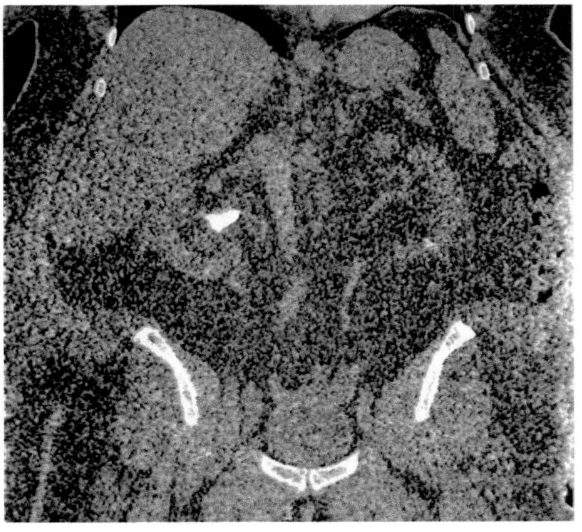

Fig. 5.2 shows a high BMI patient of 66 kg/m^2

the patient. Even supine PCNL patients need to be lifted to position a bag under the flank of the operated side.

- Glaucoma—Postoperative visual loss after surgery in the prone position has an estimated incidence of 0.01–1%. Although spinal surgery poses the greatest risk, it has been reported in other operations. Narrow-angle glaucoma (in addition to ischaemic heart disease, smoking, hypertension, and polycythaemia) is a known risk factor.
- Blood-thinning medication—The perioperative use of certain medications (aspirin, clopidogrel, NSAIDs, and anticoagulants) need to be carefully considered. Some perioperative bleeding is normal but rarely it may be significant enough to need a blood transfusion (in less than 5% of cases). The use of these medications increases that risk. Patients usually need to be able to come off and stay off anticoagulants (warfarin, heparin, rivaroxaban, dabigatran, apixaban, edoxaban) and strong antiplatelet (clopidogrel, ticlopidine, prasugrel, ticagrelor) preoperatively and postoperatively to reduce the risks of intraoperative and postoperative bleeding. Haematology consultations are useful and if patients are deemed too high risk to come off their anticoagulants or strong antiplatelet medications, retrograde intrarenal surgery (RIRS) should be considered.

The following investigations are routinely performed on patients during their preoperative assessment for PCNL surgery.

- Full blood count and differential
- Renal profile
- Albumin
- Calcium
- Coagulation screen
- Group and screen
- MRSA culture screen
- Urine—microscopy and culture (MSU)

Additionally, as per national guidelines the following tests are sometimes carried out:

- ECG—If ASA1, to consider if over 65 years old. To be done in all patients ASA2 or greater, hence any cardiovascular or respiratory comorbidities, including hypertension, ischaemic heart disease.
- Lung function tests—Considered in people who are ASA grade 3 or 4 due to known or suspected respiratory disease.
- Echocardiogram—Consider resting echocardiography if the person has a heart murmur and any cardiac symptom (including breathlessness, pre-syncope, syncope or chest pain) or signs or symptoms of heart failure.

5.2 MSU and Management of UTI Preoperatively

It is imperative to check the midstream urine (MSU) results from at least 2 weeks prior to the planned surgery so that there is sufficient time to treat urinary tract infection (UTI) prior to PCNL. Untreated UTI is associated with an increased risk of urinary sepsis and septicaemia. High-risk patients with an infected staghorn stone should be electively managed and monitored in a high dependency unit postoperatively.

At the induction of surgery gentamicin or a suitable antibiotic should be administered. In higher risk patients, a further two doses of i.v.

antibiotic is usually given. Stone fragments should be sent for culture and sensitivity testing in infected cases.

Antibiotics treat bacteria in the urine but usually cannot treat bacteria inside an infected stone or penetrate the bacterial biofilms on a stent. Bacteria are released from an infected stone or a stent during an operation and a longer course of antibiotics postoperatively should be considered.

5.3 Patient Preparation

To ensure patients are prepared for surgery, the following should be considered and managed:

- The patient's understanding of and consent to the procedure and share in the decision-making process
- An explanation of the options for anaesthesia, an opportunity to ask questions and agreement to the anaesthetic technique proposed
- Preoperative fasting, the proposed pain relief method, expected sequelae and possible major risks (where appropriate)
- A plan for the perioperative management of anticoagulant drugs, diabetic drugs and other current medications
- A process of medicines reconciliation by a pharmacist or pharmacy technician should be in place preoperatively
- The documentation of details of any discussion in the anaesthetic record

5.4 Postoperative Critical Care Management

The decision to admit a patient electively to critical care after surgery is subjective most of the time. The rationale of admission after elective PCNL surgery supposes that ICU admission can be preventive, which is not necessarily true. Many complications and risk factors discussed above have their roots in the pre-operative and operative period and, therefore, cannot be prevented by ICU admission. However, there are some patients where a higher dependency care is beneficial.

It is generally accepted that all patients with 5% or greater 30-day perioperative mortality should be admitted for postoperative monitoring but given that for this type of surgery mortality risk is lower, one looks towards other indicators. Patients with respiratory co-morbidities raised BMI and spinal injuries are at greater risk of postoperative pulmonary complications so may need ventilatory support, chest physio and early mobilization facilitated by greater nursing care. Patients with cardiac co-morbidities may need more rigorous blood pressure monitoring or cardiac telemetry to earlier diagnose, manage or treat any potential cardiac events. Patients with infected stones are prone to septic events so may benefit to more frequent monitoring to detect signs of sepsis and quicker treat any potential postoperative infections.

The need for postoperative critical care is significantly higher in males, elderly, patients with poor preoperative risk morbidity stratification scores, preexisting medical illness, major intra-operative hemorrhage, hypotension requiring inotropic support, perioperative respiratory problems and patients who suffer trauma (lung/bowel).

5.5 Planning and Safety Meeting

A weekly multidisciplinary meeting involving urologists, radiologists, microbiologists, nephrologists, specialist nurses and the team is useful to assess upcoming PCNL cases, especially complex patients. The patients' cases and circumstances, blood and urine results are checked. Imaging is reviewed to decide on tract access and whether an up to date CT KUB scan may be valuable. Complex patients are optimized, and a decision is made regarding elective admission to a high dependency unit postoperatively. These meetings help to familiarise the team with patients, ensure a smooth hospital journey and avoid unnecessary last minute surprises and cancellations.

Summary Points

- Principle is delivery of safe and appropriate surgery and anaesthesia
- Preoperative assessment to optimise patients in order to improve outcomes and reduce perioperative risk
- MSU results must be checked and UTI treated prior to PCNL
- High-risk patients must be assessed by a consultant anaesthetist and considered for elective admission to a high dependency unit postoperatively
- Consult a haematologist for patients to come off anticoagulation and antiplatelet treatment and agree on a bridging plan preoperatively and postoperatively
- Multidisciplinary planning meetings are useful to optimise safety and ensure a smooth hospital journey for the patient

Positioning During PNL

6

András Hoznek

6.1 Evolution of Positioning Techniques: Historical Background

In 1929, Dos Santos described the technique of lumbar aortography [1]. This consisted of the oblique insertion of a puncture needle in prone position with an entry point lateral to the vertebral column. The procedure allowed performing renal arteriography helping the diagnosis of kidney tumors. In the following years, lumbar aortography became quite popular and was routinely used. With the patient in the prone position for a translumbar aortogram, Willard Goodwin unintentionally inserted a needle into a hydronephrotic kidney [2]. This gave him the idea of antegrade pyelography and trocar nephrostomy in hydronephrosis [3]. Hence, from the late 1970s, puncturing the kidney during percutaneous nephrolithotomy was based on these previous experiences in the prone position [4].

Classical prone nephrolithotomy consists of two distinct operative steps: placement of a ureteric catheter in the lithotomy position followed by a second positioning in the prone position to create percutaneous access to the kidney and the nephroscopy itself (Figs. 6.1 and 6.2). However, this way of proceeding presents the inconvenience of the necessity of repositioning an intubated and perfused patient. Moreover, in many patients, general anesthesia in the prone position is not tolerated or contraindicated. In morbidly obese patients, the respiration reservoir is restricted because of increased baseline intra-abdominal pressure. This is aggravated in the prone position because of abdominal compression. Narrowing the inferior vena cava results in a decrease in venous return and in cardiac preload.

In 1987, Valdivia Uria reported a new method of patient positioning in the supine position [5]. After ureteric catheterization in the lithotomy position, the patient is repositioned with both legs in extension with an inflatable air bag under the lumbar region, and the ipsilateral arm is placed across the thorax (Figs. 6.3 and 6.4).

Later, this technique was improved by Ibarluzea in the Galdakao hospital [6]. This consists of a modified lithotomy position with the ipsilateral leg extended and the contralateral abducted and flexed. With the exception of this difference, it reproduces the principles of Valdivia (Figs. 6.5 and 6.6). This innovation is known worldwide as the "Galdakao-modified supine Valdivia position" (GMSV). Progressively this modification became increasingly popular. Actually, it allows accessing the urinary tract not only through an anterograde percutaneous route

A. Hoznek (✉)
Service d'Urologie CHU Henri Mondor, Créteil, France
e-mail: andras.hoznek@aphp.fr

G. Zeng, K. Sarica (eds.), *Percutaneous Nephrolithotomy*,
https://doi.org/10.1007/978-981-15-0575-1_6

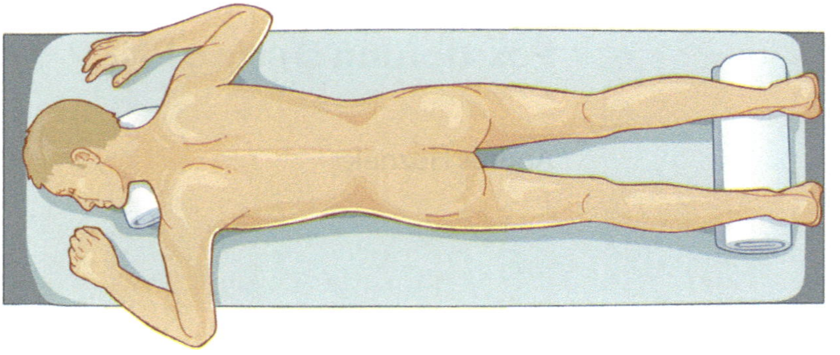

Fig. 6.1 Prone position for PCNL: superior view

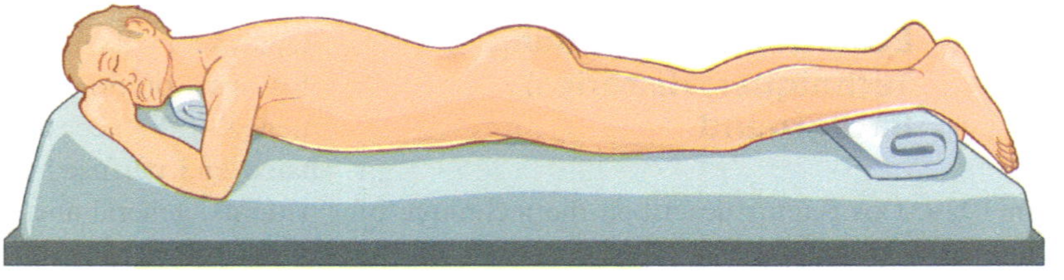

Fig. 6.2 Prone position for PCNL: lateral view

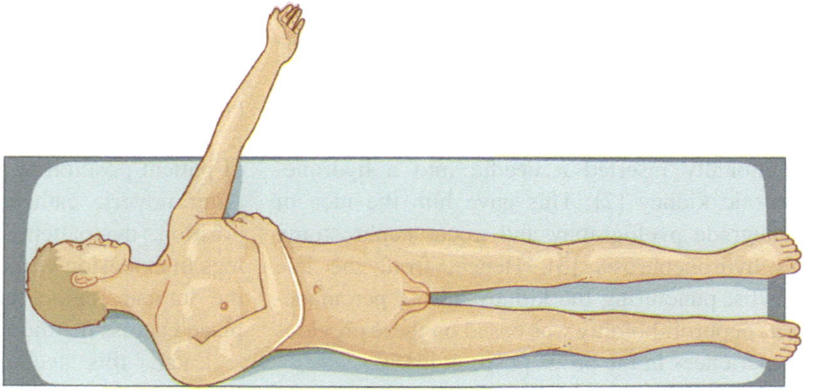

Fig. 6.3 Supine valdivia position: superior view

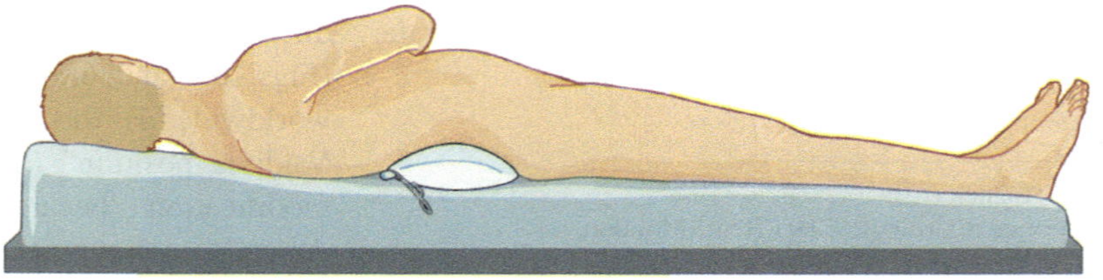

Fig. 6.4 Supine valdivia position: lateral view

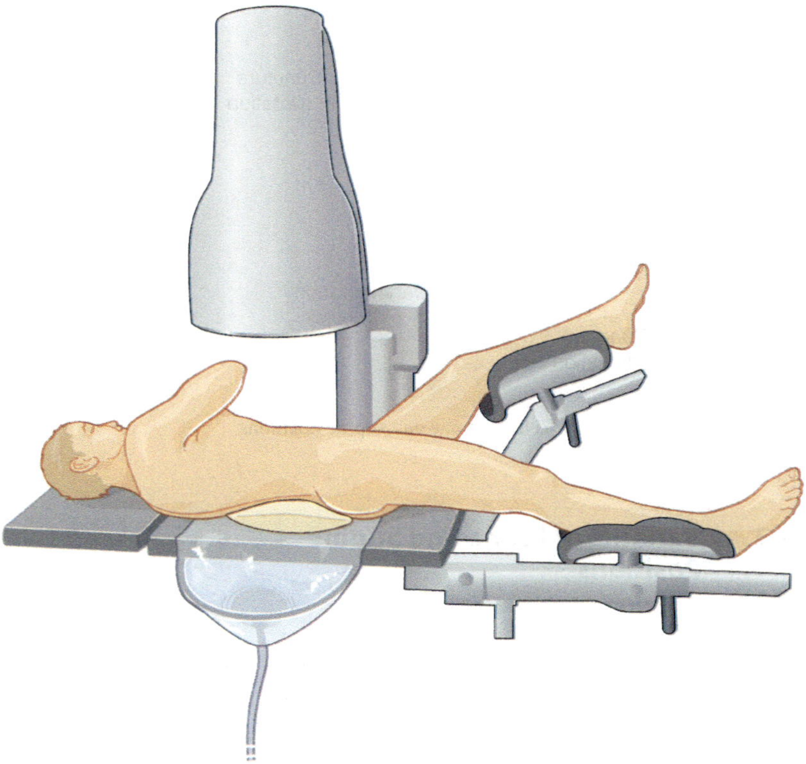

Fig. 6.5 Galdakao-modified supine Valdivia positon (GMSV)

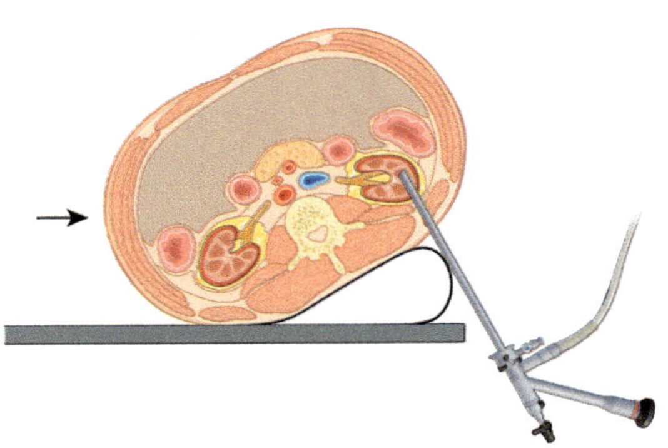

Fig. 6.6 In the GMSV position, the patient is pulled to the border of the table to avoid instrument collisions

but also via the ureter in the retrograde approach. In addition, two surgeons can work in tandem and perform several tasks simultaneously, opposed to the prone position which usually follows a sequential order.

With the development of flexible instruments, a combination of transurethral and percutaneous routes became possible. This led to the concept of "endoscopic combined intra-renal surgery" (ECIRS), popularized by Scoffone and Cracco [7]. The GMSV position also eliminates the necessity of repositioning the patient who needs to be draped only once. All these characteristics are supposed to shorten operative room occupation time (Fig. 6.7).

However, for many years, the majority of urologists remained faithful to the classical prone position [8]. According to the worldwide prospective study of the Clinical Research Office of the Endourology Society including 5803 patients, 80.3% of still performed the prone PCNL instead of the supine in 2011.

Both for prone and supine positioning, alternatives were proposed to improve ergonomics and outcomes.

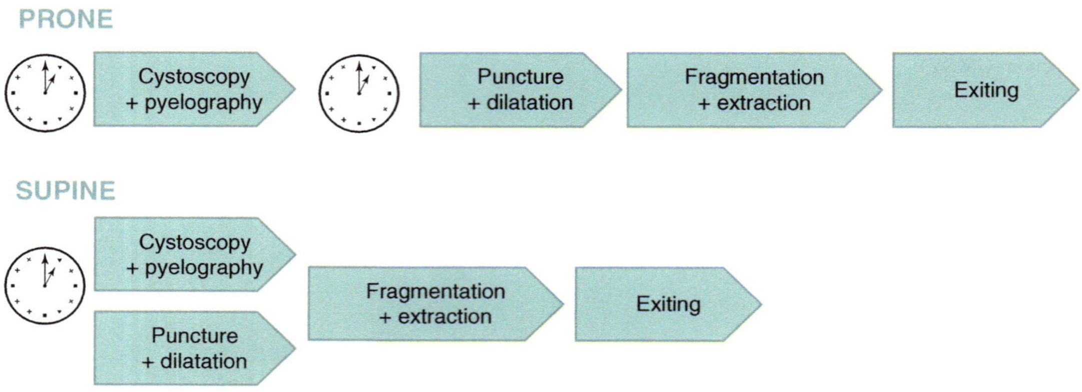

Fig. 6.7 Organigram of PCNL in prone and supine positions

6.2 Variants of Prone and Supine Positions

6.2.1 Prone Variants

Endoscopic combined intra-renal surgery is also possible in the prone position. For this purpose, the reverse lithotomy position [9] and prone split leg position were developed [10] (Fig. 6.8). Using flexible instruments, the bladder and upper urinary tract are accessed even if this can be less ergonomic.

The prone flexed position modifies the anatomical relationships of kidney, thorax and adjacent organs [11] (Fig. 6.9). The kidney is displaced caudally in the retroperitoneum providing improved access to the upper pole, often reducing the necessity of supracostal puncture. It was reported that 45% fewer supra-11th rib punctures are required to reach the superior calyx. In addition, the distance between the iliac crest and the 12th rib increases, creating more working space. However, this position impairs the patient's respiration, decreases cardiac index and compresses the inferior vena cava.

6.2.2 Lateral Positions

In morbidly obese patients, Kerbl suggested PCNL in lateral decubitus in 1994 [12]. The advantage is that in the lateral position, the pendulous abdomen moves sideways.

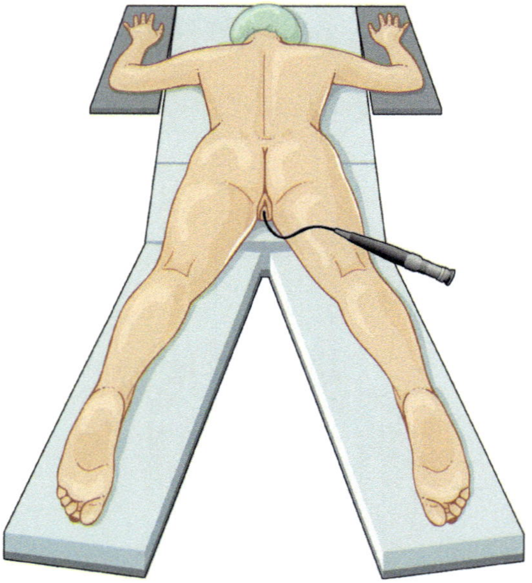

Fig. 6.8 Prone split leg position

However, this position also necessitates a separate time for retrograde ureteric catheterization in the lithotomy position and repositioning in lateral decubitus. In addition, in this position the kidney is projected on the vertebra during fluoroscopy making the puncture and identification of residual fragments difficult.

Bart's technique is a hybrid position that consists of tilting the pelvis 45° with the shoulders perpendicular to the operating table [13]

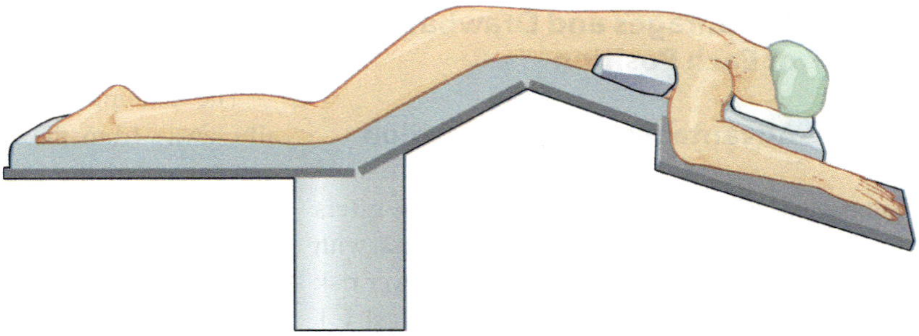

Fig. 6.9 Prone flexed position

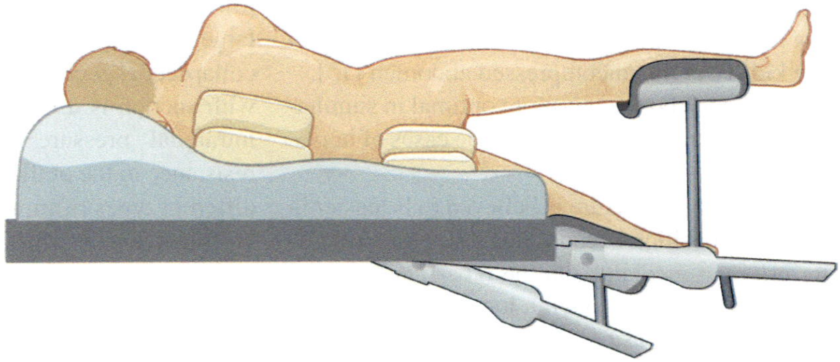

Fig. 6.10 Bart's position

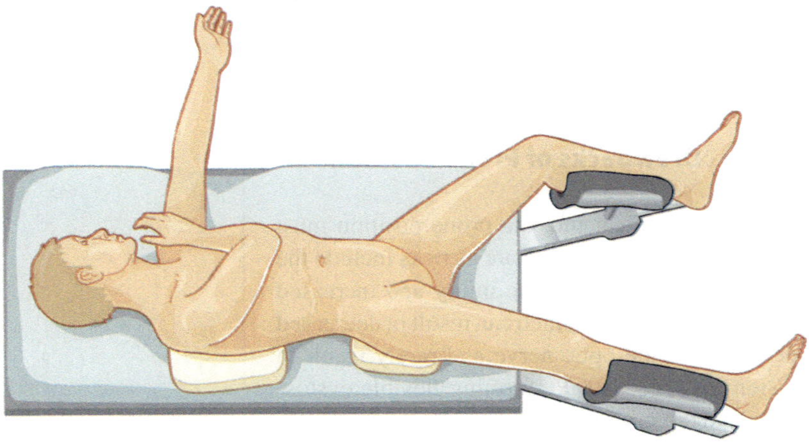

Fig. 6.11 Bart's flank free position

(Fig. 6.10). It requires only one positioning but results in a torque of the vertebral column.

6.2.3 Supine Variants

Besides the already mentioned Valdivia and GMSV positions, these basic techniques also underwent some minor modifications. One of the most popular is the Bart's flank free position in which the lumbar region is free; the patient is only slightly tilted by using a saline bag under the rib cage and a gel pad under the pelvis [14]. It is suggested that this position exposes the flank better than with other supine positions (Fig. 6.11).

6.3 Advantages and Drawbacks of Each Position

6.3.1 Advantages of Prone Position

Supporters of prone position argue that it offers larger surface area for percutaneous access with more medial access and, in principle, a lower risk of visceral injury. According to anatomical CT studies, despite more anterior puncture during the supine position, the risk of colon perforation is not increased because the bowel floats away from the kidney in the uncompressed abdomen [15].

The prone position is more optimal in simultaneous bilateral PCNL and in some cases of horseshoe kidney.

Upper pole puncture is believed to be easier in the prone position because it is located more posteriorly and medially. On the other hand, access to the upper pole through a lower calix puncture has been found easier [16]. In a prospective study including 45 patients, Sofer found that access to the upper calix through a lower pole puncture was possible in 20% of prone and 80% of supine percutaneous nephrolithotomies.

6.3.2 Drawbacks of Prone Position

Rolling the patient into the prone position must be undertaken with great care as risks include the potential for cervical spine injury and increased periorbital pressure, which can result in decreased perfusion to the optic nerve and rarely result in vision loss [17, 18]. Performing flexible cystoscopy and ureteroscopy is challenging in the prone position. Handling of the ureteric catheter necessitates specific precautions with respect to surgical asepsis.

6.3.3 Advantages of Supine Position

The supine position offers to the surgical team a great versatility. Simultaneous antegrade and retrograde access to the urinary tract is easy and comfortable. It also makes possible combining laparoscopy and endourology.

The abdominal wall is punctured more laterally, away from the lumbar muscles; therefore, movements of the endoscope are less restricted. The nephrostomy tube is better tolerated when the patient is lying on his back. The puncture of anterior calices is easier with a better puncture angle.

Horizontal direction of the tract maintains lower pressure which can be a drawback with large Amplatz because the collecting system is collapsed, especially if ultrasound fragmentation with suction is used. However, this reduction in intrarenal pressure counterbalances increased resistance to the outflow of irrigation fluid during different types of miniaturized PCNL. Wash out of fragments is easier because of the pending direction of the Amplatz. During mini-perc, the vacuum cleaner effect is more efficient (Figs. 6.12 and 6.13).

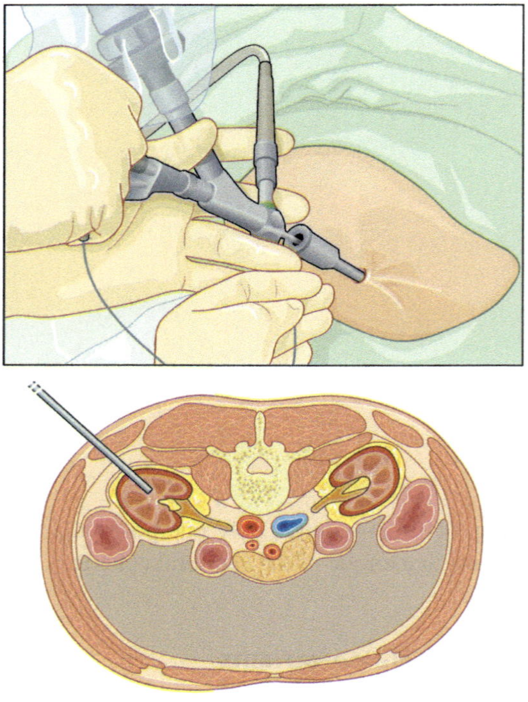

Fig. 6.12 The tract in prone position is oblique leading to slight increase in renal pressure

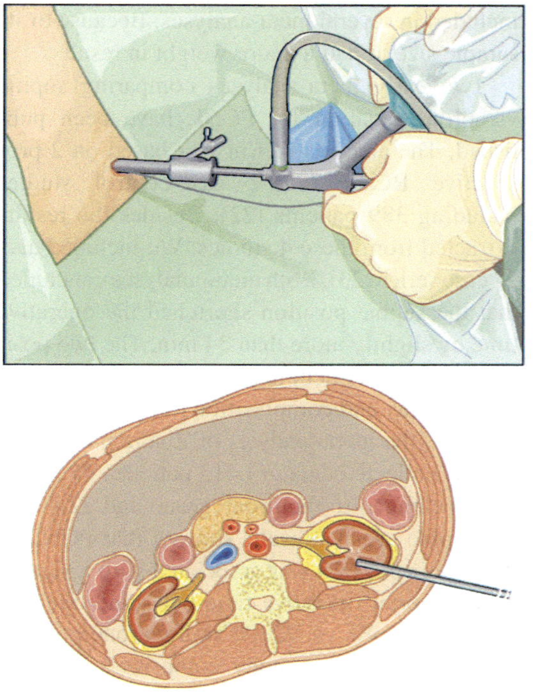

Fig. 6.13 In the supine position, stone clearance is more optimal and vacuum cleaner effect more efficient

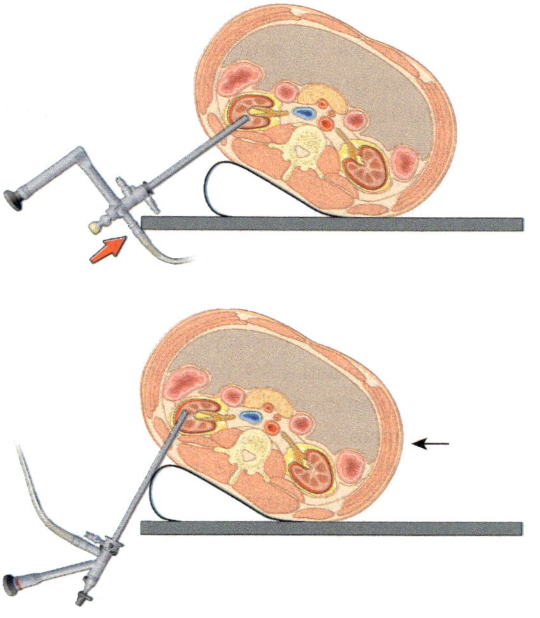

Fig. 6.14 Improper nephroscope design and patient positioning in the middle of the table result in instrument collisions. With modern nephroscopes and the patient pulled to the border of the table, fewer collisions occur

6.3.4 Drawbacks of Supine Position

In the beginning, many concerns were formulated relative to the supine position. The main criticism of the supine position is that the flank is not fully exposed, which makes access to the posterior and medially lying upper pole more difficult and provides less availability for multiple accesses.

The operating table and the patient's hips might also restrict instrument manipulation. Therefore, the choice of the nephroscope is fundamental. In older scopes, the light cable and the optical cable are located in the 6 and in the 12 o'clock positions on the instrument. In more recent nephroscopes, the optical and light cables and the irrigation line are connected in the same direction, thus limiting collisions. The patient should also be pulled to the border of the operative table (Fig. 6.14). This somewhat limits the feasibility of the supine position in some operative rooms equipped with integrated endoscopic-radiologic tables. On these tables, the patient must remain in the middle.

The absence of abdominal compression leaves the kidney more mobile, which can make dilatation of the tract more challenging. This difficulty can be overcome by the through and through the passage of the guidewire.

6.4 Review of the Literature

The clinical research office of the Endourology Society conducted a prospective multicentre study including 5775 PCNL patients from 96 centres worldwide [8, 19]. The conclusions of this ambitious project had a major impact on the opinion of urologic community for many years [20]. At the time of the study, the novel supine position was performed only in 19.7% while the majority of urologists remained faithful to the classical prone position corresponding to 80.3% of cases.

Stone-free rate was superior in the prone group with 77% of patients vs. 70.2% in the supine group ($p < 0.001$). However, the method evaluating residual fragments was dissimilar in the two groups: more patients had postoperative computed tomography in the supine group and the method of evaluation was not mentioned in a larger proportion of patients treated prone.

But the better results in the prone group had also a price in terms of complications. Transfusions were necessary in 6% of patients in the prone group and 4.3% in the supine group. A possible explanation of higher transfusion rate and superior stone-free rate might be a more radical treatment strategy in the prone group. Upper pole puncture was more frequent in the prone group with 11.4% of cases and only 4.0% in supine position. Multiple punctures were used in 9.0% in prone and 4.1% in supine cases. Both upper pole and multiple punctures increase the risk of bleeding.

Complications graded Clavien 2 or more were less frequent in supine group with 7.2% of patients vs. 10% in the prone group. This lower complication rate in the supine position is especially noteworthy as there were more high-risk patients in the supine group. In the prone and supine positions 54.7% vs. 46.8% were ASA1 and 33.4% vs 42.1% were ASA2, respectively.

The conclusions of the CROES study about operative time merit special attention and should be interpreted with caution. Mean operative time was significantly shorter in patients operated in the prone position with 82.7 min and 90.1 min. However, this result is rather misleading. Actually, operative time was defined as puncture to exit [21]. As a result, one of the main advantages of the supine technique, which is single positioning, was simply ignored by the CROES study. Yet, the time necessary to perform ureteric catheterization in the lithotomy position, turning the patient prone, second prepping and draping necessitates at least 20–30 min even in well-organized teams.

The critical analysis of the CROES study is important because later on its data were also included in several meta-analyses. Because of its sample size, it had a major weight in results.

Two early meta-analyses comparing supine vs. prone position for PCNL have been published. The analysis of Liu was based on 2 prospective RCTs and 2 case-control studies including 389 patients [22]. Besides the results extracted from these 4 studies, Wu included also 27 case series [23]. Both meta-analyses concluded that the supine position shortened the operative time by slightly more than 24 min. The two positions were equivalent to stone-free rate, length of hospital stay and complication rate.

Later, the meta-analysis of Zhang based on 9 studies collected data of 6413 patients. 77.3% of them belonged to the prone group and 22.7% to the supine group. Results showed that PCNL in the supine position was associated with a significantly shorter operative time but stone-free rate was only 72.9% vs. 77.3% in the prone position [24]. However, this study comprised only two randomized trials: one was a prospective non-randomized study and six were retrospective studies with no randomization. Data from the CROES database provided 86.3% of the data.

Presently, the highest evidence level available arises from a recent meta-analysis including exclusively randomized studies [25]. Fifteen studies were selected collecting data from 1474 patients.

Stone-free rate was 78.1% (574/735) in the supine group and 80.0% (591/739) in the prone group; the difference is non-significant. Operative time was slightly but significantly shorter in the supine group with a mean weighted difference of 12.02 min. There was no difference in transfusion rate, urinary fistula, and thoracic complications. However, the risk of fever was significantly higher in the prone group. Hospital stay was similar. But again, the limitation of this meta-analysis is the heterogeneity of reporting among different studies. Other factors than the difference in patient positioning may have an impact on results: puncture and fragmentation techniques, definition of operative time and stone-free rate.

6.5 Conclusion

The main goal of percutaneous nephrolithotomy is to clear the kidney of as much stone as possible in a minimally invasive way. Today, the prone position is no more the exclusive way to do percutaneous nephrolithotomy. There is no clear evidence supporting the superiority of either the prone or supine position regarding stone-free rate, complications and morbidity. Nevertheless, an increasing number of publications admit an advantage of the supine position in terms of operative time.

Yet, the final decision as to the position of the patient belongs to the surgeon according to his personal preference, experience, training and his operative environment. The most important is to do a good job and feel comfortable.

References

1. Dos Santos RLA, Pereira-Caldos J. L'artériographie des membres de l'aorte et de ses branches abdominales. Soc Natl Chir Bull Meme. 1929;55:587–601.
2. Goodwin WE. A memoir of percutaneous access to the kidney (antegrade pyelography and percutaneous nephrostomy). J Endourol. 1991;5:4.
3. Goodwin WE, Casey WC, Woolf W. Percutaneous trocar (needle) nephrostomy in hydronephrosis. J Am Med Assoc. 1955;157:891–4.
4. Castaneda-Zuniga WR, Clayman R, Smith A, Rusnak B, Herrera M, Amplatz K. Nephrostolithotomy: percutaneous techniques for urinary calculus removal. AJR Am J Roentgenol. 1982;139:721–6.
5. Valdivia Uria JG, Lachares Santamaria E, Villarroya Rodriguez S, Taberner Llop J, Abril Baquero G, Aranda Lassa JM. [Percutaneous nephrolithectomy: simplified technic (preliminary report)]. Arch Esp Urol. 1987;40:177–80.
6. Ibarluzea G, Scoffone CM, Cracco CM, Poggio M, Porpiglia F, Terrone C, et al. Supine Valdivia and modified lithotomy position for simultaneous anterograde and retrograde endourological access. BJU Int. 2007;100:233–6.
7. Scoffone CM, Cracco CM, Cossu M, Grande S, Poggio M, Scarpa RM. Endoscopic combined intrarenal surgery in Galdakao-modified supine Valdivia position: a new standard for percutaneous nephrolithotomy? Eur Urol. 2008;54:1393–403.
8. Valdivia JG, Scarpa RM, Duvdevani M, Gross AJ, Nadler RB, Nutahara K, et al. Supine versus prone position during percutaneous nephrolithotomy: a report from the clinical research office of the endourological society percutaneous nephrolithotomy global study. J Endourol. 2011;25:1619–25.
9. Lehman T, Bagley DH. Reverse lithotomy: modified prone position for simultaneous nephroscopic and ureteroscopic procedures in women. Urology. 1988;32:529–31.
10. Grasso M, Nord R, Bagley DH. Prone split leg and flank roll positioning: simultaneous antegrade and retrograde access to the upper urinary tract. J Endourol. 1993;7:307–10.
11. Ray AA, Chung DG, Honey RJ. Percutaneous nephrolithotomy in the prone and prone-flexed positions: anatomic considerations. J Endourol. 2009;23:1607–14.
12. Kerbl K, Clayman RV, Chandhoke PS, Urban DA, De Leo BC, Carbone JM. Percutaneous stone removal with the patient in a flank position. J Urol. 1994;151:686–8.
13. Moraitis K, Philippou P, El-Husseiny T, Wazait H, Masood J, Buchholz N. Simultaneous antegrade/retrograde upper urinary tract access: Bart's modified lateral position for complex upper tract endourologic pathologic features. Urology. 2012;79:287–92.
14. Bach C, Goyal A, Kumar P, Kachrilas S, Papatsoris AG, Buchholz N, et al. The Barts 'flank-free' modified supine position for percutaneous nephrolithotomy. Urol Int. 2012;89:365–8.
15. Tuttle DN, Yeh BM, Meng MV, Breiman RS, Stoller ML, Coakley FV. Risk of injury to adjacent organs with lower-pole fluoroscopically guided percutaneous nephrostomy: evaluation with prone, supine, and multiplanar reformatted CT. J Vasc Interv Radiol. 2005;16:1489–92.
16. Sofer M, Giusti G, Proietti S, Mintz I, Kabha M, Matzkin H, et al. Upper calyx approachability through a lower calyx access for prone versus supine percutaneous nephrolithotomy. J Urol. 2016;195:377–82.
17. Addla SK, Rajpal S, Sutcliffe N, Adeyoju A. A simple aid to improve patient positioning during percutaneous nephrolithotomy. Ann R Coll Surg Engl. 2008;90:433–4.
18. Miano R, Scoffone C, De Nunzio C, Germani S, Cracco C, Usai P, et al. Position: prone or supine is the issue of percutaneous nephrolithotomy. J Endourol. 2010;24:931–8.
19. de la Rosette J, Assimos D, Desai M, Gutierrez J, Lingeman J, Scarpa R, et al. The Clinical Research Office of the Endourological Society percutaneous nephrolithotomy global study: indications, complications, and outcomes in 5803 patients. J Endourol. 2011;25:11–7.
20. Kamphuis GM, Baard J, Westendarp M, de la Rosette JJ. Lessons learned from the CROES percutaneous nephrolithotomy global study. World J Urol. 2015;33:223–33.
21. Yamaguchi A, Skolarikos A, Buchholz NP, Chomon GB, Grasso M, Saba P, et al. Operating times and bleeding complications in percutaneous nephrolithotomy: a comparison of tract dilation methods in 5,537 patients in the Clinical Research Office of the Endourological

Society Percutaneous Nephrolithotomy Global Study. J Endourol. 2011;25:933–9.
22. Liu L, Zheng S, Xu Y, Wei Q. Systematic review and meta-analysis of percutaneous nephrolithotomy for patients in the supine versus prone position. J Endourol. 2010;24:1941–6.
23. Wu P, Wang L, Wang K. Supine versus prone position in percutaneous nephrolithotomy for kidney calculi: a meta-analysis. Int Urol Nephrol. 2011;43(1):67–77.
24. Zhang X, Xia L, Xu T, Wang X, Zhong S, Shen Z. Is the supine position superior to the prone position for percutaneous nephrolithotomy (PCNL)? Urolithiasis. 2014;42:87–93.
25. Li J, Gao L, Li Q, Zhang Y, Jiang Q. Supine versus prone position for percutaneous nephrolithotripsy: a meta-analysis of randomized controlled trials. Int J Surg. 2019;66:62–71.

7 Anesthesia

Wenqi Wu

7.1 Introduction

Percutaneous nephrolithotomy (PCNL), a minimally invasive procedure, was used for the removal of upper urinary tract stone. It was initially started in the 1950s but widely used in 1976 [1], and has now become the primary treatment for multiple, large kidney stone or staghorn stone [2]. PCNL has the advantages of being minimally invasive and less painful and providing a quick recovery. Because of the better control of breathing and the ability to make patients more comfortable, general anesthesia with endotracheal intubation is more frequently performed in patients with PCNL [3]. Several changes have taken place to modify the procedure and lower the analgesic requirements, complications, and hospitalization duration in the last two decades. Nowadays, PCNL can be performed after the administration of general, epidural, or local anesthesia. The anesthesia method used during the operation is mainly determined by the patient's condition. It is crucial to choose an anesthetic method with high safety and good effect. The patient's safety will be threatened if an anesthesia-related problem occurs during surgery. Insufficient anesthesia will increase the pain and impact the safety and effect of surgery.

7.2 Part I: Preoperative Assessment and Treatment

Patients with kidney stones have different preoperative conditions, since upper urinary tract stones are able to result in renal function damage, accompanied by water and electrolyte disorder and acid-base imbalance. Also, cardiovascular system, metabolism, and hematopoietic system abnormalities are closely connected with it. In addition, upper urinary tract stone is often associated with urinary tract infections, which contributes to the intraoperative and postoperative fever, chills, vomiting, and even urinary sepsis [2]. PCNL has special requirements for position and equipment. Before anesthesia, appropriate anesthesia methods and anesthetics should be selected according to the condition and special requirements of the operation. It is very important to evaluate the condition and provide the suitable treatment to improve the patient's condition, in order to ensure the safety of the operation, reduce postoperative complications, and recover the patient quickly. To understand the general condition of patients and evaluate the important organ functions such as heart, lung, liver, kidney, and brain are important to prepare for the anesthesia. Giving full consideration to intraoperative and

W. Wu (✉)
Department of Urology and Guangdong Key Laboratory of Urology, The First Affiliated Hospital of Guangzhou Medical University, Guangzhou, China

G. Zeng, K. Sarica (eds.), *Percutaneous Nephrolithotomy*,
https://doi.org/10.1007/978-981-15-0575-1_7

postoperative complications and providing the requirements for full preparation are critical.

7.2.1 Age

All age groups of patients may present for PCNL. Elderly patients may have many accompanying comorbidities such as ischemic heart disease, respiratory dysfunction, and diabetes, while young children may be uncooperative.

7.2.2 Nutrition

Malnutrition, hypoproteinemia, and anemia significantly reduce the tolerance of anesthesia and postoperative anti-infective capacity. For patients with the above conditions, enteral nutrition should be added as much as possible preoperatively. Parenteral nutrition and blood transfusion should be a supplement when necessary, also pay attention to maintaining water, electrolyte, and acid-base balance. Hemoglobin and hematocrit are able to reflect the general situation of anemia, dehydration, and blood volume. There is a risk of shock during anesthesia if the hemoglobin of the adult patient is less than 80 g/L. Patients over 70 years of age should pay more attention to the correction of anemia. Urinary tract stone patients with renal insufficiency are always accompanied by anemia due to the decline of erythropoietin. For infants younger than 3 months, preoperative hemoglobin should exceed 100 g/L; for those older than 3 months, it should be at least 90 g/L.

7.2.3 Hypertension

The safety of anesthesia in patients with hypertension is determined by the extent of damage of organs such as brain, coronary artery, heart, and renal function. One of the key points of preoperative preparation is to preserve the stability of blood pressure. Nowadays, scholars agree with the idea that using antihypertensive drugs during the day of surgery is conducive to maintaining the stability of blood pressure. Patients with diastolic blood pressure exceeding 90 mmHg should be treated with antihypertensive drugs. Surgery should be performed after achieving normal blood pressure or when blood pressure is reduced by 20%. For patients with diastolic blood pressure exceeding 110 mmHg, antihypertensive drugs must be continued until the morning of surgery to prevent acute injury such as heart failure or cerebrovascular accident due to severe blood pressure fluctuations during surgery. The use of vasopressor is effective against intraoperative hypotension. For patients with hypertension accompanied by kidney damage, comprehensive consideration should be given to the choice of anesthetic type and dosage. For patients with hypertension combined with myocardial ischemia, the treatment of myocardial ischemia should be strengthened. Surgery should be postponed for patients with recent myocardial ischemia.

7.2.4 Cardiovascular Diseases

Echocardiography should be performed to understand cardiac structural changes and cardiac function when the preoperative electrocardiogram suggests ST-segment changes or cardiac hypertrophy. Selective radionuclide angiography can be used to understand the condition of coronary artery if necessary. Patients with arrhythmia should have 24-h Holter monitoring and echocardiography to understand the degree of arrhythmia and cardiac function. For patients taking nonsteroidal anti-inflammatory drugs (NSAIDs), for example aspirin, it should be discontinued at least 5–10 days before surgery and resumed 48–72 h after surgery. Other kinds of NSAIDs should be deactivated for at least 48 h prior to surgery. For patients who have not stopped using these drugs, it is necessary to check the clotting time to become normal before surgery. Many patients with kidney stones are accompanied by renal insufficiency. For patients requiring dialysis, surgeon and anesthesiologist should fully understand the method and time of hemodialysis, especially the heparinized dialysis. In addition, coagulation function needs to be closely monitored. Heparin-free or low-molecular-weight heparinized dialysis is better. Hemorrhage is one of the common complications of PCNL. Patient's coagulation function is the primary factor to prevent the hemorrhage. To sew or coagulate hemostasis like open surgery is impracticable; thus, coagulation function is very important.

7.2.5 Respiratory Diseases

Preoperative treatment of patients with respiratory diseases includes quitting smoking, control of acute and chronic lung infections, and use of effective antibiotics 3 days before surgery. Patients with chronic obstructive pulmonary disease (COPD) or bronchi wheezing; the bronchodilator such as aminophylline and salbutamol should be provided. Patients with frequent asthma attacks can be treated with adrenal cortex and asthma medication. Patients with pulmonary heart disease and heart failure need to use digitalis, diuretics, oxygen, and pulmonary vascular resistance drugs to control the situation. Pre-anesthesia is mainly administered in small doses. Generally, respiratory function can be significantly improved after the therapy mentioned above. Because the PCNL surgery needs to be performed in the prone position, respiratory management and monitoring should be better performed especially during the anesthesia of such patients. The use of intraspinal block increases the risk of restriction of circulation or breathing because the prone position restricts the dilation of the chest. Patients with respiratory diseases are more likely to suffer from dyspnea; thus, general anesthesia with endotracheal intubation is preferred for them to strengthen respiratory management.

7.2.6 Renal Function Assessment

Glomerular filtration rate is an objective indicator of glomerular filtration function and is often used clinically to assess the renal function. Inhibition of anesthetics, surgical trauma, hypotension, or dehydration can cause the decline of the blood supply to kidney and produce nephrotoxic substances, which may cause the temporary decline of renal function. This phenomenon is more common in patients with renal insufficiency. The key point of protecting the kidney function is to ensure the blood supply to kidney and protect the glomerular filtration rate. The following points are important to protect the renal function. Firstly, ensuring adequate blood volume is an effective method to prevent kidney ischemia. Secondly, avoiding using vasoconstrictors as far as possible. Thirdly, providing enough intravenous rehydration to ensure the urine volume. Furosemide could be used if necessary. Additionally, avoiding the use of nephrotoxic drugs is important. Last but not the least, urinary tract infections should be prevented and controlled. Patients with severe renal insufficiency require hemodialysis treatment to improve their condition before surgery. The volume and speed of fluid infusion should be strictly controlled during the operation. The operation time of this kind of patients should be strictly controlled, too. The two-stage surgery could be used.

It is necessary to evaluate renal function by intravenous pyelogram (IVP), dimercaptosuccinic acid (DMSA), or diethylenetriaminepentaacetic acid (DTPA) scan [4]. DMSA is an imaging tool to assess renal morphology and structure. DTPA renal scan is used to evaluate the blood supply, renal function, and excretion of urine. This test can be used to understand what percentage each kidney contributes to the total function. There is no indication for performing PCNL with a nonfunctional kidney. Nephrectomy would be a preferable operation. Being aware of the existing comorbidities in the perioperative period could reduce complications and mortality.

7.2.7 Infection

The acute infection should be controlled preoperatively.

7.3 Part II: Preparation and Medication Before Anesthesia

The anesthesiologist should carefully understand the patient's personal history, past history, allergy history, therapeutic medication history, previous surgical anesthesia history, and current operation status before PCNL, including smoking and alcohol consumption, pregnancy, allergies, use of illegal drugs, antihypertensive drugs, and antibiotics, level of blood sugar and glucocorticoids, etc. Which kind of anesthesia methods and drugs have been used in the past should be understood. Anesthesiologist should talk with the surgeon to find out the difficulty of this operation. In addition, it is necessary to communicate with the patient preoperatively to explain the anesthesia and eliminate the patient's tension and anxiety.

7.3.1 Physical Examination Related to Anesthetic Operation and Examination of Anesthetic Condition

1. The examination of general anesthesia with endotracheal intubation:
   (a) The range of mobility of head and neck is between 90° and 165°. If mobility of head is tilted back less than 80°, the operation of intubation would be difficult.
   (b) The mouth opening involves three transverse fingers. Normally, the tongue and jaw spacing is no less than three transverse fingers. Patients with tongue and jaw spacing less than two transverse fingers often prevent the placement of laryngoscopy.
   (c) Anesthesiologist should pay more attention to whether there is thyroid mass pressing the trachea, the stenosis situation of trachea, also be careful of the laryngeal edema, laryngeal submucosal hematoma, acute laryngitis, etc. Patients with difficulty in endotracheal intubation need to be equipped with fiber-optic bronchoscope.
2. The examination of spinal functions should be carried out for patients who intend to receive spinal anesthesia:
   (a) Check the clarity of puncture marks.
   (b) Be careful of the spine disease and malformation.
   (c) Check the infection condition of puncture point.
   (d) Check whether there is bleeding disease, bleeding tendency, or anticoagulant treatment.
   (e) Understand the history of frequent headaches.
   (f) Check whether there is recessive myelopathy.

If the above conditions are present, spinal anesthesia should be prohibited in order to avoid the occurrence of severe complications such as total spinal anesthesia, aggravation of myelopathy, formation of intravertebral hematoma, secondary paraplegia caused by intravertebral infection, and pyogenic granuloma.

7.3.2 Examination of Drug Treatment

For patients with complicated conditions who have received a series of drug treatments before surgery, the interaction between certain drugs and anesthetic drugs should be considered before anesthesia, and the use of drugs should be determined. For example, the use of digitalis, insulin, corticosteroids, antiepileptics, and antihypertensive drugs should be continued until the day of surgery. Some CNS restrain drugs like barbiturate, monoamine oxidase inhibitor, and tricyclic antidepressant, should be stopped before the operation. Antihypertensive drugs such as reserpine will lead to intraoperative hypotension, and should be stopped 7–14 days before surgery.

7.3.3 Gastrointestinal Preparation

The emptying of gastrointestinal tract in selective surgery is preferred. The purpose is to prevent accidents such as pulmonary infection or asphyxia caused by esophageal reflux, vomiting, aspiration, etc. The prone position is used most of the time during PCNL surgery and we need to place a thick pad on the patient's abdomen to achieve the purpose of compressing the patient's abdomen, which is more likely to cause symptoms such as nausea and vomiting. The gastric emptying time is usually 4–6 h; for this reason, adults usually stop drinking and fasting at least 8 h or even 12 h before anesthesia. Children are made to fast for at least 8 h, and water is forbidden for 4 h. The importance of prohibiting drinking and fasting should be clearly explained to patients or their families.

7.3.4 The Preparations for Accidents During the Operation

Patients with anemia or the difficult case with a long operation time should be given a full consideration in the preparation of red blood cells and fresh frozen plasma. Patients with hypertension and heart disease should be prepared with vasodilators, cardiotonic drugs, adrenaline, and so on. Asthma patients need to prepare anti-asthmatic drugs, adrenaline, glucocorticoids, etc. Patients with upper urinary tract infection need to be prepared with antibiotics, glucocorticoids, etc. Renal dysfunction patients should get attention for the renal function protection. Diuretics and dopamine would be useful. Endotracheal intubation supplies should be prepared when spinal anesthesia is used. Endotracheal intubation should be used to assist breathing during surgery if necessary. Patients with a higher puncture position need to be alerted to the possibility of pneumothorax. We also need to prepare ephedrine and atropine to prevent the decrease of heart rate and blood pressure. PCNL is easy to result in retroperitoneal and peritoneal effusion after surgery, which is able to inhibit breathing.

7.3.5 Premedication

Some sedative analgesic drugs can be given to the patients before anesthesia to reduce their psychological burden and nervousness, and improve the anesthetic effect, which is called pre-anesthesia administration. In this way, we can significantly reduce the doses of anesthetics and improve the patient tolerance to anesthetics by inhibiting the cerebral cortex and subcortical and limbic system, which could induce the consciousness relaxation, emotional stability, and forgetting effect. It could improve pain threshold to make up for some anesthesia methods' analgesia insufficiency. Finally, we can ensure that the airway patency and circulatory system function could be stabled by reducing autonomic and sympathetic nerve activity, catecholamine release, antagonizing histamine, and gland secretion activity.

We usually used benzodiazepines and anticholinergic drugs as pre-anesthesia medications. For example, midazolam, which belongs to antianxiety drug, is usually used to relieve the nervous fear and pain stress response effectively. And if patients were infants, we need to use the anesthesia mask. In addition, these drugs also have an effect on the prevention of myocardial ischemia caused by anxiety in adults. The main side effect is temporary inattention, induced hallucinations, interference with normal cognitive perception, and subtle motor skills. So we must have to use them in the right way, and we adopted intramuscular injection of 0.05–0.07 mg/kg 20–60 min before induction of anesthesia; for the elderly, the drug doses should be appropriately reduced. We also used anticholinergic drugs because they can keep the airway for intubation dry; atropine and scopolamine can also prevent bradycardia caused by laryngeal stimulation, laryngeal spasm, and hypoxia.

7.4 Part III: Anesthetic Choices for Percutaneous Nephrolithotomy

PCNL is a well-established procedure for the removal of kidney stone, which can be performed under general anesthesia, regional anesthesia, or local anesthesia. Regional anesthesia includes epidural anesthesia, spinal anesthesia, spinal-epidural anesthesia, and paravertebral anesthesia.

7.4.1 General Anesthesia

General anesthesia is a preferred choice of urologists and anesthesiologists for PCNL due to the better control of patients' breathing. Also, it is more appropriate to control the tidal volume during percutaneous access puncture, thus reducing the risk of injury to the pleura and lungs, prolonging anesthesia, and improving patients' comfort. Furthermore, the urologist could make multiple punctures with minimal discomfort due to the long operation time when the patients with large stone burden. The defect of general anesthesia includes the risk of atelectasis, postoperative nausea and/or vomiting, drug reactions, and vascular and neurological complications [5, 6]. The most common neurological complication is the trauma of the brachial plexus and spine under general anesthesia when the patient is in prone position [7]. Additional risks of general anesthesia involve intraoperative awareness, stress response, extubation response, and postoperative agitation [8]. Moreover, it is difficult and time consuming to change position during the PCNL under general anesthesia. Obviously, this will increase the risk of complications in the case of the elderly and obese patients. Besides, the risk of extended ileus and deep vein thrombosis should be valued because of the restrictive mobility under general anesthesia. For several specific cases, general anesthesia should be recommended.

7.4.1.1 Neurologic or Cardiovascular Abnormity

Neurologic and cardiovascular status should be evaluated carefully before anesthetic choices. For patients with neurologic or cardiovascular abnormity, general anesthesia should be recommended to decrease injury.

7.4.1.2 Pediatric Patients

Most pediatric patients are unable to maintain stillness during needle puncture, which can expose the neural structures to traumatic injury, as well as raised intracranial pressure. Therefore, general anesthesia should be recommended for pediatric patients.

7.4.1.3 Elderly Patients

Most elderly patients have abnormal cardiopulmonary function; therefore general anesthesia should be recommended to control patient breathing and improve patient comfort.

7.4.1.4 Upper Pole Punctures

For patients with upper pole puncture, general anesthesia should be recommended because it permits the control of respiratory movements, which is essential to minimize the risk of pulmonary complications.

7.4.2 Regional Anesthesia

Regional anesthesia includes epidural anesthesia, spinal anesthesia, spinal-epidural anesthesia, and paravertebral anesthesia. Compared with general anesthesia, both spinal and combined spinal-epidural anesthesia have been proved to be effective [9–11].

Compared to spinal anesthesia, segmental epidural anesthesia has a lot of merits such as hemodynamic stability, rapid recovery, patient satisfaction, postoperative analgesia, and reduced incidence of postoperative nausea and vomiting [12]. In the meantime, patients under segmental epidural anesthesia can take a prone position without much assistance, which could shorten the operation time and reduce operative assistance effectively. However, segmental epidural anesthesia has significant disadvantages in supplementing general anesthesia requirements, with intraoperative discomfort, unprotected airways, and likelihood of patient movement [13].

Several studies have demonstrated that PCNL under regional anesthesia offers some advantages compared with general anesthesia such as decreased overall analgesia requirements, cost-effectiveness, lower postoperative pain and complication, and avoidance of side effects from multiple medications during general anesthesia [10, 11, 14, 15]. Additionally, in PCNL operations performed with spinal anesthesia, when the patient is awake under the first access, the risk of limb or nerve damage may be minimized during positioning. In addition, early mobilization can be achieved during the postoperative period [7, 16]. Compared with local infiltration anesthesia, regional anesthesia may be more effective in controlling intraoperative pain and allows for a transition to open surgery if necessary [17].

Several issues may be related to the techniques of regional anesthetic. Firstly, a relatively high block is required to eliminate all pain of kidney. Secondly, a vasovagal response would occur due to the expansion of the renal pelvis during the operation, which is not always prevented by regional anesthesia. Regional anesthesia is a more feasible choice only if the surgical team is highly specialized and the uncomplicated case is met. Also, there are several absolute contraindications to regional anesthesia, such as patient refusal, localized sepsis, and an allergy to the planned drugs. Besides, there are several relative contraindications to regional anesthesia.

7.4.2.1 Neurologic Abnormity

Neurologic abnormity should be carefully evaluated, such as myelopathy or peripheral neuropathy, spinal stenosis, spine surgery, multiple sclerosis, and spina bifida.

7.4.2.2 Cardiac Abnormity

Cardiac abnormity should be carefully evaluated, such as aortic stenosis or fixed cardiac output and hypovolemia.

7.4.2.3 Hematologic Abnormity

Hematologic abnormity should be carefully evaluated, such as thromboprophylaxis and inherited coagulopathy.

7.4.2.4 Systematic Infections

Systematic infection should be carefully evaluated before anesthetic choices.

7.4.3 Local Anesthesia

With the improvement of technique and experience, and the requirement of shortening hospitalization time, many urologists are interested in performing PCNL under local anesthesia, which is equally safe. The elderly have better tolerance under local anesthesia [18]. PCNL performed under local infiltration anesthesia in a selected group of patients is feasible and provides satisfactory clinical outcomes. It has its own merit in the form of less postoperative pain, less blood loss, and early recovery and discharge, thereby reducing the stay in the hospital. Furthermore, local anesthesia can be administered to patients who are not suitable for general anesthesia or regional anesthesia. Local anesthetic, for example lidocaine, can be delivered into the access tract by using an 8.3-Fr anesthetic injection catheter with multiple side holes or with a dual-lumen ureteral access catheter [18] or using a 23-gauge spinal needle with injection along the access tract to the renal capsule. The presence of pain during PCNL may be a main limitation factor for the use of local anesthesia for PCNL. Several methods can be used for the prevention of severe pain.

7.4.3.1 Enough Local Anesthetic

The key to the prevention of severe pain is using enough local anesthetic along the entire tract from the skin to the capsular puncture site and the underlying parenchyma.

7.4.3.2 Controlled Water Pressure

The pain during PCNL is mainly caused by the dilatation of the renal capsule and parenchyma. Therefore, controlling the water pressure of the pelvis is an additional pain reduction method.

7.4.3.3 Preoperative Communications

Preoperative communication is also important for good perioperative cooperation, which can raise the pain threshold of patients during the procedure.

7.4.3.4 Perioperative Analgesics

Proper administration of perioperative analgesics can improve the tolerance of patients.

7.4.3.5 Excellent Techniques

It is recommended that PCNL under local infiltration anesthesia should be performed by a urologist with excellent PCNL technique.

7.5 Part IV: Intraoperative Anesthesia Management

On the basis of ensuring analgesia and sedation of the patient, intraoperative anesthesia should monitor the respiratory and circulatory function and body temperature, analyze the cause of the change, and protect the renal function.

7.5.1 Anesthesia Effect and Depth

The anesthesia plane is so high that it causes respiratory and circulatory inhibition. The anesthesia depth monitoring index should be observed during the operation, including blood pressure, heart rate, pulse and sweating, and tears and pupil changes. In shallow anesthesia, the sympathetic nerve is excited, but the situation is opposite in deep anesthesia. At present, better indicators for monitoring the anesthesia depth are bispectral index (BIS) and auditory evoked potential index (AAI). BIS can reflect the changes of blood concentration of anesthetic sedatives and the depth of sedative hypnosis. AAI is sensitive to the foresight conversion process.

7.5.2 Respiratory Function Monitoring

When the intraspinal anesthesia plane is too high, respiratory movement may stop in severe cases. If the patient uses intravenous anesthesia medicine, the physician should pay attention to the effect of oral secretions on respiration, and timely sucking to prevent airway obstruction. For general anesthesia with endotracheal intubation, the position of tracheal catheter should be given attention during posture change to prevent the catheter from protruding or bending. It is also important to note that the surgeon is prone to damaging the pleura during the selection of high puncture and fistulostomy, which will result in pneumothorax, dyspnea, and weakened pneumothorax side auscultation breath sound.

7.5.3 Cyclic Function Monitoring

7.5.3.1 Blood Pressure Monitoring

Blood pressure is a routine monitoring item during anesthesia, which has very important clinical significance. Blood pressure and cardiac output are directly related to peripheral vascular resistance. Maintaining normal blood pressure can ensure blood perfusion of various organs and tissues.

7.5.3.2 Electrocardiogram (ECG) Monitoring

ECG monitoring is an essential monitoring item for any surgical anesthesia. It can dynamically reflect the changes of heart rate, heart rhythm, and myocardial ischemia, and timely determine whether there is arrhythmia or myocardial ischemia. When the patients have myocardial ischemia or severe arrhythmia during surgery, patients may complain of discomfort such as chest tightness and difficulty in breathing.

7.5.3.3 Central Venous Pressure (CVP) Monitoring

Monitoring CVP can assess blood volume, right heart function, and cardiac preload. Rapid fluid replacement can be performed through the central venous catheter when there is hemorrhage during operation. The normal value of CVP is 5–12 cmH_2O. The surgeon can judge the blood volume and cardiac function according to the CVP and the change of blood pressure.

7.5.4 Body Temperature Monitoring

During hypothermia, the inhibitory effect of all anesthetics is enhanced, and the recovery of patients is delayed. For patients with general anesthesia with endotracheal intubation, hypothermia also affects the metabolism, excretion, enzyme activity of muscle relaxants, and neuromuscular sensitivity. Therefore, sedation, analgesic anesthetics, and muscle relaxants should be reduced accordingly. It is necessary to closely observe the body temperature change in PCNL. When the operation time is long, the physiological saline for flushing needs to be warmed, and the room temperature should be controlled at 26 °C.

7.5.5 Anesthesia and Perioperative Kidney Protection

We should follow the principle of choosing drugs that have the least impact on circulation, metabolism, controllability, and short-term efficacy for renal insufficiency patients. When intraoperative spinal anesthesia is selected, the plane should be controlled below T5 as much as possible. Analgesic and sedative drugs that have less influence on hemodynamics should be selected to avoid hypotension and damaged renal perfusion. Low-dose dopamine is recognized as a drug that maintains circulation stability, increases renal blood flow, and effectively dilates renal blood vessels. The key to perioperative kidney protection is maintaining adequate renal perfusion and urine output.

In addition, a rapid quantitative analysis of blood glucose needs to be done on patients with diabetes during operation. General routine intraspinal anesthesia monitoring includes blood pressure, heart rate, ECG, respiratory rate, and pulse oxygen saturation (SpO_2). General anesthesia with endotracheal intubation also needs to monitor end-tidal carbon dioxide ($PETCO_2$), airway pressure, tidal volume, minute ventilation, and anesthetic gas concentration.

7.6 Part V: Intraoperative Complication

Complications related to vital signs may occur during surgery. Some complications are caused by surgical procedures. Intraoperative anesthetic may also lead to complications. Therefore, the anesthesiologists need to pay close attention to vital signs of patients and be ready to deal with complications effectively.

7.6.1 Hypotension

The average arterial pressure should not be lower than 20% of its baseline value [19]. Blocked sympathetic nervous system caused by intraoperative spinal cord block can contribute to hypotension and bradycardia. When the position of patients changes to prone position, with elevated level of anesthesia, hypotension is more likely to occur. In severe cases, hypotension causes insufficient cerebral blood supply and the patients present with nausea, vomiting, pallor, restlessness, and other symptoms. To settle the dilemma, supplementing the blood volume is the first choice. Vascular pressure drugs like ephedrine should be used when still under hypotension after supplementing the blood volume and position adjustment [20]. Deep anesthesia during general anesthesia with endotracheal intubation can also lead to a decrease in blood pressure. It is necessary to adjust the depth of anesthesia and supplement the blood volume. Severe bleeding can also lead to lower blood pressure. Blood loss can be estimated according to the volume, color, and depth of the kidney irrigation fluid during surgery. If intraoperative hemorrhage is considered, hemostatic drugs and blood volume expansion therapy should be given immediately. In severe cases, the operation should be terminated, and further treatment such as embolization or open surgery should be considered. Placement of working sheath is easy to cause the vagus nerve reflex of the kidney, resulting in a decrease in blood pressure and heart rate. It is usually improved by using a small amount of ephedrine or atropine.

7.6.2 Respiratory Depression

Respiratory depression mainly occurs in regional anesthesia. The prone position of PCNL requires padding abdomen, which can cause diaphragm to elevate, affecting the patient's breathing to a certain extent [21]. If the anesthesia plane is too high, thoracic spinal nerve block would cause intercostal muscle paralysis, aggravating respiratory depression with decreased tidal volume. And patients should breathe using an oxygen mask to maintain hemodynamic stability. Rescue measures such as artificial respiration through endotracheal intubation and maintenance of circulation need to be implemented immediately when respiratory arrest, drop in blood pressure, and sudden cardiac arrest occur. For patients with pulmonary insufficiency or obesity, general anesthesia with endotracheal intubation should be chosen to avoid respiratory depression during operation.

7.6.3 Nausea and Vomiting

The reasons of nausea and vomiting are as follows: the cerebral hypoxia caused by hypotension, increased gastrointestinal peristalsis resulting from vagal hyperactivity, and parasympathetic reflex during surgical traction. Once intraoperative nausea and vomiting occur, it is necessary to figure out whether the anesthesia plane is too high or blood pressure drops. If necessary, application of antiemetic drugs such as tropisetron should be considered.

7.6.4 Intraoperative Shivering

Toxic effect of anesthesia drug and urosepsis infection both can lead to intraoperative shivering [22]. The presence of urinary tract infection should be considered if preoperative urinary tests indicate elevated white blood cells, and preoperative antibiotic therapy should be used [2]. Dexamethasone can also be considered to prevent sepsis during surgery. Continuous irrigation with cold normal saline can also lead to hypothermia and shivering. It is worth noting that endotracheal intubation in patients with general anesthesia does not shiver after the use of muscle relaxants.

7.6.5 Rinse Solution Extravasation

PCNL requires constant irrigation under pressure of normal saline during the operation, resulting in some irrigation fluid entering into the retroperitoneum and around the kidneys and forming effusion. If the fistula sheath is out of the kidney, the extravasation will be more serious. Patients with spinal anesthesia often complain of swelling pain in the renal area on the puncture side and dyspnea in severe cases. Careful attention should be paid to the amount of saline irrigation during the operation. The risk of overabsorption of irrigation fluid is inherent in this technique. Intraoperative monitoring of inflow and outflow should be performed, with attention to maintaining low intracavitary pressure. In a complex case, peritoneal extravasation was reported, leading to hyperinfection with metabolic acidosis, reflex intestinal obstruction, and peritonitis. The furosemide dehydration treatment can be given for patients with a small amount of washing fluid extravasation, and the surgery should be terminated as soon as possible for pateints with serious effusion. Patients with severe effusion can be punctured and drained under the guidance of ultrasound, and the changes of blood electrolytes should be treated in time [23].

7.6.6 Tracheal Tube Prolapse

Patients with general anesthesia with endotracheal intubation may change their position during surgery. As the patient moves from lithotomy to prone position, the surgeon and anesthesiologist should communicate. The anesthesiologist is responsible for protecting the patient's neck and head. The surgeon is responsible for protecting the patient's limbs and torso. Therefore, anesthesiologists are required to pay special attention to the depth of endotracheal intubation, not too deep or too shallow; fix the catheter; avoid the catheter distortion; and auscultate before and after the change of position to ensure the correct position of the catheter. Effective ventilation volume, airway pressure, $PETCO_2$, and SpO_2 should be monitored during anesthesia. If insufficient ventilation, too high airway pressure, or oxygenation disorder occurs, the cause should be quickly identified: whether catheter prolapse, overpenetration, or torsion has occurred, or whether the expansion of the thoracic cage is severely restricted due to the change of patient's position.

7.6.7 Low Temperature

Intraoperative hypothermia is defined as a temperature less than 35 °C, and the amount of lavage fluid greater than 20 L is associated with intraoperative hypothermia. Hypothermia is easy to occur during continuous saline perfusion, and intraoperative temperature should be monitored, especially in patients with chills, when oxygen consumption increases more than three times. Measures to maintain warmth and deal with chills should be taken in time to prevent chills caused by cold, myotonia or restlessness, and hypoxemia caused by cold. Therefore, maintaining warmth during PCNL surgery is very important. Building a heating blanket is an effective preventive measure, but it comes at a cost. The use of preheated saline in a heating tank is a simple precaution. In the process of PCNL, the use of warm perfusion solution can significantly reduce hypothermia, postoperative average score, and chills. Therefore, warm water irrigation is recommended [22].

7.6.8 Soft-Tissue or Peripheral Nerve Injury

To avoid tissue or peripheral nerve damage, itinerant nurses can apply Vaseline to patients after anesthesia to prevent skin damage. During surgery and anesthesia, patients should always be checked for changes in posture and support points to avoid serious complications. Avoid the overheight of the foot frame at the lithotomy position, and put a soft pad on the foot frame to prevent common peroneal nerve injury or arteriovenous embolism. In prone position, pay attention to the compression of the eyeball or supraorbital nerve. When the patient needs to raise his/her hands to the sides of his/her head, pay attention to the injury caused by excessive abduction of brachial plexus nerve. Long period of low head during operation is likely to cause congestion and edema in neck and face. Therefore, shortening the operation time and protecting the patient's skin, tissues, organs, and nerves are good protective measures.

7.7 Part VI: Postoperative Anesthesia Management

7.7.1 Postoperative Analgesia

PCNL is one of the primary treatments for renal calculi, and it is also one of the common minimally invasive surgeries in urology. PCNL is safe and effective for patients with renal calculi. Nevertheless, the trauma is inevitable in the process of establishing puncture channels. Indwelling nephrostomy tube are seen postoperatively for most patients. Some patients may have complicated renal calculi in which the stones are removed with multi-tract PCNL. Multiple nephrostomy tube are indwelling after surgery, which will become the main cause of early postoperative pain. Surveys have shown that early postoperative pain affects patients' recovery and feelings, and postoperative pain is closely related to the occurrence of complications. Hence, early postoperative analgesia in clinical practice can improve patients' postoperative feelings and promote early activities of getting out of bed and intestinal peristalsis. Postoperative analgesia plays a positive role in patients' recovery after PCNL.

Traditionally, patient-controlled analgesia (PCA) can be used after PCNL, which can be separated into two implementation approaches:

epidural controlled analgesia (PCEA) and intravenous controlled analgesia (PCIA). PCEA was diluted to 100 mL with ropivacaine (0.125 mg/mL) + sufentanil (0.4 μg/mL), background infusion volume was 2 mL/h, controlled infusion single dose was 0.5 mL, and locking time was 15 min. In addition to traditional methods, a large number of recent studies have demonstrated that the following methods can also effectively relieve postoperative pain in patients. Intercostal nerve block: after the removal of calculi by a single-tract PCNL, intercostal nerve block is performed under the guidance of ultrasound or transmitted X-ray. The needle is passed below the rib margin, and continued to be inserted about 2–3 mm along the lower edge of the rib. If no blood is obtained when the needle is aspirated, 0.5% bupivacaine 20 mL is injected into the neurovascular sheath with epinephrine. This method can effectively control the early postoperative pain of PCNL (within 6 h) and improve the postoperative health-related quality of life (HRQL) of patients. It is an economical and a safe postoperative analgesic method [24–27]. The infiltration anesthesia of nephrostomy tract: after the removal of calculi, the patient is given local infiltration anesthesia around the nephrostomy tract under the X-ray guidance. It should be noted that the depth of anesthesia is consistent with the puncture sheath, which is to ensure the infiltration of local anesthetics to the subcutaneous tissue, muscle, and renal capsule surface. In patients undergoing tubeless PCNL, the wound can be strapped with a tight occlusive dressing after local anesthesia. 1.5 mg/kg of 0.25% bupivacaine is used in the method, and it can relieve the pain of patients after PCNL and greatly reduce the need for additional analgesics [28]. Subarachnoid anesthesia before general anesthesia: the patient is placed in lateral decubitus position, subarachnoid anesthesia is performed by the anesthesiologist, and 0.3–0.5 mg morphine sulfate is administered intrathecally. This method can significantly reduce the use of postoperative analgesics, promote patients to get out of bed as soon as possible, effectively relieve postoperative pain, and reduce postoperative nausea [9]. Thoracic paravertebral block: at the end of PCNL, the anesthetist performed paravertebral space puncture at T10, T11, and T12, respectively, with 4 mL 5% levobupivacaine. Patients were very satisfied with the effect of this method, and it had less side effect on intestinal function than the above methods [29].

Adverse reactions and management of postoperative analgesia: (1) Urinary retention: it is a common complication of epidural analgesia. Opioids also cause urinary retention. (2) Pruritus: it is a common adverse reaction when opioids are given epidurally, which can be relieved by antihistamine. (3) Nausea and vomiting: it is related to surgery and use of opioid. Adding haloperidol to PCA solution can reduce the incidence of nausea and vomiting. (4) Dizziness: it is mainly caused by sedatives.

Whether it is the traditional postoperative analgesia method or the continuously exploring analgesia method, both of them can effectively alleviate the pain of patients after PCNL; the latter can also reduce the occurrence of some complications. In addition, postoperative analgesia reduces the length of stay in hospital and the cost of treatment. Most patients benefit from early postoperative pain management after PCNL. However, the choice and method of PCNL postoperative analgesia do not have unified guidelines. With the continuous development of ERAS, postoperative analgesia will become an indispensable part of PCNL perioperative management.

7.7.2 Postoperative Nausea and Vomiting (PONV)

PONV is a common postoperative complication. About 30–40% of the patients may have nausea and vomiting after the operation, and some patients may have this complication after the hospital. Several factors lead to the occurrence of PONV, including side effects of anesthetic drugs, type of surgical procedure, operative time, and individual conditions of patients (such as age, weight, gender, and a history of motion sickness). The mechanism of PONV may be related to dopamine, 5-HT_3, opioid, and cholinergic receptors. PONV can occur independently or with other symptoms such as retching, which may cause serious consequences, such as aspiration pneumonia, wound dehiscence and bleeding, dehydration, and electrolyte disorder. It is important for urologists and anesthesiologists to note that nausea may be an early sign of postoperative hypotension, especially after spinal and epidural anesthesia. Once the patient encounters these troubles, the satisfaction of patients during postoperative recovery will be seriously affected, and the length of stay and treatment cost will be increased; this can even be a menace in life.

About the treatment of PONV, current studies have shown that selective 5-hydroxytryptamine receptor 3 (5-HT_3) antagonists can effectively control PONV. The alternative drugs and dosages include ondansetron 4 mg, granisetron 0.01–0.04 mg/kg, and dolasetron 12.5 mg, among which granisetron can be combined with dexamethasone to produce a synergistic effect to reduce the incidence of PONV. In addition, oral aprepitant (Emend®) 40 mg before anesthesia induction may be used to prevent PONV. Yet, it is still controversial whether prophylactic medication is needed for all patients to prevent PONV, which needs to be evaluated in combination with multiple PONV risk factors.

7.7.3 Postoperative Septic Shock

Postoperative septic shock is one of the most serious complications after PCNL. The incidence rate is only 0.3–1%. However, the mortality is 66–80%, which should get attention from the urologist [30]. Some patients had symptoms of infection because of infectious renal calculi. They had fever, chills, elevated white blood cells in urine, and positive urine culture before surgery. For these patients, antibiotic should be given before PCNL, which is the key ingredient to prevent postoperative septic shock. Nevertheless studies have shown that septic shock may also occur after PCNL in some patients without symptoms of infection and negative urine culture before PCNL. The reason may be that bacteria and endotoxin are released from the interstices of stone during the process of lithotripsy, which triggers a systemic inflammatory response. When the intrapelvic pressure increases to a level, bacteria and endotoxin flow back into the blood to induce postoperative SIRS, and eventually cause postoperative septic shock [31, 32]. The occurrence of postoperative septic shock is related to many factors, including positive urine culture, gender (the incidence rate of female is higher than that of male), renal insufficiency, high perfusion pressure during the process of PCNL, staghorn stone, diabetes, infectious calculi, indwelling catheter, preoperative obstruction, long operative time, etc. Septic shock may be manifested by intraoperative or postoperative chills, fever, hypotension, elevated heart rate, elevated white blood cells, increased neutrophils, and abnormal blood coagulate function in severe cases. Septic shock associated with calculi often occurs within 6 h after surgery, and physicians need to be cautious in its diagnosis.

Postoperative septic shock is a critical urgent complication, with high mortality. If any signal indicates that it may occur, treatment measures should be taken immediately. The treatment mainly includes three aspects. (1) Antibiotic therapy: begin empirical antibiotic treatment immediately to control infection via intravenous route. The antibiotics, which have wide antimicrobial spectrum and huge strength, should be chosen at first. Then change the drug which is sensitive to pathogenic microorganism according to the susceptibility testing. Sufficient dose is required for the treatment, which includes combination commonly of two or more antibiotics. (2) Fluid infusion: replenish blood volume by intravenous fluids, and maintain electrolyte and acid-base balance. Generally, 4–5% sodium bicarbonate can be used. The dosage is 400 mL/day for mild shock and 600–900 mL/day for severe shock. The dosage can be adjusted according to PH to prevent microcirculation stasis. Physicians need to deal with related complications positively, such as ARDS, renal insufficiency, gastrointestinal symptoms, and DIC [33].

7.7.4 Postoperative Cognitive Dysfunction (POCD)

Postoperative cognitive dysfunction (POCD) refers to brain dysfunction in patients without mental abnormalities before surgery, which are caused by various factors in the perioperative period, and are manifested by decreased level of consciousness and varying degrees of impairment in attention, memory, and reaction time. At present, most studies believe that there is a temporary (1–7 days after surgery) cognitive function decline, and some long-term (1–6 months) cognitive function deterioration [34].

The reasons why PCNL results in cognitive dysfunction mainly include the following: (1) Operative factors: PCNL requires a lot of flushing fluid, which may lead to hypothermia. During the operation, the position of lithotomy should be followed by continuous prone position. If the surgery lasts for a long time, it is easy to lead to low blood pressure, respiratory inhibition, and hypoxia. In addition, the vagus nerve is easily stimulated when the surgeon performs renal puncture, which causes reflex bradycardia and induces hypotension. As the central nerve cells are very sensitive to hypoxia, hypotension and hypoxia cause decreased release of neurotransmitters and induce hypoxemia, leading to postoperative psychological and mental damage in patients. (2) Release of inflammatory mediators: inflammatory mediators can be released by lymphocytes to activate the immune system in the surgery. In addition, in the process of lithotripsy, some infectious stones may also cause inflammatory reaction, leading to increased release of inflammatory mediators, which have direct or indirect effects on brain function. Animal studies have shown that POCD is associated with increased levels of inflammatory mediators [35, 36]. (3) Effects of anesthetic drugs: studies have found that general anesthetic drugs have toxic effects on neurons in developing rats. It can induce the release of inflammatory cytokines to enhance the apoptosis of brain neurons. The scopolamine used before PCNL had obvious symptoms. Atropine could significantly reduce the ability of number recalling. Benzodiazepines could significantly affect cognitive function, and both propofol and isoflurane anesthesia could affect the neuromotor function of patients. Postoperative analgesia pump at the same time can also produce some side effects. The side effects of the tramadol medication include emotional change, activity change, and cognitive change. The adverse reactions of lornoxicam include drowsiness, dizziness, paresthesia, and other symptoms. The patient's symptoms disappeared automatically after the withdrawal of the analgesia pump. (4) Acid-base imbalance and electrolyte disorder: PCNL procedure needs a lot of flushing fluid, which may lead to electrolyte disorder. Additionally, the use of diuretics causes electrolyte disorders. Some patients with preoperative renal dysfunction may have metabolic acidosis and electrolyte disorder. If physicians do not take any timely treatment to correct acid-base imbalance and electrolyte disorder, it is easy to cause mental disorders.

Treatment: (1) Strengthen perioperative management: correct electrolyte disorder and acid-base imbalance before surgery, correct hypoproteinemia and hypoxemia, and strengthen psychological counseling before surgery. (2) Strengthen intraoperative anesthesia management: maintain smooth respiratory function and stable circulation, and maintain the homeostasis of the body. (3) Sedative treatment: it is better to choose hypnotic sedative drugs, like short-acting benzodiazepines which have less hypotension or cardiac side effects, for patients who still have mental abnormalities, mental disorders, amnesia syndrome, or personality changes of different degrees within several months after the operation. Chlorpromazine and almitrine raubasine (duxil) treatment can be given, and the symptoms will gradually improve. (4) Oxygen absorption and detection of blood oxygen saturation, maintaining $SpO_2 > 95\%$, are also important. (5) Closely monitor the change of vital signs, and give extreme care to prevent accidental injury.

References

1. Fernstrom I, Johansson B. Percutaneous pyelolithotomy. A new extraction technique. Scand J Urol Nephrol. 1976;10(3):257–9.
2. Chen D, Jiang C, Liang X, Zhong F, Huang J, Lin Y, et al. Early and rapid prediction of postoperative infections following percutaneous nephrolithotomy in patients with complex kidney stones. BJU Int. 2019;123(6):1041–7. https://doi.org/10.1111/bju.14484.
3. Malik I, Wadhwa R. Percutaneous nephrolithotomy: current clinical opinions and anesthesiologists perspective. Anesthesiol Res Pract. 2016;2016:9036872. https://doi.org/10.1155/2016/9036872.
4. Taylor AJ. Quantitation of renal function with static imaging agents. Semin Nucl Med. 1982;12(4):330–44.
5. Kuzgunbay B, Turunc T, Akin S, Ergenoglu P, Aribogan A, Ozkardes H. Percutaneous nephrolithotomy under general versus combined spinal-epidural anesthesia. J Endourol. 2009;23(11):1835–8. https://doi.org/10.1089/end.2009.0261.
6. Karacalar S, Bilen CY, Sarihasan B, Sarikaya S. Spinal-epidural anesthesia versus general anesthesia in the management of percutaneous nephrolithotripsy. J Endourol. 2009;23(10):1591–7. https://doi.org/10.1089/end.2009.0224.
7. Mehrabi S, Karimzadeh SK. Results and complications of spinal anesthesia in percutaneous nephrolithotomy. Urol J. 2010;7(1):22–5.
8. Bajwa SJ, Kaur J, Singh A. A comparative evaluation of epidural and general anaesthetic technique for renal surgeries: a randomised prospective study. Indian J Anaesth. 2014;58(4):410–5. https://doi.org/10.4103/0019-5049.138975.
9. Andreoni C, Olweny EO, Portis AJ, Sundaram CP, Monk T, Clayman RV. Effect of single-dose subarachnoid spinal anesthesia on pain and recovery after unilateral percutaneous nephrolithotomy. J Endourol. 2002;16(10):721–5. https://doi.org/10.1089/08927790260472863.
10. Gonen M, Basaran B. Tubeless percutaneous nephrolithotomy: spinal versus general anesthesia. Urol J. 2014;11(1):1211–5.
11. Mehrabi S, Mousavi ZA, Akbartabar TM, Mehrabi F. General versus spinal anesthesia in percutaneous nephrolithotomy. Urol J. 2013;10(1):756–61.
12. Nandanwar AS, Patil Y, Wagaskar VG, Baheti VH, Tanwar HV, Patwardhan SKA. Comparison of efficacy of segmental epidural block versus spinal anaesthesia for percutaneous nephrolithotomy. J Clin Diagn Res. 2015;9(8):C1–4. https://doi.org/10.7860/JCDR/2015/14091.6301.
13. Parikh DA, Patkar GA, Ganvir MS, Sawant A, Tendolkar BA. Is segmental epidural anaesthesia an optimal technique for patients undergoing percutaneous nephrolithotomy? Indian J Anaesth. 2017;61(4):308–14. https://doi.org/10.4103/0019-5049.204247.
14. Cicek T, Gonulalan U, Dogan R, Kosan M, Istanbulluoglu O, Gonen M, et al. Spinal anesthesia is an efficient and safe anesthetic method for percutaneous nephrolithotomy. Urology. 2014;83(1):50–5. https://doi.org/10.1016/j.urology.2013.08.064.
15. Movasseghi G, Hassani V, Mohaghegh MR, Safaeian R, Safari S, Zamani MM, et al. Comparison between spinal and general anesthesia in percutaneous nephrolithotomy. Anesth Pain Med. 2014;4(1):e13871. https://doi.org/10.5812/aapm.13871.
16. Aravantinos E, Karatzas A, Gravas S, Tzortzis V, Melekos M. Feasibility of percutaneous nephrolithotomy under assisted local anaesthesia: a prospective study on selected patients with upper urinary tract obstruction. Eur Urol. 2007;51(1):224–7; discussion 228. https://doi.org/10.1016/j.eururo.2006.06.027.
17. Pu C, Wang J, Tang Y, Yuan H, Li J, Bai Y, et al. The efficacy and safety of percutaneous nephrolithotomy under general versus regional anesthesia: a systematic review and meta-analysis. Urolithiasis. 2015;43(5):455–66. https://doi.org/10.1007/s00240-015-0776-2.
18. Dalela D, Goel A, Singh P, Shankhwar SN. Renal capsular block: a novel method for performing percutaneous nephrolithotomy under local anesthesia. J Endourol. 2004;18(6):544–6. https://doi.org/10.1089/end.2004.18.544.
19. Bijker JB, van Klei WA, Kappen TH, van Wolfswinkel L, Moons KG, Kalkman CJ. Incidence of intraoperative hypotension as a function of the chosen definition: literature definitions applied to a retrospective cohort using automated data collection. Anesthesiology. 2007;107(2):213–20. https://doi.org/10.1097/01.anes.0000270724.40897.8e.
20. Charlson ME, MacKenzie CR, Gold JP, Ales KL, Topkins M, Shires GT. Preoperative characteristics predicting intraoperative hypotension and hypertension among hypertensives and diabetics undergoing noncardiac surgery. Ann Surg. 1990;212(1):66–81. https://doi.org/10.1097/00000658-199007000-00010.
21. Edgcombe H, Carter K, Yarrow S. Anaesthesia in the prone position. Br J Anaesth. 2008;100(2):165–83. https://doi.org/10.1093/bja/aem380.
22. Vorrakitpokatorn P, Permtongchuchai K, Raksamani EO, Phettongkam A. Perioperative complications and risk factors of percutaneous nephrolithotomy. J Med Assoc Thail. 2006;89(6):826–33.
23. Dore B. [Complications of percutaneous nephrolithotomy: risk factors and management]. Ann Urol (Paris). 2006;40(3):149–60.
24. Honey RJ, Ghiculete D, Ray AA, Pace KT. A randomized, double-blinded, placebo-controlled trial of intercostal nerve block after percutaneous nephrolithotomy. J Endourol. 2013;27(4):415–9. https://doi.org/10.1089/end.2012.0418.
25. Ozkan D, Akkaya T, Karakoyunlu N, Arik E, Ergil J, Koc Z, et al. Effect of ultrasound-guided intercostal nerve block on postoperative pain after percutaneous nephrolithotomy: prospective randomized controlled

study. Anaesthesist. 2013;62(12):988–94. https://doi.org/10.1007/s00101-013-2253-z.
26. Jonnavithula N, Pisapati MV, Durga P, Krishnamurthy V, Chilumu R, Reddy B. Efficacy of peritubal local anesthetic infiltration in alleviating postoperative pain in percutaneous nephrolithotomy. J Endourol. 2009;23(5):857–60. https://doi.org/10.1089/end.2008.0634.
27. Gokten OE, Kilicarslan H, Dogan HS, Turker G, Kordan Y. Efficacy of levobupivacaine infiltration to nephrostomy tract in combination with intravenous paracetamol on postoperative analgesia in percutaneous nephrolithotomy patients. J Endourol. 2011;25(1):35–9. https://doi.org/10.1089/end.2010.0346.
28. Shah HN, Shah RH, Sodha HS, Khandkar AA, Gokhale A. A randomized control trial evaluating efficacy of nephrostomy tract infiltration with bupivacaine after tubeless percutaneous nephrolithotomy. J Endourol. 2012;26(5):478–83. https://doi.org/10.1089/end.2011.0465.
29. Ak K, Gursoy S, Duger C, Isbir AC, Kaygusuz K, Ozdemir KI, et al. Thoracic paravertebral block for postoperative pain management in percutaneous nephrolithotomy patients: a randomized controlled clinical trial. Med Princ Pract. 2013;22(3):229–33. https://doi.org/10.1159/000345381.
30. Michel MS, Trojan L, Rassweiler JJ. Complications in percutaneous nephrolithotomy. Eur Urol. 2007;51(4):899–906; discussion 906. https://doi.org/10.1016/j.eururo.2006.10.020.
31. Scherz HC, Parsons CL. Prophylactic antibiotics in urology. Urol Clin North Am. 1987;14(2):265–71.
32. Zhong W, Zeng G, Wu K, Li X, Chen W, Yang H. Does a smaller tract in percutaneous nephrolithotomy contribute to high renal pelvic pressure and postoperative fever? J Endourol. 2008;22(9):2147–51. https://doi.org/10.1089/end.2008.0001.
33. Liu C, Zhang X, Liu Y, Wang P. Prevention and treatment of septic shock following mini-percutaneous nephrolithotomy: a single-center retrospective study of 834 cases. World J Urol. 2013;31(6):1593–7. https://doi.org/10.1007/s00345-012-1002-2.
34. Jorm AF, Christensen H, Korten AE, Henderson AS, Jacomb PA, Mackinnon A. Do cognitive complaints either predict future cognitive decline or reflect past cognitive decline? A longitudinal study of an elderly community sample. Psychol Med. 1997;27(1):91–8.
35. Kohl BA, Deutschman CS. The inflammatory response to surgery and trauma. Curr Opin Crit Care. 2006;12(4):325–32. https://doi.org/10.1097/01.ccx.0000235210.85073.fc.
36. Lucas SM, Rothwell NJ, Gibson RM. The role of inflammation in CNS injury and disease. Br J Pharmacol. 2006;147 Suppl 1:S232–40. https://doi.org/10.1038/sj.bjp.0706400.

Principles of a Perfect Puncture for Percutaneous Nephrolithotomy

8

David B. Bayne and Thomas L. Chi

8.1 Introduction

First reported in 1976 [1], percutaneous nephrolithotomy (PCNL) has replaced open surgery for large renal stones [2]. Initially described using fluoroscopic guidance in the prone position, contemporary approaches have expanded to now include ultrasound, computed tomography, and endoscopic guidance techniques in multiple patient positions. Regardless of the approach, crucial to successful PCNL is the accurate placement of the percutaneous access needle into the renal calyx of choice [3]. Here we review the various options for approaching the perfect renal puncture for PCNL.

8.2 Instrumentation

8.2.1 Needle

We recommend the use of an 18 gauge needle (Fig. 8.1). More narrow needles may deform as they traverse long lengths of tissue while wider needles may increase the risk of trauma or bleeding. When using ultrasound guidance, an echogenic tip version of the puncture needle can improve needle visibility. The needle should have an inner stylet that once removed allows for passage of urine, injection of contrast or air, and passage of a guidewire through the needle and into the collecting system.

8.2.2 C-Arm

Performing a fluoroscopy-guided puncture requires fluoroscopic equipment. Ideally the fluoroscopic machinery is mobile with rotational capacity, allowing for the visualization of the needle and collecting system in multiple planes.

8.2.3 Ultrasound

The best probe for guiding punctures is a curved array 3.5–5 MHz abdominal transducer probe for optimal visualization of the kidney (Fig. 8.1). Probes exist in many shapes and sizes for specialized usage. With higher-frequency transducers, greater imaging resolution is achieved but at the cost of lesser tissue penetration. With high-frequency probes, imaging depth is not long enough to visualize the kidney, especially when the patient is obese and the renal access tract is long. Doppler functionality can be used for visualization and avoidance of vessels in the puncture

D. B. Bayne (✉) · T. L. Chi
Urology, University of California, San Francisco, San Francisco, CA, USA
e-mail: David.Bayne@ucsf.edu; tom.chi@ucsf.edu

G. Zeng, K. Sarica (eds.), *Percutaneous Nephrolithotomy*,
https://doi.org/10.1007/978-981-15-0575-1_8

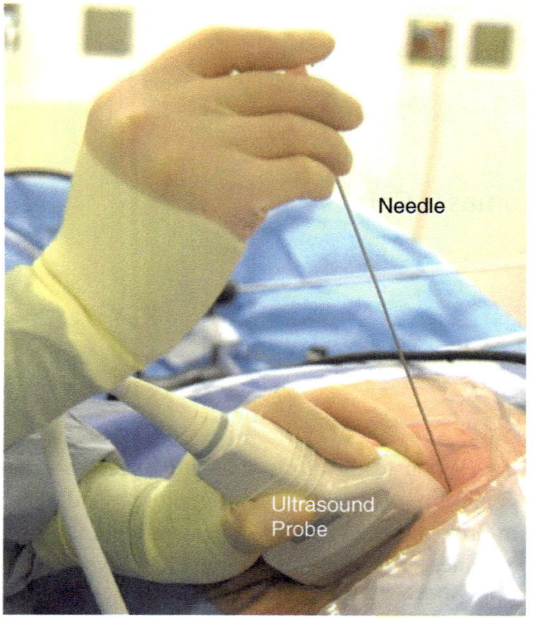

Fig. 8.1 Images of renal access needle and ultrasound probe

path though B mode ultrasound is the most frequently used imaging modality for renal access.

8.2.4 Guidewire

Many types of wire can be used for establishing access, including hydrophilic, super stiff, and hybrid wires. We have found that a J-tipped moveable core guidewire is ideal for maintaining puncture access once the needle is in the collecting system. The J-shaped tip minimizes risk of collecting system perforation and compared to other wires offers a balance of stiffness, maneuverability, and cost. Guidewires are inserted through the needle and into the collecting system and needle puncture and used as a placeholder for renal tract dilation.

8.2.5 Exchange Catheter

Both ultrasound and fluoroscopic guidance benefit from placement of a 5-French exchange catheter prior to starting the puncture. For fluoroscopic guidance, retrograde contrast injection into the collecting system allows visualization of renal anatomy. For ultrasound guidance it can facilitate hydrodistention of the collecting system via retrograde infusion of saline through the exchange catheter. While some advocate the use of a ureteral occlusion balloon for these purposes, in our experience, an open-ended exchange catheter without a balloon is more than adequate.

8.3 Fluoroscopy-Guided Puncture

There are many approaches to fluoroscopic guidance for percutaneous renal access. These techniques require retrograde insertion of a ureteral catheter for the purpose of retrograde radiological contrast injection. Patients can be in the prone or supine position, but this is limited by the specific fluoroscopy technique chosen.

8.3.1 Monoplanar Access

The monoplanar fluoroscopic guidance technique involves placement of the needle over the skin to calculate the angle of needle entry in the horizontal plane, and surgeon experience is used to dictate needle angle in the vertical plane combined with active fluoroscopic guidance [4]. The surgeon is able to deduce that the needle is not in the correct location if the needle tip goes beyond the calyx of choice. This is done in the prone position.

8.3.2 Biplanar Access in Long Axis

Long-access biplanar axis incorporates the same placement of the needle over the skin to calculate needle entry angle in the horizontal plane. In this case, the surgeon rotates the C-arm with a surgical clamp attached to the anterior drapes to determine the depth of the needle. If the needle is in between the collecting system and the clamp then it is superficial to the collecting system. If the clamp is above the collecting system it is too deep to the target [5].

8.3.3 Biplanar Access: Perpendicular "Bull's Eye" Technique

The "bull's eye" technique requires placing the C-arm at initially in the anterior-posterior orientation with the patient in the prone position. This positioning is used to select the target calyx. Once the target calyx is selected, the C-arm is rotated 30° towards the surgeon. This allows for the surgeon to line up the needle directly in line with the target calyx. The needle is then advanced in line with the C-arm generating a "bull's eye" or "eye of the needle." To judge for depth, the C-arm is rotated back into the anterior-posterior position as this informs a surgeon as to whether or not the needle has been advanced too far or not far enough to reach the collecting system [6]. Once the needle is thought to be in the appropriate position, the stylette is removed, and the position in the collecting system is confirmed with aspiration of urine.

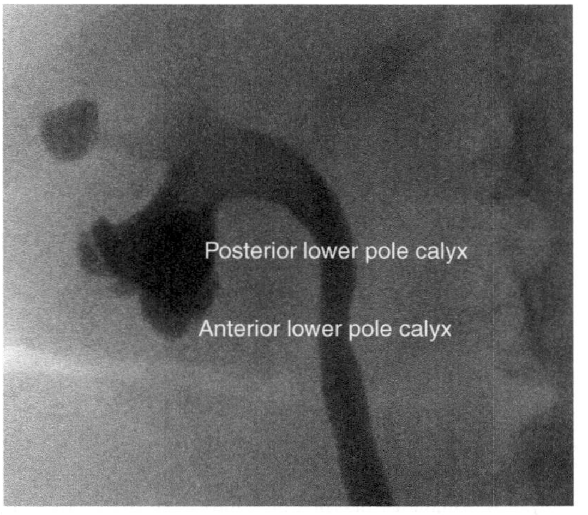

Fig. 8.2 Retrograde pyelogram of left kidney in prone position; in this case the lower pole posterior calyx is the target calyx

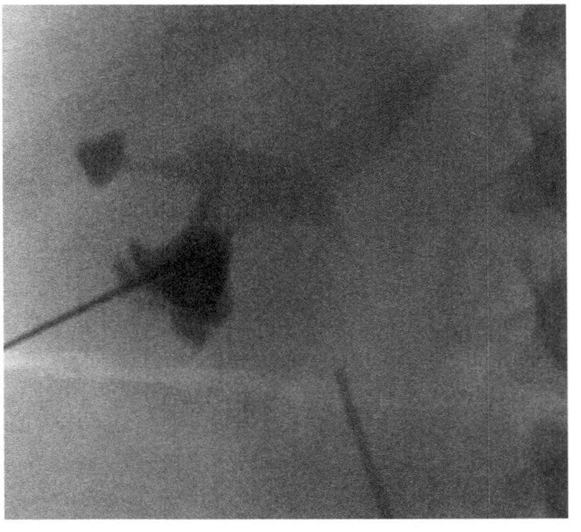

Fig. 8.3 Anterior/posterior image of needle entry into posterior lower pole calyx

8.3.4 Triangulation

The triangulation technique is also traditionally described in the prone position; in this technique an equilateral triangle is created after generating the first point over the target calyx with the C-arm in the anterior-posterior position. The second point is generated over the target calyx when the C-arm is rotated at 30°. The last point forms an equilateral triangle going lateral and cephalic to the first and second points. As the needle is advanced, the C-arm is rotated between 0 and 30° (Figs. 8.2, 8.3, and 8.4). The needle is gradually inserted into the target calyx of choice, and C-arm images are checked to confirm the appropriate course of the needle [7].

8.3.5 Supine Positioning

For fluoroscopic puncture, triangulation and biplanar access techniques can be applied in the supine position. Rana et al. describe using a small towel roll to elevate the ipsilateral flank by 20°, lateralizing the kidney and allowing for the lower calyx to be positioned at an angle perpendicular to the operating table. The C-arm is then used to visualize the passage of the needle into the desired calyx at a puncture site 1 cm above the posterior axillary line [8].

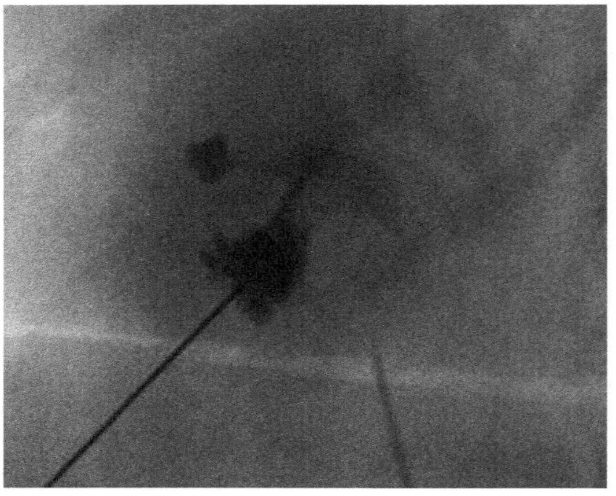

Fig. 8.4 Image of needle entry into lower pole posterior calyx with C-arm rotated 30° from anterior/posterior plane, confirming entry at appropriate depth in target calyx

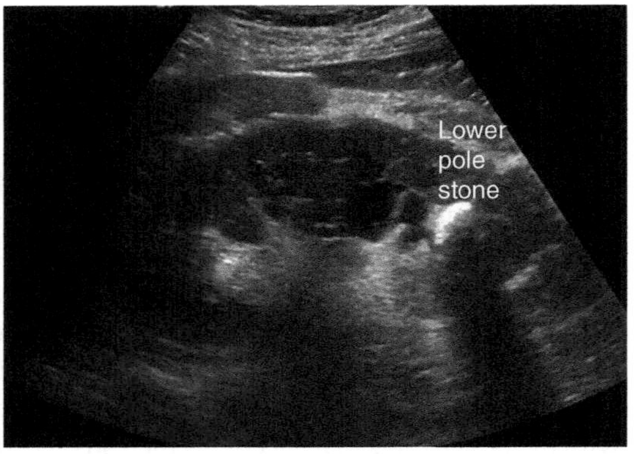

Fig. 8.5 Single stone in hydronephrotic kidney

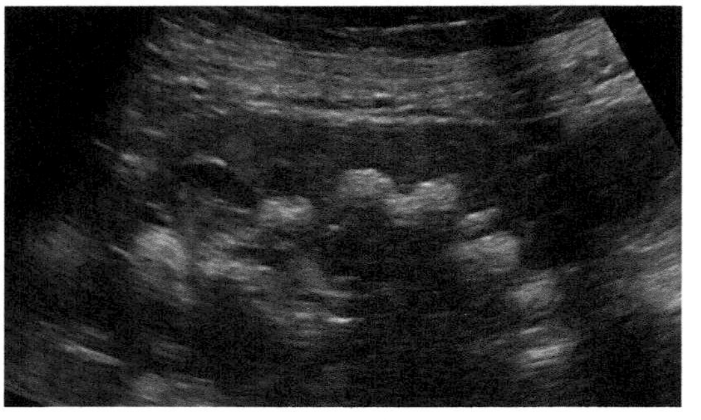

Fig. 8.6 Staghorn stone in kidney without hydronephrosis

8.4 Ultrasound-Guided Puncture

Ultrasound-guided percutaneous nephrolithotomy has been described in both Asia and Europe and has recently gained popularity in the United States. The advantages of ultrasound-guided percutaneous nephrolithotomy are that it limits radiation exposure to the patient and to the physician, has been described as being a lower cost modality compared to fluoroscopy [9], allows for visualization of surrounding viscera that are not readily apparent on fluoroscopic images, and allows for the potential to do simultaneous Doppler imaging to ascertain vascular anatomy [10]. Most importantly, its adoption is associated with a shorter learning curve compared to the use of fluoroscopy, allowing for more urologists to take control of renal access over interventional radiologists (Figs. 8.5 and 8.6). Wider adoption of ultrasound for percutaneous renal access amongst urologists has been limited by lack of formal training opportunities in renal ultrasonography. Ultrasound-guided renal access is dependent on the ability to obtain clear renal imaging as reflected by increased difficulty obtaining accurate or clear ultrasound imaging in patients with very high body mass index [11]. After achieving competence in the principles of renal ultrasound imaging, the two needle control techniques described below can be applied to achieving accurate renal puncture.

8.4.1 Longitudinal Plane Approach

Ultrasound-guided percutaneous nephrolithotomy has been described by visualizing needle entry in the longitudinal plane of the ultrasound probe. As described in fluoroscopic guidance an 18-gauge needle is used to achieve access. Usage of an echogenic tip on the needle will help with improved visualization of the entire needle under ultrasound guidance. With the longitudinal approach, the surgeon should obtain a sagittal view of the kidney, bringing the target calyx toward one side of the imaging screen or the other (usually the right side for the lower pole and the left side for upper pole or

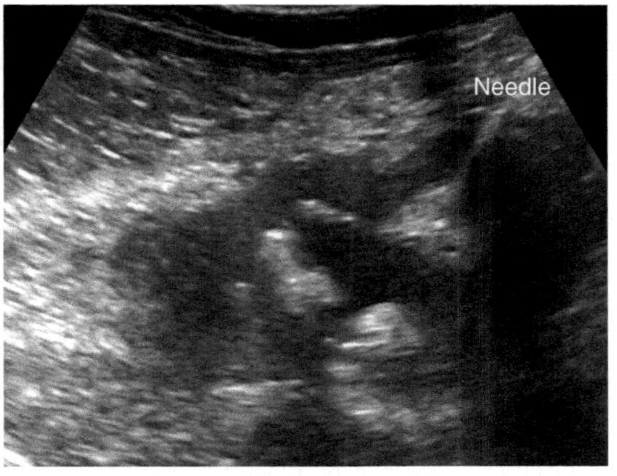

Fig. 8.7 Ultrasound image of needle entry into target calyx

mid-kidney) to shorten the distance from the skin to the target and prevent an extremely shallow angle of entry into the skin. Once this image is fixed in place, the goal should be maintaining visualization of the entire kidney and continued visualization of the entire length of the needle as the needle is advanced into the target calyx (Fig. 8.7). It is important to take the correct angle using an end on calyceal approach. This prevents taking an oblique angle making surgery difficult as this would cause the working probe to be limited by the patient's iliac crest in the prone position [12].

8.4.2 Transverse Plane Approach

Ultrasound-guided percutaneous nephrolithotomy has also been described using the transverse plane of the ultrasound probe. The skin is punctured orthogonal to the long axis of the probe using the access needle. With this approach, the surgeon should sweep the ultrasound probe back and forth in order to visualize the needle tip as it is advanced into the target calyx. Because the entire length of the needle cannot be visualized in this imaging plane it is very important to advance the needle gradually and continuously reestablish the image of the tip of the needle as the probe is swept back and forth to watch it enter into the target calyx.

8.5 Computed Tomography

Computed-tomography-guided percutaneous nephrolithotomy has been described in select cases of patients with anatomical anomalies, allowing for the visualization and avoidance of surrounding abdominal viscera relative to the target calyx [13]. For example, a transgluteal CT-guided approach has been utilized to achieve access in pelvic horseshoe kidney [14]. While portable "O-arms" are available to provide CT capability in the operating room, for the most part utilizing CT guidance relies on collaboration with the interventional radiology team to obtain renal access with this imaging modality. In these cases where access is obtained by partner services, an important principle is clear communication and direct guidance of the radiology team to identify which calyx should be entered to maximize stone clearance ability during PCNL. Without such an integrated approach, suboptimal renal access may result in increased bleeding and complication rates, lower stone clearance rates, and potentially higher need for secondary procedures.

8.6 Retrograde Visualization

Endoscopic combined intrarenal surgery (ECIRS) employs antegrade and retrograde access to the upper urinary tract, allowing for retrograde visualization of antegrade puncture [15]. Retrograde visualization of percutaneous renal puncture (Endovision puncture) offers several important advantages. By directly visualizing the needle enter through the target papilla, it allows the operator assurance of the exact puncture location. It limits need for fluoroscopy as one is able to visualize the steps of dilation endoscopically rather than relying on only fluoroscopic guidance. It also allows for easier placement of the security guide wire through the percutaneous tract down the ureter and out of the urethra for a through and through control of the urinary tract [15, 16]. There is some evidence to suggest that this approach may reduce high-grade complication rates [17] and facilitate stone clearance given the ability to approach stones in both a retrograde and antegrade fashion [18]. ECIRS also facilitates simultaneous stone removal to be done in the presence of ipsilateral ureteral stones, contralateral smaller stones capable of being cleared with ureteroscopy, conduit instrumentation, retained ureteral stents, and any surgery where it is necessary to have both retrograde and antegrade access.

During ECIRS, prior to puncture the patient is scoped retrograde with ureterorenoscopy and the ipsilateral ureter is visualized. If ureteral stones are encountered they are treated with laser fragmentation. If the ureter is cleared of stones, a ureteral access sheath can be placed and a ureteroscope placed through the access sheath. Once the scope is in the collecting system, it allows for retrograde injection of contrast through the scope to assist in fluoroscopic puncture.

8.6.1 Positioning

8.6.1.1 Galdakao-Modified Supine Valdivia (GMSV) Position

The supine patient position typically described for ECIRS is the Galdakao-modified supine Valdivia (GMSV) position [19]. In this position the patient lies supine with a saline bag or bolster under the operative flank. This props the patient up where the operative flank is elevated facilitating puncture access to the kidney. The patient's legs are positioned in stirrups with the contralateral leg well abducted and the ipsilateral leg either extended or slightly elevated in the modified lithotomy position. This allows for instrumentation and access of the urinary tract through the urethra. This position offers several advantages as the patient can be accessed from the retrograde and antegrade positions without need for re-positioning. This is particularly useful for patients with urinary diversions that need to be scoped through their conduits, or patients with ureteral pathology such as ureteral stones or ureteral structures with simultaneous renal stones requiring treatment. It is also a comfortable position from an anesthesiologist's perspective for airway management.

8.6.1.2 Prone Split Leg

In this position, patients are placed prone with padded rolls under the thorax and upper abdomen with the genitalia at the bottom of the standard table. The lower extremities are then placed on two padded adaptors level with the operative table and split up to 45° [20]. This position allows for retrograde instrumentation of the urethra while the patient is in the prone position and localization of the ureteral orifice of choice for placement of a guidewire. Depending on the need for retrograde intervention, an access sheath and a flexible scope can be placed to facilitate stone clearance [21]. This offers advantages of improved space to access the kidney relative to the supine position.

8.7 Retrograde Puncture

8.7.1 Lawson Retrograde Endoscopic-Guided Nephrostomy Access

Lawson first described retrograde puncture through the kidney to the skin in 1983 [22]. With subsequent improvement in endoscopic technology, some have gone back to this method citing improved endoscopic visualization and needle control making it a safer option now compared to its original application in the 1980s. This has been described with fluoroscopic supplementary guidance. Once the desired calyx is selected on retrograde fluoroscopic visualization, the working port of the ureteroscope is used to advance the Lawson nephrostomy needle catheter through the target calyx. Fluoroscopy is employed to ensure that the needle stays straight as it is advanced. Once the needle is seen tenting the skin, an incision is made over the needle with a scalpel. The needle is grasped and pulled out of the body, leaving the Lawson wire coming from the ureteroscope out through the skin. After removal of the ureteroscope, there is full control of the GU tract with wire access from the kidney down through the urethra. Dilation is then performed over the wire [23]. While this approach obviates the need to master antegrade image-guided placement of a needle into the target calyx, its limitations include the possible inability to use the upper or lower pole for calyceal access for many cases.

8.8 Calyceal Location Considerations for Puncture

Traditionally, ideal access is obtained at the fornix of the renal calyx, splitting the midline of the renal papilla to minimize vessel injury and bleeding [24]. Blood vessels course through the kidney like spokes on a wheel, branching into smaller caliber sizes going centrally to peripherally in the kidney. Entry into the calyceal fornix has, therefore, always been thought of as the safest location to enter the collecting system with minimal risk for bleeding. While some challenged this approach by showing safe outcomes with infundibular puncture [25], the calyceal approach is still thought of as the ideal entry point.

The decision as to whether to perform an upper pole versus mid kidney versus lower pole puncture is dependent on multiple factors. For example, a large proximal kidney stone maybe more susceptible to access via an upper pole puncture. The upper pole provides a straight path to access the proximal ureteral stone whereas a lower pole puncture requires making a sharp turn from the lower pole into the renal pelvis and down to the proximal ureteral stone. On the other hand, a lower pole puncture may provide the ideal access point to fragment a lower pole stone. In the case of staghorn stones, upper and lower pole punctures may allow for complete access of the staghorn stone as opposed to mid kidney punctures which may require steep turns to access upper or lower pole fragments. The mid kidney can provide a "best of all worlds" access into the kidney and can be used with good effect. Regardless of the actual puncture used, the guiding principle should be obtaining access to the calyx that provides the easiest path to stone removal in the straightest fashion possible.

Despite the choice of an ideal initial puncture location, there may be elements of the stone not easily accessible, requiring additional punctures. This must be pursued with caution, however, as multiple puncture tracts may predict for decrease in renal function as a consequence of surgery [26, 27].

8.9 Patient Position Considerations

Maximal access to an upper pole puncture typically will dictate a prone patient position. In the prone position, the access can be placed medially in a manner not possible with supine positioning. Although upper pole punctures can be achieved in the supine position, the prone position allows for a more ergonomic access to the upper pole with a more posterior access point than typically facilitated by a supine position.

Lower pole and mid kidney access can be achieved in either the supine or prone position with equivalent efficacy. Retrograde access of the lower urinary tract can also be achieved when the patient is positioned supine or prone. The supine position may be more familiar for urologists who are used to performing transurethral surgery from the dorsal lithotomy position. In the prone position, with practice, retrograde access can be obtained without special positioning equipment, though split leg splitter bars have been described to allow for easier retrograde access into the upper collecting system [20].

Obese patients can be positioned in both the supine and prone positions. Longer tracts have been described in the supine position. For the majority of patients, whether obese or not, this increase in length is not a barrier to gaining supine access to the kidney.

8.10 Special Circumstances

8.10.1 Horseshoe Kidney

Percutaneous nephrolithotomy has been demonstrated successfully in horseshoe kidneys in numerous studies [28, 29]. Classically an upper pole posterior calyceal approach is preferred, and as such the patient in the prone position provides what is thought to be ideal access to the posterior upper pole. With ultrasound guidance, it has been demonstrated that mid and lower kidney calyces can also provide adequate access into the kidney.

8.10.2 Pediatrics

Percutaneous access has been shown to be safe and effective in pediatric patients. In order to minimize radiation exposure, which is a particular concern in this population, we recommend ultrasound guidance for access.

8.10.3 Obesity

Obese patients present specific challenges for percutaneous nephrolithotomy when considering airway management with complex positioning [30]. However, skin to stone distance has not been demonstrated as a factor in determining success and complications in fluoroscopy-guided PCNL [31, 32]. For ultrasound-guided procedures, some studies have shown documented increased difficulty for achieving accessing in these patients but that these difficulties can be overcome with experience [11]. To successfully perform PCNL in obese patients, experienced urologists working in concert with an experienced anesthesia team is critical.

8.10.4 Spinal Deformity

Spinal deformities can make imaging and positioning during percutaneous access challenging. These patients must be approached on a case by case basis as ultrasound may be difficult in some patients due to shadowing from the spine. On the other hand, fluoroscopic guidance may be equally challenging due to difficulty with positioning and C-arm placement. Patients with spinal deformities do have higher rates of complications and lower stone-free rates with PCNL [33]. Nevertheless successful access has been documented in these patients when in the hands of experience and expertise [34, 35]. When a safe access window to the kidney is obscured by body protrusions, liver, lung, spleen, and bowel, CT-guided access is often the best option.

8.11 Conclusion

The surgeon has numerous options to achieve percutaneous access for the purpose of percutaneous nephrolithotomy. There is no specific single technique to achieve the perfect puncture. The most important principle to keep in mind is accurate needle placement into a calyceal target appropriately positioned for stone removal. Matched to that principle, the surgeon should be familiar with multiple options available to him or her including ultrasound guidance, fluoroscopic guidance, prone or supine positioning, retrograde endoscopic combined visualization, or retrograde needle access. Surgeons must tailor their practice specific to their skills and the patient on a case-by-case basis.

References

1. Fernström I, Johansson B. Percutaneous pyelolithotomy: a new extraction technique. Scand J Urol Nephrol. 1976;10(3):257–9.
2. Alivizatos G, Skolarikos A. Is there still a role for open surgery in the management of renal stones? Curr Opin Urol. 2006;16(2):106–11.
3. Knoll T, Daels F, Desai J, Hoznek A, Knudsen B, Montanari E, Scoffone C, Skolarikos A, Tozawa K. Percutaneous nephrolithotomy: technique. World J Urol. 2017;35(9):1361–8.
4. Hatipoglu NK, Bodakci MN, Penbegül N, Bozkurt Y, Sancaktutar AA, Atar M, Söylemez H. Monoplanar access technique for percutaneous nephrolithotomy. Urolithiasis. 2013;41(3):257–63.
5. Hoznek A, Ouzaid I, Gettman M, Rode J, De La Taille A, Salomon L, Abbou CC. Fluoroscopy-guided renal access in supine percutaneous nephrolithotomy. Urology. 2011;78(1):221–4.
6. Sharma G, Sharma A. Determining site of skin puncture for percutaneous renal access using fluoroscopy-guided triangulation technique. J Endourol. 2009;23(2):193–6.
7. Sharma G, Sharma A. Determining the angle and depth of puncture for fluoroscopy-guided percutaneous renal access in the prone position. Indian J Urol. 2015;31(1):38.
8. Rana AM, Bhojwani JP, Junejo NN, Bhagia SD. Tubeless PCNL with patient in supine position: procedure for all seasons?—with comprehensive technique. Urology. 2008;71(4):581–5.
9. Hudnall M, Usawachintachit M, Metzler I, Tzou DT, Harrison B, Lobo E, Chi T. Ultrasound guidance reduces percutaneous nephrolithotomy cost compared to fluoroscopy. Urology. 2017;103:52–8.
10. Agarwal M, Agrawal MS, Jaiswal A, Kumar D, Yadav H, Lavania P. Safety and efficacy of ultrasonogra-

phy as an adjunct to fluoroscopy for renal access in percutaneous nephrolithotomy (PCNL). BJU Int. 2011;108(8):1346–9.
11. Bayne DB, Usawachintachit M, Tzou D, Taguchi K, Shindel A, Chi TL. Increasing body mass index steepens the learning curve for ultrasound-guided percutaneous nephrolithotomy. Urology. 2018;120:68–73.
12. Chu C, Masic S, Usawachintachit M, Hu W, Yang W, Stoller M, Li J, Chi T. Ultrasound-guided renal access for percutaneous nephrolithotomy: a description of three novel ultrasound-guided needle techniques. J Endourol. 2016;30(2):153–8.
13. Matlaga BR, Shah OD, Zagoria RJ, Dyer RB, Streem SB, Assimos DG. Computerized tomography guided access for percutaneous nephrostolithotomy. J Urol. 2003;170(1):45–7.
14. Mullins RJ, Dauw CA, Borofsky MS, York N, Patel AA, Lingeman JE. Transgluteal CT-guided percutaneous renal access for percutaneous nephrolithotomy in a pelvic horseshoe kidney. J Endourol Case Rep. 2015;1(1):27–9.
15. Scoffone CM, Cracco CM, Cossu M, Grande S, Poggio M, Scarpa RM. Endoscopic combined intrarenal surgery in Galdakao-modified supine Valdivia position: a new standard for percutaneous nephrolithotomy? Eur Urol. 2008;54(6):1393–403.
16. Miano R, Scoffone C, De Nunzio C, Germani S, Cracco C, Usai P, Tubaro A, Kim FJ, Micali S. Position: prone or supine is the issue of percutaneous nephrolithotomy. J Endourol. 2010;24(6):931–8.
17. Marguet CG, Springhart WP, Tan YH, Patel A, Undre S, Albala DM, Preminger GM. Simultaneous combined use of flexible ureteroscopy and percutaneous nephrolithotomy to reduce the number of access tracts in the management of complex renal calculi. BJU Int. 2005;96(7):1097–100.
18. Cracco CM, Scoffone CM. ECIRS (endoscopic combined intrarenal surgery) in the Galdakao-modified supine Valdivia position: a new life for percutaneous surgery? World J Urol. 2011;29(6):821–7.
19. Ibarluzea G, Scoffone CM, Cracco CM, Poggio M, Porpiglia F, Terrone C, Astobieta A, Camargo I, Gamarra M, Tempia A, Valdivia Uria JG. Supine Valdivia and modified lithotomy position for simultaneous anterograde and retrograde endourological access. BJU Int. 2007;100(1):233–6.
20. Grasso M, Nord R, Bagley DH. Prone split leg and flank roll positioning: simultaneous antegrade and retrograde access to the upper urinary tract. J Endourol. 1993;7(4):307–10.
21. Hamamoto S, Yasui T, Okada A, Taguchi K, Kawai N, Ando R, Mizuno K, Kubota Y, Kamiya H, Tozawa K, Kohri K. Endoscopic combined intrarenal surgery for large calculi: simultaneous use of flexible ureteroscopy and mini-percutaneous nephrolithotomy overcomes the disadvantageous of percutaneous nephrolithotomy monotherapy. J Endourol. 2014;28(1):28–33.
22. Lawson RK, Murphy JB, Taylor AJ, Jacobs SC. Retrograde method for percutaneous access to kidney. Urology. 1983;22:580.
23. Kaler KS, Parkhomenko E, Lin CY, Valley ZA, Kim WK, Okhunov Z, Patel RM, Landman J. A new twist on an old technique: Lawson retrograde endoscopic-guided nephrostomy access for percutaneous nephrolithotomy in prone split-leg position. J Endourol Case Rep. 2018;4(1):190–4.
24. Sampaio FJ. Anatomic background for intrarenal endourologic surgery. J Endourol. 1992;6(5): 301–4.
25. Kyriazis I, Kallidonis P, Vasilas M, Panagopoulos V, Kamal W, Liatsikos E. Challenging the wisdom of puncture at the calyceal fornix in percutaneous nephrolithotripsy: feasibility and safety study with 137 patients operated via a non-calyceal percutaneous track. World J Urol. 2017;35(5):795–801.
26. Gorbachinsky I, Wood K, Colaco M, Hemal S, Mettu J, Mirzazadeh M, Assimos DG, Gutierrez-Aćeves J. Evaluation of renal function after percutaneous nephrolithotomy—does the number of percutaneous access tracts matter? J Urol. 2016;196(1):131–6.
27. Hyams ES, Shah OD. Risk of renal function deterioration after percutaneous nephrolithotomy in patients with baseline renal insufficiency. J Urol. 2008;179:432.
28. Symons SJ, Ramachandran A, Kurien A, Baiysha R, Desai MR. Urolithiasis in the horseshoe kidney: a single-centre experience. BJU Int. 2008;102(11):1676–80.
29. Satav V, Sabale V, Pramanik P, Kanklia SP, Mhaske S. Percutaneous nephrolithotomy of horseshoe kidney: our institutional experience. Urol Ann. 2018;10(3):258–62.
30. El-Husseiny T, Moraitis K, Maan Z, Papatsoris A, Saunders P, Golden B, Masood J, Buchholz NP. Percutaneous endourologic procedures in high-risk patients in the lateral decubitus position under regional anesthesia. J Endourol. 2009;23(10): 1603–6.
31. Gonulalan U, Akand M, Coban G, Cicek T, Kosan M, Goktas S, Ozkardes H. Skin-to-stone distance has no impact on outcomes of percutaneous nephrolithotomy. Urol Int. 2014;92(4):444–8.
32. Zhou X, Sun X, Chen X, Gong X, Yang Y, Chen C, Yao Q. Effect of obesity on outcomes of percutaneous nephrolithotomy in renal stone management: a systematic review and meta-analysis. Urol Int. 2017;98(4):382–90.
33. Mitchell S, Gurung PM, Choong S, Morris T, Smith D, Woodhouse C, Philp T. Percutaneous nephrolithotomy and spina bifida: complex major stone surgery? J Endourol. 2018;32(3):205–12.
34. Goumas-Kartalas I, Montanari E. Percutaneous nephrolithotomy in patients with spinal deformities. J Endourol. 2010;24(7):1081–9.
35. Wang S, Zhang X, Xiao B, Hu W, Chen S, Li J. Ultrasound guided percutaneous nephrolithotomy for upper urinary tract calculi in patients with spinal deformity: a decade's experience. BJU Int. 2019;124(1):109–15.

9 Tract Dilation During PNL

Thomas Knoll

9.1 Introduction

There are two major steps of percutaneous nephrolithotomy (PNL): the puncture of the kidney and the subsequent dilatation to establish the percutaneous tract. In the past decades, three concepts have been used: the Alken metal telescope bougies [1], Amplatz fascial dilators and single-step dilators [5] and the balloon dilation [6]. Most surgeons choose the method of access according to their experience and preference. Some series and meta-analyses have addressed this issue and may give advice in the selection process. However, other factors as imaging for access have a significant impact on outcome and might influence outcome data for dilation.

9.2 Successful Dilation

9.2.1 Single-Step Vs. Metal Dilators

Amjadi et al. compared sequential metal dilators with single-step dilation and could not demonstrate a difference in safety [2]. A study by Joel reported a slightly higher perforation of Amplatz dilators after balloon failures, indicating difficult situations [11]. Data from Safak et al. showed a higher perforation rate of Amplatz dilators vs. balloon dilators [16].

A meta-analysis of Dehong et al. compared single step vs. metal telescope dilators and could not demonstrate a difference in outcome (stone free rate) [8]. Another comparable systematic review by Li confirmed this finding of almost 100% successful dilatation in both groups [13]. Both groups concluded that factors other than the dilation method as method of puncture, location and number of tracts might have more impact on the outcome of the procedure.

Scar tissue in recurrent interventions may negatively influence tract dilation. Most authors report better results for metal dilators in such situations and consider them as the method of choice when scarring is present. Especially balloon dilation is limited in hard perirenal tissue (Joel et al.) [11]. But even single-step dilation can be frustrating as underlined by a study of Ziaee et al. [17] where single-step dilation had a failure rate of 7% while metal dilation was possible in all cases what is in accordance to a study of Lojanapiwat [14].

9.2.2 Operative Time

Many surgeons assume a shorter operative (OR) time with balloon compared to sequential dilation

T. Knoll (✉)
Department of Urology, Klinikum Sindelfingen-Böblingen, University of Tuebingen, Tuebingen, Germany
e-mail: t.knoll@klinikverbund-suedwest.de

G. Zeng, K. Sarica (eds.), *Percutaneous Nephrolithotomy*, https://doi.org/10.1007/978-981-15-0575-1_9

methods but the systematic review of Dehong et al. could not show a difference in OR time between Amplatz and balloon dilations [8]. However, after exclusion of the series of Gönen that included patients after open renal surgery, OR time was in favor of balloon dilation [10].

It is quite difficult to compare the available literature as no standard PNL tract size exists. While some urologists use 30 or 32 French access, others consider 24–26 French as standard. The size of the tract clearly affects OR time as smaller tracts require more extensive stone disintegration.

9.2.3 Fluoroscopy Time

Single-step dilation was first reported by Frattini et al. [9]. They demonstrate a shorter fluoroscopy time when comparing with balloon and metal dilation. However, stone volume was higher in the metal dilator group, why shorter fluoroscopy (and OR) times might be biased by more difficult case selection. Furthermore, the measured OR time was defined very different by authors, so interpretation shall be done carefully. However, a shorter fluoroscopy time seems to be a logical consequence of one-shot dilation, a fact that was shown by most series [2, 16, 17].

9.3 Complications

When comparing single step vs. metal telescope dilation, the analysis of Dehong showed a lower hemoglobin drop for single step vs. telescope while the analysis of Li could not demonstrate significant difference [8, 13]. Same findings were shown for blood transfusion rates. When comparing Amplatz vs. balloon dilations, the decrease in hemoglobin was in favor of the balloon dilation. The results of the CROES Global PNL Study, however, were in contrast to these systematic reviews [3, 7, 12]. In this large data collection of >5000 consecutive PNLs, balloon dilation resulted in a higher transfusion rate. It is under discussion whether this finding was a result of the type of access (more fluoroscopy guidance in the balloon group compared to more ultrasound guided access in the telescopic dilator group) or more complex stone situations.

In the series of Li et al., no statistical difference was seen in transfusion rates when comparing single step with sequential dilation [13]. Again, data should be interpreted carefully. Most studies report blood loss by comparing pre- vs. postoperative difference of red blood cells, which is a very imprecise value that is highly affected by fasting status and fluid infusions. Transfusion rates are, therefore, more reliable, but vary largely, indicating that many factors predict outcome, like stone volume, technique and surgeon's skills.

9.4 New Advances

The advantage of sequential dilators, mainly the Alken telescope dilators, is the ability to dilate even scarred perirenal tissue after prior surgery. In contrast, standard nephrostomy balloons allow maximum insufflation pressures of 17–20 ATM, which is not enough for successful dilation in 10–15% of the cases. New systems with up to 30 ATM may overcome this drawback. Several authors have worked on minor modifications of the existing three concepts [4, 15].

9.5 Costs

Only few studies have evaluated the costs of the different dilation concepts. Frattini et al. estimated the costs of a nondisposable metal dilator set in with 500€ while an Amplatz single-step dilator may cost 60€ and a balloon dilator 300€ [9]. Clearly, the nondisposable stainless-steel metal dilators outperform the disposable devices. It has to be mentioned that metal single-step dilators are available mainly for miniaturized accesses and may have comparable cost efficacy like the Alken metal dilators.

9.6 Summary

The three standard techniques for dilation of the percutaneous tract for nephrolithotomy are all viable options. Differences have been shown for OR time, fluoroscopy time, complications and costs. However, such differences are small and heterogeneous protocols do not allow clear conclusions. Therefore, the chosen technique is usually based on the surgeon's personal preference.

References

1. Alken P, Hutschenreiter G, Gunther R, et al. Percutaneous stone manipulation. J Urol. 1981;125:463.
2. Amjadi M, Zolfaghari A, Elahian A, et al. Percutaneous nephrolithotomy in patients with previous open nephrolithotomy: one-shot versus telescopic technique for tract dilatation. J Endourol. 2008;22:423–5.
3. Andonian S, Scoffone CM, Louie MK, et al. Does imaging modality used for percutaneous renal access make a difference? A matched case analysis. J Endourol. 2013;27:24–8.
4. Baldwin DD, Maynes LJ, Desai PJ, et al. A novel single step percutaneous access sheath: the initial human experience. J Urol. 2006;175:156–61.
5. Castaneda-Zuniga WR, Clayman R, Smith A, et al. Nephrostolithotomy: percutaneous techniques for urinary calculus removal. AJR Am J Roentgenol. 1982;139:721–6.
6. Clayman RV, Castaneda-Zuniga WR, Hunter DW, et al. Rapid balloon dilatation of the nephrostomy track for nephrostolithotomy. Radiology. 1983;147:884–5.
7. De La Rosette J, Assimos D, Desai M, et al. The clinical research office of the endourological society percutaneous nephrolithotomy global study: indications, complications, and outcomes in 5803 patients. J Endourol. 2011;25:11–7.
8. Dehong C, Liangren L, Huawei L, et al. A comparison among four tract dilation methods of percutaneous nephrolithotomy: a systematic review and meta-analysis. Urolithiasis. 2013;41:523–30.
9. Frattini A, Barbieri A, Salsi P, et al. One shot: a novel method to dilate the nephrostomy access for percutaneous lithotripsy. J Endourol. 2001;15:919–23.
10. Gonen M, Turan H, Ozturk B, et al. Factors affecting fever following percutaneous nephrolithotomy: a prospective clinical study. J Endourol. 2008;22:2135–8.
11. Joel AB, Rubenstein JN, Hsieh MH, et al. Failed percutaneous balloon dilation for renal access: incidence and risk factors. Urology. 2005;66:29–32.
12. Labate G, Modi P, Timoney A, et al. The percutaneous nephrolithotomy global study: classification of complications. J Endourol. 2011;25:1275–80.
13. Li Y, Yang L, Xu P, et al. One-shot versus gradual dilation technique for tract creation in percutaneous nephrolithotomy: a systematic review and meta-analysis. Urolithiasis. 2013;41:443–8.
14. Lojanapiwat B. Previous open nephrolithotomy: does it affect percutaneous nephrolithotomy techniques and outcome? J Endourol. 2006;20:17–20.
15. Pathak AS, Bellman GC. One-step percutaneous nephrolithotomy sheath versus standard two-step technique. Urology. 2005;66:953–7.
16. Safak M, Gogus C, Soygur T. Nephrostomy tract dilation using a balloon dilator in percutaneous renal surgery: experience with 95 cases and comparison with the fascial dilator system. Urol Int. 2003;71:382–4.
17. Ziaee SM, Karami H, Aminsharifi A, et al. One-stage tract dilation for percutaneous nephrolithotomy: is it justified? J Endourol. 2007;21:1415–20.

Intracorporeal Lithotripsy During PCNL

10

Xiaofeng Gao, Ziyu Fang, Hao Dong, Fei Xie, Chaoyue Lu, and Zeyu Wang

10.1 Introduction

Percutaneous nephroscope surgery began in the 1940s. In 1941, Rupol and Brown used an endoscopic instrument to remove the residual stones from a percutaneous approach after open surgery. In 1955, Goodwin first performed percutaneous nephrostomy and successfully relieved hydronephrosis. In 1976, Fernstrom and Johannson were successful in extracting stones from the kidney through PCNL for the first time [1].

Since then, due to continuous improvements in surgical techniques and equipment, PCNL has evolved into an effective method for treating stones larger than 2 cm, with a lower overall incidence of complications. Effective stone removal and evacuation is one of the key steps in PCNL. Some small stones can be removed with special grasping forceps, but many large stones cannot be removed through PCNL. Therefore, effective lithotripters are needed for PCNL in different situations.

Lithotripters can be roughly divided into rigid and flexible types. Rigid lithotripters include pneumatic lithotripters and ultrasonic lithotripters, and flexible lithotripters include electrohydraulic (EHL) and lasers. In the process of PCNL, the fragmentation of most stones is usually performed by rigid lithotripters such as pneumatic and ultrasonic lithotripters, while flexible lithotripters are mainly used for stones that are difficult to be reached through rigid lithotripters. All rigid lithotripters have an energy-generating handheld device, and the probe can provide energy to fragment stones. Compared to rigid lithotripters, flexible instruments are less efficient, but they have the advantages of creating less percutaneous channels [2]. With the development of rigid and flexible lithotripsy, the efficiency of PCNL is significantly improved.

10.2 Rigid Lithotripters

10.2.1 Pneumatic Lithotripters

10.2.1.1 Mechanism

When the pneumatic ballistic lithotripters work, the probe breaks the stone by using the mechanical energy which imitates the industrial air hammer. The compressed air produced during the function of pneumatic lithotripsy strikes the probe repeatedly, and the probe strikes the stones in pulse. The air comes either from the hospital's air pipe or from a portable tank, which is then transferred to the handheld device.

X. Gao (✉) · Z. Fang · H. Dong · F. Xie
C. Lu · Z. Wang
Department of Urology, Changhai Hospital, Second Military Medical University, Shanghai, China

G. Zeng, K. Sarica (eds.), *Percutaneous Nephrolithotomy*,
https://doi.org/10.1007/978-981-15-0575-1_10

10.2.1.2 Advantages and Disadvantages

This approach has the advantages of reducing the risk of thermal damage to the urothelium, fast lithotripsy, and high efficiency and can crush stones of various components. Its successful rate of fragmentation for ureteral calculi of various components is 73~100% [3–8]. Pneumatic ballistic lithotripters can still work even though the operation vision is not very clear, and it is simple to operate and maintain a low cost. Thus, it can be used as a basic and regular equipment. Its disadvantages include relatively high retropulsion rate and easy to isolate the stone fragments. It has been reported that the stone retropulsion rate for ureteroscopic lithotripsy ranges from 2 to 17%. This is caused by the inability to limit stone movement in the ureter [9]. After lithotripsy, the stone fragments can be removed by a gripper or suction of ultrasonic devices [10]. The pneumatic lithotripters are inflexible and require nephroscope with straight working channels.

10.2.1.3 Technique Tips

Our experience for ballistic lithotripsy is fixing the stone slightly at the front of the sheath and starting lithotripsy from the corner or edge of the stone with a short and intermittent method of continuous percussion, which can improve the efficiency. The stones are easy to move in the larger space of renal collection system, which makes it more difficult to crush. For optimal use, stones should be fixed to the urothelium in order to reduce the displacement of the stones away from the probe. When hitting against the stone, prolonged force exposure increases the risk of ureteral perforation. For the removal of large stones, repeated in and out of the channel is needed. As the probe cannot be bended, it only suits for rigid endoscope. During lithotripsy, it is better to gently put the probe on stone and try to grasp the rhythm of breaking stone. Urologists should have a holistic view for lithotripsy and find out the most suitable pressure point of the stone. The staghorn stone can be fragmented from the corner of the stone and then crushed one by one. Smaller stone can be directly washed out (suitable for 11~20F channel) with pulse perfusion. We do not recommend the use of pneumatic lithotripters in flexible ureterscopy, as it is easy to cause damage to the scope in the course of operation.

10.2.2 Ultrasonic Lithotripters

In 1953, ultrasonic vibration was first reported to break kidney stones [11].

Researchers invented the “Aachen model,” which lays the foundation for the current ultrasonic lithotripsy. The principle remains the same although the technology has been improved a lot.

10.2.2.1 Mechanism

Current is passed through piezoelectric ceramic crystals, generating ultrasonic waves and making it to resonate at 23–25 kHz. When the probe touches the stone, it causes the stone to resonate and to be fragmented. But the damage will be minimal when the probe comes into direct contact with the tissues because of the lack of resonance in the tissues [12].

The ultrasonic probe connects with a suction device, and only when the lithotrite is activated, the suction device will be activated. In order to optimize visualization, removal of small debris, and irrigation, the best pressure should be kept at 60–80 cm H_2O. Ultrasound does not work well for all types of stones. The components of the stone may affect the lithotripsy time taken for the stone to be completely crushed. Some harder stones such as cysteine and calcium oxalate monohydrate stones are very difficult to be crushed. Furthermore, the size, density, and surface characteristics of the stones are also important. The small, low-density stones with a rough surface can be fragmented more rapidly while the large and smooth ones are hard to be broken [13, 14].

10.2.2.2 Advantages and Disadvantages

One of the advantages is its ability to fragment and remove stones at the same time by using the larger caliber ultrasound probes. Furthermore, repeated studies have shown that ultrasonic lithotripsy is effective when treating the stone through the percutaneous approach. The stone-free rate ranges from 84 to 100% [15, 16]. Ultrasound probes are also exceedingly safe. An animal testing has been conducted to confirm the safety of ultrasonic lithotripsy. Researchers placed the probe on the urothelium of the rabbit bladder and found that only a little mucosal edema occurred. Similarly, experiments in the canine model also showed minimal histological changes [17]. However, if the continuous suction of irrigation fails, the probe is likely to damage the tissue due to overheating. Therefore, users should pay attention to the adequacy of suction. Again, the disadvantage of this probe is its limitation in dealing with ureteral stone.

10.2.2.3 Technique Tips

The sound frequencies of these waves are higher than the human auditory threshold, which pass through the probe to make the tip vibrating and then touch the stone and cause the mechanical fragmentation. This requires direct contact with the stone. The lumen of the ultrasonic probe is hollow, which can suck out the stone debris. The piezoelectric ceramic crystal will also be cooled by the evacuated liquid through the handpiece, providing the best operating temperature [10]. The size of these probes ranges from 2.5 to 6.0 F. The smallest one has no hollow lumen, so inhaling debris is not allowed. Ultrasonic lithotrite needs to contact the stone closely in order to work effectively. During the contact, stones are usually needed to be fixed in a place to improve efficiency, although some small fragments can be sucked to the tip of the probe.

If the stones are hard (e.g. calcium oxalate monohydrate stones and calcium phosphate brushes stones), it is better to fragment these hard stones into some small pieces first, make them smaller than the diameter of the sheath, and then use the grasping forceps to remove these pieces. For softer stone like magnesium ammonium phosphate stone, we usually try to remove large parts with ultrasonic equipment and use the suction to remove all the small fragments. It is important to put the probe as close to the stone as possible to maintain the intraoperative negative pressure, and it will also reduce the stone migration.

10.2.3 Combination of Ultrasonic and Pneumatic Lithotripters

For over 30 years, ultrasonic and pneumatic intracorporeal lithotripters have been favored for percutaneous nephrolithotripsy. Ultrasonic lithotripters, although are relatively inefficient at fragmenting hard stones, provide the advantage of concurrent suction, often eliminating the need for manual endoscopic extraction. Conversely, pneumatic lithotripters, which are not typically equipped with suction control, have proven superior at fragmenting stones of many types. However, subsequent retrieval of fragments can be proven to be both tedious and time-consuming. In recent years, one of the developments of intracorporeal lithotripsy in PCNL is the emergence of double-modality lithotripters. It consists of traditional ultrasonic components and ballistic components. The purpose of this dual lithotrite is to integrate the advantages of ultrasonic and ballistic devices and improve the efficiency of lithotripsy and stone-free rate.

10.2.3.1 Advantages and Disadvantages

Large stones with infection can be treated by lithotrite with negative pressure suction system, which has the advantages of two different technologies of ultrasonic lithotripsy and pneumatic ballistic lithotripsy. Large and hard stones are first fragmented by pneumatic lithotripsy and then evacuated by ultrasonic lithotripsy, so that it can reduce the intrarenal pressure and improve the safety of the treatment of stones with infection and the efficiency of the lithotripsy, and the combination lithotripters also perform well with minimally invasive nephroscope.

10.2.3.2 Technique Tips

After the percutaneous channel is established, minimally invasive nephroscope is placed through the channel to enter the renal collecting system for observation. And lithotripsy is performed for stone removal and evacuation. During the whole operation, the visual field must be kept clear. The blood clot that obscured the field of vision should be removed by simple grasping forceps or sucked out with a syringe. For the turbid urine which was caused by infection, repeated suction by negative pressure suction device will make the vision clear. When the renal collection system is examined, the angle of nephroscope should be rotated and swung to observe the kidneys in all directions. When we use the double-modality lithotrite with standard nephroscope, it could relieve the high pressure of the renal pelvis, which is beneficial to avoid the absorption of toxins and pyrogen in the process of lithotripsy, thereby reducing the incidence of sepsis, fluid extravasation, and complications of perirenal infection.

10.3 Flexible Lithotripters

10.3.1 Electrohydraulic Lithotripter

Electrohydraulic lithotripter (EHL) is the first extracorporeal lithotripter which was introduced in 1975 for the treatment of kidney stones. It was invented by an engineer named Yutkin in 1955 [12].

10.3.1.1 Mechanism

The electric current creates a spark through an insulating area between two electrodes. Sparks can produce water vapor around the electrode, forming cavitation bubbles that produce shock waves during the expansion process. This shock wave has no focus, so the stones are needed to be put precisely at the location of the shock wave [12].

EHL is relatively flexible compared with ultrasound and pneumatic lithotripsy. It can be used with flexible or rigid cystoscope, ureteroscope, or nephroscope for lithotripsy throughout the urinary system.

10.3.1.2 Advantages and Disadvantages

In terms of effective stone fragmentation, EHL is usually used to fragment ureteral stones [18]. In addition, the EHL lithotripter is very cheap. The generator is about 1200 dollars, with 200 dollars per disposable probe [19]. In one case, one or two probes may be used. If stones are harder such as calcium oxalate monohydrate, more probes may be used. The biggest drawback of EHL may be its damage to the urothelium because of the impact of rapidly expanding cavitation bubble on the tissue. So, EHL is not recommended in the narrow space of the ureter. However, since the application of holmium laser in PCNL, EHL has become less popular due to its less versatility than holmium laser. Holmium laser has the ability of breaking all types of stones, while EHL laser can hardly break hard stones [20].

10.3.1.3 Technique Tips

The use of electrohydraulic lithotripsy should follow certain principles. The users should check the tip of the probe before inserting it into the endoscope. The tip of the probe should be smooth and the internal and external insulating layer should be intact. During ureteroscopic examination, 1.6–1.9 F of smaller probe is used. Ideally, the probe should be kept away from the distal end of the endoscope at a distance of 2–5 mm. In this way, the scope was protected. The target stone should be clearly visible before the EHL is put into use. Furthermore, the probe of EHL should be kept 1 mm away from the surface of the stone with suitable energy setting. When the stone fragments are small enough, they can be retrieved with a grasper. It is not recommended to crush debris at a size of less than 2 mm, because this may cause potential damage to the surrounding urinary tract tissues [21].

10.3.2 Laser Lithotripters

The energy of the laser is generated by a stimulated atom, which then produces electrons in turn. The electrons can release energy in the shape of a discontinuous light energy. These properties of lasers enable it to transmit a quantity of energy in a very focused way. Laser has become the most popular way in intracorporeal lithotripsy [18]. Mulvany reported the application of Ruby laser in the management of urinary stone in 1968 [22]. But it was also reported that Ruby laser can generate excessive heat when fragmenting the stone. So, it was hard for clinical use. Since then, many other lasers such as coumarin green pulse dyes, alexandrite, and neodymium lasers are introduced. Different kinds of lasers are named according to the substances that excite to produce focused light energy. Coumarin laser is a liquid laser medium with green coumarin dye, which is the first pulsed dye laser used in clinic [23]. The alexandrite laser is made of alexandrite minerals. The medium of the neodymium:yttrium aluminum garnet (Nd:YAG) laser is a crystal seeded with neodymium ions. The FREDDY (frequency-doubled double-pulse Nd:YAG laser) technology is a more efficient, lower-priced laser used for lithotripsy. It consists of two different wavelengths of lasers, one is infrared light of 1064 nm and the other is green light of 532 nm. The mechanism of action is that the laser energy hits the stone through the optical fiber, indicating that the green light is partially absorbed by the stone surface, and plasma is formed. After the plasma reabsorbs the invisible infrared light, the shock wave was generated, and in that way the stone could be fragmented [24, 25]. This is a kind of mechanical energy which provides a lower incidence of soft tissue damage than the holmium laser, because the tissue can easily absorb these waves. It is effective for almost all types of stones, except for harder stones [26, 27]. In vitro studies show that the stone fragmentation rate of FREDDY laser is significantly higher than that of holmium laser. One drawback of Freddy lithotripsy is that it is possible for stone retropulsion. An in vitro study shows that Freddy laser produced greater stone retropulsion than holmium laser [28]. With the development of science and technology, holmium:yttrium aluminum garnet (YAG) has become the most commonly used laser gradually.

10.3.2.1 Holmium: YAG Laser

Holmium laser lithotripsy was first reported in 1995 [29], it has become the gold standard for lithotripsy in the current guidelines [30]. The laser wavelength is 2140 nm and the pulse duration is about 250~350 μs. It is much longer than the pulsed dye laser. Compared with other lithotripters, holmium laser is considered to be the most effective lithotrite. In recent years, holmium laser has become the main research field with the aim of improving the ablation of stones, while reducing the incidence of complications.

10.3.2.2 Mechanism

The holmium laser-generated pulse that causes the stone to break is mainly based on these mechanisms. First, the photoacoustic effect is generated by forming cavitation bubbles at the end of the fiber, which generates a shock wave when collapsed, causing the stone to break [31, 32]. Second, holmium laser causes stone vaporization and dissociation through a photothermal mechanism. Holmium laser is mainly absorbed by water, and it produces little damage to the tissue. Since the tissue is mainly composed of water, most energy is absorbed on the tissue surface, and the thermal damage area associated with laser ablation is about 0.5~1.0 mm [33].

10.3.2.3 Advantages and Disadvantages

The advantages of holmium laser include effective fragmentation for all types of stones with different composition, and wide utilization in all endoscopic instruments. It causes only minimal damage to the mucosa because the laser has high absorption in water [34]. Holmium laser can crush stones in both anterograde and retrograde ways. Furthermore, holmium laser can fragment stone into very small pieces that can be easily removed from the collection system, thereby reducing the need for manual removal [35]. Holmium laser not only has high lithotripsy efficacy but also has the ability of cutting and coagulating soft tissue. It is commonly used for endourologic procedures. The laser fiber can be used in flexible nephroscope. So, it can also be used to treat other upper urinary tract diseases such as ureteropelvic junction stricture and upper tract tumor. In addition, holmium laser is also desirable for struvite stones because of its heat radiation. The disadvantages include its potential thermal injury to the mucosa when it directly touches the tissue and the relatively high cost. Furthermore, the larger fibers such as 365 μm and 500 μm fibers show retropulsion that cannot be ignored [36].

10.3.2.4 Technique Tips

Holmium laser is simple to use. Surgeons only need to put the fiber connecting to the stone surface before the laser is engaged. Maintaining a clear field of vision is necessary to avoid perforation. Because holmium laser can cut metal, care must be taken when approaching the guide wire or basket [37, 38]. In addition, the laser fiber should extend out of the tip of the endoscope at least 2 mm, in order to reduce damage to the lens or the channels. It can also damage the urothelium, so trying to avoid drilling past the stone with the laser fiber is important. Our experience showed that although holmium laser does not have the function of ultrasonic adsorption of stone fragments, the working sheath can make up for this defect. During the operation, the working sheath is simply placed over the crushed stone, or place the dilated sheath against the calyces, and the stone fragments can be quickly washed out of the body by hanging bag irrigation. Furthermore, the use of retrograde water irrigation will accelerate the evacuation of stone fragments from the sheath.

After percutaneous nephrolithotomy, calculus remains mainly because nephroscopy cannot enter the renal calices where residual stone is located. For small calculi that are visible but not accessible by nephroscopy, holmium laser can be used to split the mucosa of the calix and then the stones will be touched. For some residual stones, which could not be found with the nephroscope but could be located by ultrasonography or fluoroscopy, the flexible instruments are needed.

The total power output equal to the pulse energy multiply by the pulse frequency. Urologist can set different power to fragment the stone by adjusting these parameters. Low pulse energy is recommended at the beginning of treatment. The first holmium laser was low-powered laser (<20 W) because of the limitation of setting the pulse energy and pulse frequency [39]. Stones can be dusted into very small fragments by setting low pulse energy and high pulse frequency [39]. In 2007, Jou and his colleagues reported their experience of using high pulse energy (3.0 J) in PCNL for large renal stones. They concluded that the holmium laser can fragment all types of stones with different composition and dust stone with minimal retropulsion [36].

Sun and his colleagues assessed the efficiency and safety of the 70 W holmium laser (3.5 J × 20 Hz) in PCNL for kidney stones. They concluded that such high-power laser improved the efficiency of lithotripsy by fragmenting stones rapidly, which changed the traditional international concept of laser lithotripsy, improved the lithotripsy efficiency, and became the main method in treating large and complicated stones [40].

10.4 Recent Innovations

10.4.1 Moses Effect

Recently, Lumenis has developed a new technology for the Lumenis Pulse TM 120H laser system, where the laser pulse can separate with the water and then deliver the energy to the surface of target stone. This is called the "Moses effect." In this mode, a large quantity of energy produces a steam bubble, and it can separate the water, and then the remaining energy is transmitted to the stone through a steam bubble. Elhilali and his colleagues evaluated the Moses effect through both in vitro and in vivo experiments [41]. In vitro model showed less stone retropulsion in the Moses mode. Compared with the regular mode, Moses mode achieved a significantly higher ablation volume (1.6 fold, $P < 0.001$). In vivo experiment also proved the reduction of stone retropulsion in the porcine kidney. They demonstrated that the Moses technology could be more efficient, with reduced stone retropulsion and much safer lithotripsy. Ibrahim and his colleagues highlighted these findings through a stone simulator. They compared the crushing efficiency of traditional holmium lasers and Moses models. Using Moses model, the time for fragmentation and dust removal in Moses model is significantly shorter than the holmium laser. The stone retropulsion is also significantly reduced [42]. Mullerad and his colleagues reported the initial clinical experiences using the new technology. They asked the urologists to fill a questionnaire immediately after each ureteroscopic examination. They compared the procedures. Surgeons give their opinions of Moses technology ($n = 23$)

compared to conventional lithotripsy (n = 11). The working time and energy usage of laser are collected from Lumenis 120H. In all, Moses laser technology shows satisfying stone fragmentation with less time in clinical applications [32].

In terms of cost analysis, Stern and his colleagues showed a special report. They concluded that for all sizes of stones, the Moses system has an increased price of 292.36 dollars compared to the standard Holmium system. In particular, for stones >10 mm, the price of Moses technology increased by 253.16 dollars. Although the operating time with Moses system is shorter, it does not show any advantage in terms of cost due to the high cost of laser fiber and the software [43].

10.4.2 Thulium Fiber Laser

Despite these beneficial effects of holmium laser, a promising competitor is a new superpulse thulium fiber laser (TFL). This TFL technology has been remained for about 20 years [44]. Since 2005, a detailed feasibility study has been carried out for TFL lithotripsy [45]. However, all these studies were performed with previous TFLs. The superpulse TFL is very different from the previous TFLs. It has a high power of 500 W while the previous TFLs have only 100 W [46]. The main emission line of TFL (1940 nm) is approximately equal to the strong water absorption peak [47]. A few years ago, TFL effectiveness had been shown in stone lithotripsy and prostate surgery. However, it has recently attracted interest since the introduction of a superpulse model for TFL. In in vitro experiments, TFL has been shown to fragment higher stone volumes, and the retropulsion is less [48]. In addition, studies have shown that the use of thinner laser fibers can significantly produce more stone dust without generating significant heat. Initial experience of application of TFL for urolithiasis has been reported [49]. Martov AG and his colleagues proved that the Thulium Laser System "Urolaz" has significantly improved the effectiveness of upper urinary tract endoscopic intervention and significantly reduced the possibility of intraoperative trauma and postoperative complications. Still, more and more researches are needed to assess the efficiency and safety of this newly developed technology.

10.5 Conclusion

Both rigid and flexible lithotripters are effective to carry out percutaneous lithotripsy. When choosing a lithotripter to deal with urinary stones, the doctor should consider the patient's kidney anatomy, the location of the stones, and the planned procedure of surgery. The current lithotripters offer a number of options for urologists, and it is necessary for surgeons to understand the advantages and disadvantages of each type and to gain a deep understanding of its mechanisms when choosing these lithotripters. Holmium laser is considered to be the most widely used endoscopic lithotripter. Its flexibility and small diameter fibers allow it to manage stones in the ureter and renal collecting system. It also remains the preferred flexible lithotrite for its advantages of fragmenting all types of stones and its safety. Among patients undergoing PCNL, rigid lithotripters (i.e. ultrasonic lithotripsy, pneumatic lithotripsy) are safely and effectively especially in removing large stones. It should be noted that in single cases, the ideal stone-free rate can be achieved by combining a variety of different lithotripsy instruments. The generation of dual-mode ultrasound and pneumatic lithotripters provide surgeons with powerful and efficient tools for stone fragmentation and removing stones quickly. In general, the combined devices and other new technologies are promising and worth expecting, but further researches are needed to ensure whether they improve the efficiency of stone removal and evacuation.

References

1. Fernstrom I, Johansson B. Percutaneous pyelolithotomy. A new extraction technique. Scand J Urol Nephrol. 1976;10(3):257–9.
2. Williams SK, Leveillee RJ. A single percutaneous access and flexible nephroscopy is the best treatment for a full staghorn calculus. J Endourol. 2008;22(9):1835–7; discussion 9. https://doi.org/10.1089/end.2008.9795.

3. Murthy PV, Rao HS, Meherwade S, Rao PV, Srivastava A, Sasidharan K. Ureteroscopic lithotripsy using mini-endoscope and Swiss lithoclast: experience in 147 cases. J Endourol. 1997;11(5):327–30. https://doi.org/10.1089/end.1997.11.327.
4. Knispel HH, Klan R, Heicappell R, Miller K. Pneumatic lithotripsy applied through deflected working channel of miniureteroscope: results in 143 patients. J Endourol. 1998;12(6):513–5. https://doi.org/10.1089/end.1998.12.513.
5. Aghamir SK, Mohseni MG, Ardestani A. Treatment of ureteral calculi with ballistic lithotripsy. J Endourol. 2003;17(10):887–90. https://doi.org/10.1089/089277903772036208.
6. Akhtar MS, Akhtar FK. Utility of the lithoclast in the treatment of upper, middle and lower ureteric calculi. Surgeon. 2003;1(3):144–8.
7. Delvecchio FC, Kuo RL, Preminger GM. Clinical efficacy of combined lithoclast and lithovac stone removal during ureteroscopy. J Urol. 2000;164(1):40–2.
8. Hong YK, Park DS. Ureteroscopic lithotripsy using Swiss lithoclast for treatment of ureteral calculi: 12-years experience. J Korean Med Sci. 2009;24(4):690–4. https://doi.org/10.3346/jkms.2009.24.4.690.
9. Denstedt JD, Razvi H. Management of urinary calculi during pregnancy. J Urol. 1992;148(3 Pt 2):1072–4; discussion 4–5.
10. Lowe G, Knudsen BE. Ultrasonic, pneumatic and combination intracorporeal lithotripsy for percutaneous nephrolithotomy. J Endourol. 2009;23(10):1663–8. https://doi.org/10.1089/end.2009.1533.
11. Mulvaney WP. Attempted disintegration of calculi by ultrasonic vibrations. J Urol. 1953;70(5):704–7.
12. Grocela JA, Dretler SP. Intracorporeal lithotripsy. Instrumentation and development. Urol Clin North Am. 1997;24(1):13–23.
13. LeRoy AJ, Segura JW. Percutaneous ultrasonic lithotripsy. Urol Radiol. 1984;6(2):88–94.
14. Marberger M. Disintegration of renal and ureteral calculi with ultrasound. Urol Clin North Am. 1983;10(4):729–42.
15. Segura JW, Patterson DE, LeRoy AJ, Williams HJ Jr, Barrett DM, Benson RC Jr, et al. Percutaneous removal of kidney stones: review of 1,000 cases. J Urol. 1985;134(6):1077–81.
16. Segura JW, Patterson DE, LeRoy AJ, May GR, Smith LH. Percutaneous lithotripsy. J Urol. 1983;130(6):1051–4.
17. Terhorst B. [The effect of electrohydraulic waves and ultrasound on the urothelium]. Urologe A. 1975;14(1):41–5.
18. Matlaga BR, American Board of Urology. Contemporary surgical management of upper urinary tract calculi. J Urol. 2009;181(5):2152–6. https://doi.org/10.1016/j.juro.2009.01.023.
19. Zheng W, Denstedt JD. Intracorporeal lithotripsy. Update on technology. Urol Clin North Am. 2000;27(2):301–13.
20. Wu TT, Hsu TH, Chen MT, Chang LS. Efficacy of in vitro stone fragmentation by extracorporeal, electrohydraulic, and pulsed-dye laser lithotripsy. J Endourol. 1993;7(5):391–3. https://doi.org/10.1089/end.1993.7.391.
21. Denstedt JD, Clayman RV. Electrohydraulic lithotripsy of renal and ureteral calculi. J Urol. 1990;143(1):13–7.
22. Mulvaney WP, Beck CW. The laser beam in urology. J Urol. 1968;99(1):112–5.
23. Watson G, Murray S, Dretler SP, Parrish JA. The pulsed dye laser for fragmenting urinary calculi. J Urol. 1987;138(1):195–8.
24. Zorcher T, Hochberger J, Schrott KM, Kuhn R, Schafhauser W. In vitro study concerning the efficiency of the frequency-doubled double-pulse neodymium:YAG laser (FREDDY) for lithotripsy of calculi in the urinary tract. Lasers Surg Med. 1999;25(1):38–42.
25. Delvecchio FC, Auge BK, Brizuela RM, Weizer AZ, Zhong P, Preminger GM. In vitro analysis of stone fragmentation ability of the FREDDY laser. J Endourol. 2003;17(3):177–9. https://doi.org/10.1089/089277903321618752.
26. Dubosq F, Pasqui F, Girard F, Beley S, Lesaux N, Gattegno B, et al. Endoscopic lithotripsy and the FREDDY laser: initial experience. J Endourol. 2006;20(5):296–9. https://doi.org/10.1089/end.2006.20.296.
27. Yates J, Zabbo A, Pareek G. A comparison of the FREDDY and holmium lasers during ureteroscopic lithotripsy. Lasers Surg Med. 2007;39(8):637–40. https://doi.org/10.1002/lsm.20545.
28. Marguet CG, Sung JC, Springhart WP, L'Esperance JO, Zhou S, Zhong P, et al. In vitro comparison of stone retropulsion and fragmentation of the frequency doubled, double pulse nd:yag laser and the holmium:yag laser. J Urol. 2005;173(5):1797–800. https://doi.org/10.1097/01.ju.0000154341.08206.69.
29. Denstedt JD, Razvi HA, Sales JL, Eberwein PM. Preliminary experience with holmium:YAG laser lithotripsy. J Endourol. 1995;9(3):255–8. https://doi.org/10.1089/end.1995.9.255.
30. Turk C, Petrik A, Sarica K, Seitz C, Skolarikos A, Straub M, et al. EAU guidelines on interventional treatment for urolithiasis. Eur Urol. 2016;69(3):475–82. https://doi.org/10.1016/j.eururo.2015.07.041.
31. Zhong P, Tong HL, Cocks FH, Pearle MS, Preminger GM. Transient cavitation and acoustic emission produced by different laser lithotripters. J Endourol. 1998;12(4):371–8. https://doi.org/10.1089/end.1998.12.371.
32. Mullerad M, Aguinaga JRA, Aro T, Kastin A, Goldin O, Kravtsov A, et al. Initial clinical experience with a modulated holmium laser pulse-Moses Technology: does it enhance laser lithotripsy efficacy? Rambam Maimonides Med J. 2017;8(4):e0038. https://doi.org/10.5041/RMMJ.10315.
33. Wollin TA, Denstedt JD. The holmium laser in urology. J Clin Laser Med Surg. 1998;16(1):13–20. https://doi.org/10.1089/clm.1998.16.13.

34. Vassar GJ, Chan KF, Teichman JM, Glickman RD, Weintraub ST, Pfefer TJ, et al. Holmium:YAG lithotripsy: photothermal mechanism. J Endourol. 1999;13(3):181–90. https://doi.org/10.1089/end.1999.13.181.
35. Teichman JM, Vassar GJ, Glickman RD. Holmium:yttrium-aluminum-garnet lithotripsy efficiency varies with stone composition. Urology. 1998;52(3):392–7.
36. Jou YC, Shen CH, Cheng MC, Lin CT, Chen PC. High-power holmium:yttrium-aluminum-garnet laser for percutaneous treatment of large renal stones. Urology. 2007;69(1):22–5;. ; discussion 5–6. https://doi.org/10.1016/j.urology.2006.08.1114.
37. Lane BR, Singh D, Meraney A, Streem SB. Novel endourologic applications for holmium laser. Urology. 2005;65(5):991–3. https://doi.org/10.1016/j.urology.2005.01.050.
38. Freiha GS, Glickman RD, Teichman JM. Holmium:YAG laser-induced damage to guidewires: experimental study. J Endourol. 1997;11(5):331–6. https://doi.org/10.1089/end.1997.11.331.
39. Razvi HA, Denstedt JD, Chun SS, Sales JL. Intracorporeal lithotripsy with the holmium:YAG laser. J Urol. 1996;156(3):912–4.
40. Sun Y, Gao X, Zhou T, Chen S, Wang L, Xu C, et al. 70 W holmium:yttrium-aluminum-garnet laser in percutaneous nephrolithotomy for staghorn calculi. J Endourol. 2009;23(10):1687–91. https://doi.org/10.1089/end.2009.1536.
41. Elhilali MM, Badaan S, Ibrahim A, Andonian S. Use of the Moses technology to improve holmium laser lithotripsy outcomes: a preclinical study. J Endourol. 2017;31(6):598–604. https://doi.org/10.1089/end.2017.0050.
42. Ibrahim A, Badaan S, Elhilali MM, Andonian S. Moses technology in a stone simulator. Can Urol Assoc J. 2018;12(4):127–30. https://doi.org/10.5489/cuaj.4797.
43. Stern KL, Monga M. The Moses holmium system—time is money. Can J Urol. 2018;25(3):9313–6.
44. Jackson SD, Lauto A. Diode-pumped fiber lasers: a new clinical tool? Lasers Surg Med. 2002;30(3):184–90.
45. Fried NM, Irby PB. Advances in laser technology and fibre-optic delivery systems in lithotripsy. Nat Rev Urol. 2018;15(9):563–73. https://doi.org/10.1038/s41585-018-0035-8.
46. Blackmon RL, Irby PB, Fried NM. Comparison of holmium:YAG and thulium fiber laser lithotripsy: ablation thresholds, ablation rates, and retropulsion effects. J Biomed Opt. 2011;16(7):071403. https://doi.org/10.1117/1.3564884.
47. Hale GM, Querry MR. Optical constants of water in the 200-nm to 200-microm wavelength region. Appl Opt. 1973;12(3):555–63. https://doi.org/10.1364/AO.12.000555.
48. Andreeva V, Vinarov A, Yaroslavsky I, Kovalenko A, Vybornov A, Rapoport L et al. Preclinical comparison of superpulse thulium fiber laser and a holmium:YAG laser for lithotripsy. World J Urol. 2019. https://doi.org/10.1007/s00345-019-02785-9.
49. Martov AG, Ergakov DV, Guseinov MA, Andronov AS, Dutov SV, Vinnichenko VA et al. [Initial experience in clinical application of thulium laser contact lithotripsy for transurethral treatment of urolithiasis]. Urologiia. 2018;(1):112–20.

11 Tubeless PCNL

Julian Veser and Christian Seitz

11.1 Introduction

First attempts to puncture a symptomatic kidney with subsequent stone removal in a patient with nephrolithiasis were performed by Rupel and Brown in 1941. They treated a patient with solitary kidney and anuria due to an obstructive kidney stone by first inserting a 26 French catheter into the dilated kidney and after recovering they removed the stone through the initial puncture site. A 18 French catheter was left in the kidney, which was removed on the second postoperative day without any complications [1]. It then took till 1976 until the first formal percutaneous nephrolithotomy was reported by Fernstrom and Johansson, which started by subsequently dilating the access tract with Couvelair catheters up to 24 French and then waited 14 days until surgery. After successful stone removal, they placed a 16 French catheter which was removed once antegrade pyelography showed free passage down the ureter on the third postoperative day [2]. Since then PCNL has become a standard treatment modality especially for larger, more complex kidney stones. To minimize morbidity and pain, as well as shortening the hospitalization time, the technique has been modified extensively. The instruments were miniaturized to reduce damage to the tissue, the armamentarium for stone removal was revised and different exit-strategies were evaluated.

The first reported series of tubeless PCNL was published by Wickham et al. [3] in 1984 for a selected group of patients. This concept was challenged by Winfried et al. [4] 2 years later who reported prolonged hospital stay due to postoperative hemorrhage and marked urinary extravasation into the retroperitoneum or pleura in a case study of two patients following tubeless PCNL. Afterwards, placement of a nephrostomy tube for at least 24–48 h post-PCNL became a standard therapy until 1997 when Bellman et al. [5] reintroduced a modified tubeless PCNL technique including ureteral stenting. The internal drainage was placed to prevent renal obstruction due to blood clots or residual fragments, and therefore limit postoperative pain and facilitate healing of the dilatation tract. In a matched pair analysis they concluded a reduced hospital stay, lower analgesia requirements, lower overall cost and a quicker return to normal activity for the patient cohort without nephrostomy tube. While having strict inclusion criteria for the tubeless procedure, this study initiated further analysis to identify the optimal exit strategy for various PCNL techniques and different instruments. To unify the nomenclature we will further group the different techniques into "standard PCNL" with

J. Veser · C. Seitz (✉)
Department of Urology, Comprehensive Cancer Center, Medical University of Vienna, Vienna General Hospital, Vienna, Austria
e-mail: Julian.veser@meduniwien.ac.at; Christian.seitz@meduniwien.ac.at

G. Zeng, K. Sarica (eds.), *Percutaneous Nephrolithotomy*,
https://doi.org/10.1007/978-981-15-0575-1_11

nephrostomy tube, "tubeless PCNL" with ureteral stent but without nephrostomy tube and "totally tubeless PCNL" with neither ureteral stent nor nephrostomy tube.

11.2 Types of Nephrostomy Tubes

Since the first renal drainage via needles or rubber catheters, a multitude of different nephrostomy tubes were developed. Each of these tubes has unique characteristics and can serve specific purposes (see Table 11.1). To know the strength and weakness of each tube can help identifying the ideal drainage with the highest tolerability for the patient while still preventing obstruction or dislodging. The tube sizes range from 5 to 32 F, and larger tubes usually provide a better drainage in case of blood clots and residual fragments. Unfortunately nephrostomies and ureteral stents cause discomfort for the patient [6]. There are different mechanisms to prevent retention or obstruction of the drainage with some of them including a ureteral component.

11.2.1 Pigtail Catheter

Pigtail catheters are usually used for simple drainage of a dilated urinary tract and vary from 5–14 F in size. They come with or without a locking mechanism, and the circle-shaped distal tip anchors in the renal pelvis. To prevent accidental dislodgment the tube has to be fixated at the skin level with a suture or can additionally be locked with a nylon string attached to the distal tip entering the tube through the last side hole. By pulling the string the tip gets deflected into a pigtail configuration and is fixated until the nylon string is released again. The small diameter of the pigtail catheters leads to improved tolerability compared to larger tubes, enabling its use in pediatric patients or long-term access. On the other hand, the relatively small 15-G side holes are vulnerable for occlusion by blood clot or stone debris. In case of a significant larger access tract, the small diameter of the tube may not be sufficient to tamponade the tract in a case of significant bleeding. If the renal pelvis is very narrow, the pigtail catheters may be difficult to deploy because the pigtail tip requires a cavity to unfold properly, especially with the nylon string locking mechanism.

A pigtail tube is recommended after uncomplicated percutaneous renal surgery as temporary urinary drainage of an obstructed system or after pediatric surgery [7].

Table 11.1 Overview of ideal nephrostomy tubes according to the specific indication

Indication	Ideal nephrostomy tube
Drainage of obstructed system	Pigtail
Uncomplicated PCNL	Balloon, Malecot, tubeless
Problematic PCNL	Council, Kaye tamponade
Mucosal damage to UPJ or ureter	Re-entry, Endopyelotomy
Multiple tract PCNL	Circle/loop catheter

11.2.2 Balloon Retention Catheter

Balloon retention catheters have a wide range of sizes from 8 to 32 F, depending on the manufacturer and type of catheter tip. Commonly used examples are Council, Couvelaire and Foley catheters, which differ by the configuration of their catheter tip. While they are usually placed over a guide wire, the Council tip catheter is the preferred choice due to the catheters distal opening and easy advancement over the wire. In case of severe bleeding the Couvelaire tip is best suited to evacuate larger blood clots over its large side opening. To place a Foley catheter over a guide wire into the kidney, the tip has to be modified by a large-size needle first, in order to create an opening at the catheter tip. Once in place, the balloon catheter is the most effective retaining mechanism compared to the other nephrostomy types without ureteral extension. A disadvantage of this nephrostomy type is a possible obstruction of the renal calyxes caused by the balloon itself, leading to possible patient discomfort.

11.2.3 Malecot Drain

Malecot drains range in sizes (10–40 F) and modifications. They represent an alternative to balloon retention catheters with good drainage but without the risk of obstructing the renal calyxes due to their open mushroom-style tip. There are two or four wings at the distal end of the catheter which expand when placed. For removal, those wings are straightened with an inserted trocar. Compared to the previous alternatives, the Malecot retention mechanism is less secure, and the drain usually has to be fixed with a skin suture or adhesive device. There is still a risk of dislocation due to pannus movement especially in obese patients. A modification to prevent dislocation of the catheter and simultaneously drain the ureter is the reentry nephrostomy catheter. It consists of the usual Malecot nephrostomy (8–24 F) with an attached ureteral component (5–8 F, 18 cm in length). This supports excellent drainage of stone fragments or blood clot and simultaneously allows uncomplicated reinsertion in case of significant bleeding during nephrostomy tube removal. The Malecot reentry tube is ideal for complex procedures with multiple punctures, moderate bleeding and large stone burden. The ureteral extension additionally secures the drainage to the bladder, especially for antegrade stone removal and/or edema at the pyeloureteral junction (UPJ).

11.2.4 Others

For special procedures or bleeding complications, there is a variety of different nephrostomy tubes to help manage the postoperative drainage or tamponade.For multiple-access tract PCNL, *circle* or *loop nephrostomy* tubes have proven to be practical alternatives. They are inserted through one percutaneous tract and exit via another. Even in small, non-dilated collecting systems, those circle tubes offer an effective drainage and are resilient against dislocation. Additionally the material and the multiple side holes make this type of catheter more resistant to incrustation. It can be used as a long-term drainage and the design makes it easy to change the tube over a guidewire.

In case of severe bleeding of the percutaneous access tract, a *Kaye tamponade catheter* can be inserted into the access tract and functions as tamponade while simultaneously draining the renal pelvis. It consists of a 15-cm long, 36 F balloon and can also be anchored by a Malecot tip to secure its distal position in the kidney (*hemostatic Malecot tamponade catheter*).

In cases of antegrade endopyelotomy or PCNL with significant trauma of the ureteropelvic junction (UPJ) and edema, an *endopyelotomy stent* with or without external component can provide wide-diameter stenting of the UPJ. They simultaneously offer maximal drainage externally and internally, are resilient to dislocation and can easily be removed. The discomfort, especially for the stents with external component on the other hand, has been shown to be higher with possible irritation of the exit site [7].

11.3 Impact of Tube Size

Besides different types of nephrostomy tubes, there usually is a wide range of sizes to choose from. To assess the safety and patients' satisfaction there have been several studies analyzing the impact of nephrostomy tube sizes.

Cormio et al. [8] presented their results of the prospective global PCNL study from the Clinical Research Office Endourology Society (CROES), comparing procedure and outcome data according to nephrostomy tube size. There were 3968 patients included, analyzed over an 1-year period and divided into two groups, namely small-bore (SB; nephrostomy size ≤18 Fr) and large-bore (LB; nephrostomy size >18 Fr) nephrostomy. The authors concluded superiority for LB nephrostomy tubes in terms of reduced blood loss and lower overall complication rate but did not include postoperative pain or time of urinary leakage after tube removal. Simultaneously they did not match their patient populations resulting in heterogeneous patient characteristics like significantly higher use of anticoagulants and unfavorable ASA classifications in the SB nephrostomy group.

In contrast to their findings, several studies did show no effect of tube size on the risk of postoperative bleeding as well as reduced postoperative pain for small-bore nephrostomies following PCNL. Maheshwari et al. [6] compared 40 patients with either 28F nephrostomy tube or a 9F pigtail catheter placed after the procedure. They did find no statistical difference in postoperative bleeding complication but shorter hospitalization time and less urinary leakage with the smaller pigtail catheter. Similarly Pietrow et al. [9] evaluated the effect of a smaller percutaneous drainage catheter on postoperative pain and, therefore, randomized 30 consecutive patients to either a 10F pigtail catheter or a 22F Council-tip catheter for their percutaneous drainage. Their results showed lower pain scores in the immediate postoperative period with no significant change in postoperative hematocrit in the patient cohort with smaller nephrostomy tube. Beyond 6 h, the pain scores did not differ significantly. In a prospective trial by Marcovich et al. [10] no significant differences between a 24F re-entry tube, 8F pigtail catheter or a double-J stent ($N = 20$ for all groups) were found in hematocrit change, length of hospital stay or complication rates. The postoperative analog pain scores and narcotic usage were equivalent for all three groups; only the postoperative leakage showed a trend in favor of the 8F pigtail group vs. the 24F re-entry tube ($p = 0.05$). Lastly, Desai et al. [11] assessed 30 patients equally grouped into large bore (20 Fr), small bore (9 Fr) or no nephrostomy drainage following uncomplicated PCNL. As the previous studies, they did not differ in hematocrit decrease in any group, but the length of urinary leakage was significantly shorter with no nephrostomy tube (4.8 h) compared to the small bore group (13.2 h) and the large bore group (21.4 h). Additionally, postoperative pain as well as narcotic use was higher with increased tube size.

In summary, there is conflicting evidence in the postoperative hematocrit change for different nephrostomy tube sizes. But while the complication rate is rather low in both groups and there is a trend towards less morbidity and postoperative pain for smaller tubes, the use of nephrostomy sizes of 18F and smaller may be a valid alternative to large-bore drainages post-PCNL.

11.4 Tubeless PCNL

Until now, PCNL with postoperative external drainage of any kind is still the standard therapy for stone clearance of large renal stones >20 mm [12]. But as the size of the available armamentarium decreases, there are additional indications for smaller stones and a demand for less invasive procedures [13, 14]. Therefore, several randomized controlled trials and meta-analyses assessing the safety and efficacy of a tubeless PCNL technique have been published (Table 11.2). The most recent meta-analysis by Xun et al. [15] was published 2017, including 14 RCTs and involving 1148 patients. Combined results demonstrated that tubeless PCNL was significantly associated with shorter hospital stay, faster time to return to normal activity, lower postoperative pain scores, less postoperative analgesia requirements, and reduced urinary leakage. Simultaneously they reported no significant differences in postoperative hemoglobin reduction, stone-free rate, rate of postoperative fever or blood transfusion rate. As nomenclature of tubeless PCNL remains non-standardized, the tubeless population included internal or external ureteral catheters as well as totally tubeless procedures. By removing those five RCTs including totally tubeless procedures, sensitivity analysis showed similar results regarding safety and efficacy of the procedure. Another possible bias was the wide range of nephrostomy tubes sizes (8–26 F).

A prior meta-analysis by Ni et al. [16] made separate comparisons for standard and small-bore PCNL vs. tubeless PCNL. They concluded that a tubeless procedure is associated with less analgesia and a shorter hospital stay compared to any nephrostomy tube group and the return to normal activity was also diminished in comparison to the standard PCNL group. However, no significant difference was observed in the analyses concerning stone-free rate, blood transfusion

Table 11.2 Basic characteristics of included studies

	Study design	Sample size	Group design	Tube sizes	Conclusion
Tubeless					
Xun et al., 2017 [15]	Meta-analysis	1148	TL ± DJ/EUC vs. NT	8–26 F	TL has same complication rate with less side effects
Ni et al., 2011 [16]	Meta-analysis	643	TL ± DJ/EUC vs. NT	Small-bore: 8–9 F Standard: 10–26 F	TL has same complication rate with less side effects
Jiang et al., 2017 [17]	RCT	90	DJ vs. EUC vs. NT	18 F	All groups equally safe and efficacious, EUC and NT show better post-OP HRQoL scores
Chen et al., 2018 [18]	Meta-analysis	863	DJ vs. EUC	–	Less stent-related symptoms in EUC group
Gonen et al., 2009 [19]	RCT	46	DJ vs. EUC	–	Less stent-related symptoms in EUC group
Zhou et al., 2017 [20]	RCT	109	DJ vs. EUC	–	Less stent-related symptoms, less severe VUR in EUC group
Totally tubeless					
Li et al., 2019 [21]	Meta-analysis	1131	TT vs. NT	14–26 F	TT superior in operating time, hospital stay and postoperative analgesic requirement
Lee et al., 2017 [22]	Network meta-analysis	NA	TT vs. NT ± DJ/EUC	NA	TT superior in hemoglobin change, length of hospital stay, pain scores and operating time

TL tubeless, *DJ* double-J stent, *EUC* external ureteral catheter, *NT* nephrostomy tube, *TT* totally tubeless, *HRQoL* health-related quality of life score, *NA* not available, *VUR* vesicoureteral reflux

and the complication rate for any group. But again, in the first comparison of tubeless vs. standard PCNL there were several studies including totally tubeless procedures due to the lack of uniform nomenclature. With subgroup analysis excluding totally tubeless procedures, only operating time showed no longer a significant difference whereas the other results were consistent.

However, only a few of these studies did include stent-related symptoms. While the nephrostomy tube is usually removed during hospitalization, the ureteral stents were left in place up to 6 weeks. It is possible that the initially reported benefit in patients' quality of life in the tubeless but stented patient cohort is reversed with the outpatient disadvantage of stent-related discomfort. Therefore several RCTs [17, 19, 20] and one meta-analysis [18] evaluated the outcome of tubeless PCNL using two different stenting techniques: externalized ureteral catheter compared with DJ placement. The only reported difference was significantly reduced stent-related symptoms with an externalized ureteral catheter, showing that this technique is at least as feasible as double-J stenting. An alternative could be a tethered DJ stent, which avoids a second procedure for stent removal although associated with an increased risk of stent dislocation [23, 24].

Most of the studies have some kind of selection bias, excluding complicated procedures with a high risk of intra- or postoperative bleeding. The final decision on whether, or not, to place a nephrostomy tube at the conclusion of the procedure should be based on several factors including residual stones and the likelihood of a second-look procedure, intra-operative blood loss or bleeding diathesis, ureteral obstruction and solitary kidney. Accordingly, the key to effective outcome with tubeless PCNL is appropriate patient selection (Fig. 11.1).

A more conservative modification could be a combination of short-term nephrostomy tube and internal DJ stent. This allows adequate hemostasis control in the immediate postoperative phase and enables re-access in the need of second-look procedures while showing equiva-

Checklist for evaluation of nephrostomy tube placement

- presence of residual fragments
- likelihood of second look procedure
- significant intraoperative bloodloss
- urine extravasation
- ureteral obstruction
- potential persistent bacteriuria due to infected stones
- solitary kidney
- bleeding diathesis
- planned percutaneous chemolysis

Fig. 11.1 Factors to consider whether to place a nephrostomy tube according to the EAU Guidelines Urolithiasis 2019 [12]

lent results with regard to analgesic requirement, hospital stay and blood loss compared to a tubeless approach [25].

11.5 Totally Tubeless PCNL

To avoid any morbidity related to the nephrostomy tube or ureteral stent, several studies investigated the feasibility of a totally tubeless PCNL (Table 11.2). In 2004, Karami et al. [26] was the first to publish his experience in 30 selected patients undergoing totally tubeless PCNL. He concluded the tube- and stentless procedure to be a safe alternative to the standard or stented PCNL. These results were confirmed by several RCTs [22, 27–30] as well as a recent meta-analysis including 1131 patients [21], showing superiority in reduced operating time, hospital stay and postoperative analgesic requirement, without significantly more adverse events. To be mentioned, most of those studies share a carefully selected patient cohort, and there still are a number of situations requiring the consideration of nephrostomy tube placement. Factors to be considered are similar to the tubeless PCNL technique (Fig. 11.1) but may also include cases with more than two access tracts, significant perforation of the collecting system and intestinal or intrathoracic injuries. If there are residual fragments, the preexisting tract may not provide sufficient access to reach the stone during a second-look procedure. In some cases, generating a new access tract may be necessary. Alternatively to placing a nephrostomy tube, the possibility of safely managing the residual calculi by shock wave lithotripsy or retrograde intrarenal surgery should be evaluated.

To summarize, the feasibility of a totally tubeless PCNL technique has been demonstrated. In cases of uncomplicated PCNL it could even excel standard PCNL in terms of operation time, hospital stay and postoperative analgesic requirement. However the decision whether or not to place a nephrostomy tube after PCNL depends on the clinical judgment and experience of the surgeon, while inclusion criteria have not been clearly defined yet.

11.6 Tubeless in Complex PCNL

11.6.1 Multiple Tract PCNL

There is a trend towards multiple tract PCNL in complex or staghorn calculi to improve stone-free rates in fewer sessions. To assess the exit strategy in those cases, Resorlu et al. [31] retrospectively analyzed 115 patients undergoing multiple tract PCNL and categorized them into three groups. The first group had a nephrostomy tube for each tract (group 1, $n = 43$), the second group had a single nephrostomy tube placement (group 2, $n = 51$) and the third group had no nephrostomy drainage but antegrade placement of a double-J stent (group 3, $n = 21$). They did show similar results in regards of stone-free rate, operative time, average hemoglobin drop and complication rate for each group, but the average hospitalization time in the tubeless group (mean 2.1 days) was significantly shorter than that in group 1 (4.2 days) and group 2 (3.5 days). Additionally the postoperative analgesic requirement was significantly higher in group 1 compared to the single nephrostomy or tubeless group. They concluded that single nephrostomy or no external drainage following multiple tract PCNL offers a save alternative with potential advantages of decreased postoperative analgesic requirement and reduced hospitalization time.

Similar results have been shown by Agrawal et al. [32] comparing multiple-tube vs. single-tube postoperative drainage following multiple tract PCNL.

11.6.2 Tubeless in Obese Patients

To assess feasibility of tubeless PCNL in obese patients, Aghamir et al. [33] conducted a retrospective analysis of 78 morbidly obese patients (BMI >35) undergoing PCNL due to upper urinary tract calculi. Patients were randomly assigned to standard PNL with nephrostomy and ureteral stent (n = 43) and totally tubeless PNL with no ureteral stent and no nephrostomy (n = 35). While having a possible risk of intraoperative complications due to their body habitus, the results concluded that totally tubeless PCNL was leading to lower analgesic use and quicker return to normal activity compared to standard PCNL in obese patients. These findings did match with a study by Kuntz et al. [34], evaluating the impact of BMI on the outcomes of tubeless PCNL, including internal ureteric stents. In their retrospective review of 268 patients, divided into four groups based on BMI (<25, 25–29.9, 30–34.9 and ≥35 kg/m^2), no association between BMI and stone-free, or complication rate was found.Based on these findings, the use of tubeless PCNL in obese individuals can be recommended, but the level of evidence is still limited.

11.6.3 Tubeless in Children

With the introduction of smaller instruments like the 11F mini-perc, or 12F super mini PCNL (SMP) technique, alternative exit strategies after successful stone clearance in pediatric patients were evaluated [35]. Summarizing three RCTs, including 147 children, a meta-analysis comparing the outcomes of tubeless vs. standard PCNL by Nouralizadeh et al. [36] did show no differences in stone clearance rate, operative time, hemoglobin decrease, or other complications like perirenal fluid, infection or the need of a second procedure. There was a trend towards a shorter hospital stay in children undergoing tubeless PCNL, but it did not reach statistical significance. Postoperative analgesic need has not been included in this analysis partly due to heterogeneous documentation. By analyzing the individual conclusions, there was either a significant reduction in analgesic use [37, 38] or at least a reduction in psychological fear of children under 3 years of age [39]. Ozturk et al. [40] retrospectively evaluated the safety and effectiveness of totally tubeless compared to standard PCNL in preschool children. Their results indicate that totally tubeless PCNL is at least as safe and effective as standard PCNL. But the authors also highlight the importance of a proper patient selection and the need of a surgeon experienced with the procedure. Further studies including teenage children (≤18a) report similar results regarding safety and effectiveness of tubeless PCNL. They also conclude a significant reduction in analgesic use for tubeless and small bore (16F) PCNL compared to large bore nephrostomy (22F) even including supracostal access, up to two punctures, adult tract size (24F) and anomalous kidneys [41, 42].

11.6.4 Tubeless in Supracostal Access

Feasibility of tubeless PCNL with a supracostal access is still under debate with conflicting result on the complication rate. A prospective randomized trial by Shoma et al. [43] considered tubeless PCNL as a risk factor for complications in supracostal access but based on solely one patient with hemothorax after supracostal puncture in their cohort. In contrast, there are several retrospective analyses stating that tubeless supracostal PCNL provides a safe and effective alternative to the standard approach even with possible advantage of lower analgesic requirement, reduced operative time and shorter hospital stay [44–49]. Due to the lack of methodological thorough prospective RCTs, a decisive recommendation for tubeless supracostal PCNL is still pending.

11.7 Hemostatic Agents

Adequate hemostasis poses a main concern in tubeless PCNL due to the missing option to tamponade a possible bleeding with the nephrostomy tube. Therefore several RCTs evaluated the effect of different hemostatic agents on hemostasis after tubeless PCNL. The results summarized by two meta-analyses [50, 51] showed no significant improvement of complication rate like hemorrhage or urine extravasation. A further comparison of fibrin versus gelatin matrix sealing agents underlined a possible adverse outcome concerning postoperative upper tract obstruction. The study by Kim et al. [52] showed a higher obstruction rate for gelatin matrix sealants due to a dislocation of the gelatin matrix into the pyelocaliceal system and consecutive clotting of the UPJ or ureter. Combined with a relatively high cost of those hemostatic agents, further studies proving a clinical benefit are necessary before routine use after tubeless PCNL.

References

1. Rupel E, Brown R. Nephroscopy with removal of stone following nephrostomy for obstructive calculous anuria. J Urol. 1941;46:177–82.
2. Fernstrom I, Johansson B. Percutaneous pyelolithotomy. A new extraction technique. Scand J Urol Nephrol. 1976;10(3):257–9.
3. Wickham JE, Miller RA, Kellett MJ, Payne SR. Percutaneous nephrolithotomy: one stage or two? Br J Urol. 1984;56(6):582–5.
4. Winfield HN, Weyman P, Clayman RV. Percutaneous nephrostolithotomy: complications of premature nephrostomy tube removal. J Urol. 1986;136(1):77–9.
5. Bellman GC, Davidoff R, Candela J, Gerspach J, Kurtz S, Stout L. Tubeless percutaneous renal surgery. J Urol. 1997;157(5):1578–82.
6. Maheshwari PN, Andankar MG, Bansal M. Nephrostomy tube after percutaneous nephrolithotomy: large-bore or pigtail catheter? J Endourol. 2000;14(9):735–7; discussion 7–8.
7. Paul EM, Marcovich R, Lee BR, Smith AD. Choosing the ideal nephrostomy tube. BJU Int. 2003;92(7):672–7.
8. Cormio L, Preminger G, Saussine C, Buchholz NP, Zhang X, Walfridsson H, et al. Nephrostomy in percutaneous nephrolithotomy (PCNL): does nephrostomy tube size matter? Results from the global PCNL study from the Clinical Research Office Endourology Society. World J Urol. 2013;31(6):1563–8.
9. Pietrow PK, Auge BK, Lallas CD, Santa-Cruz RW, Newman GE, Albala DM, et al. Pain after percutaneous nephrolithotomy: impact of nephrostomy tube size. J Endourol. 2003;17(6):411–4.
10. Marcovich R, Jacobson AI, Singh J, Shah D, El-Hakim A, Lee BR, et al. No panacea for drainage after percutaneous nephrolithotomy. J Endourol. 2004;18(8):743–7.
11. Desai MR, Kukreja RA, Desai MM, Mhaskar SS, Wani KA, Patel SH, et al. A prospective randomized comparison of type of nephrostomy drainage following percutaneous nephrostolithotomy: large bore versus small bore versus tubeless. J Urol. 2004;172(2):565–7.
12. Türk C, Neisius A, Petřík A, Seitz C, Thomas K, Skolarikos A, EAU Guidelines on Urolithiasis. European Association of Urology Guidelines 2019 edition. Arnhem: The European Association of Urology Guidelines Office; 2019.
13. Istanbulluoglu MO, Cicek T, Ozturk B, Gonen M, Ozkardes H. Percutaneous nephrolithotomy: nephrostomy or tubeless or totally tubeless? Urology. 2010;75(5):1043–6.
14. Zilberman DE, Lipkin ME, de la Rosette JJ, Ferrandino MN, Mamoulakis C, Laguna MP, et al. Tubeless percutaneous nephrolithotomy—the new standard of care? J Urol. 2010;184(4):1261–6.
15. Xun Y, Wang Q, Hu H, Lu Y, Zhang J, Qin B, et al. Tubeless versus standard percutaneous nephrolithotomy: an update meta-analysis. BMC Urol. 2017;17(1):102.
16. Ni S, Qiyin C, Tao W, Liu L, Jiang H, Hu H, et al. Tubeless percutaneous nephrolithotomy is associated with less pain and shorter hospitalization compared with standard or small bore drainage: a meta-analysis of randomized, controlled trials. Urology. 2011;77(6):1293–8.
17. Jiang H, Huang D, Yao S, Liu S. Improving drainage after percutaneous nephrolithotomy based on health-related quality of life: a prospective randomized study. J Endourol. 2017;31(11):1131–8.
18. Chen Y, Feng J, Yue Y, Zhao Z, Deng T, Wu W, et al. Externalized ureteral catheter versus double-J stent in tubeless percutaneous nephrolithotomy for upper urinary stones: a systematic review and meta-analysis. J Endourol. 2018;32(7):581–8.
19. Gonen M, Ozturk B, Ozkardes H. Double-j stenting compared with one night externalized ureteral catheter placement in tubeless percutaneous nephrolithotomy. J Endourol. 2009;23(1):27–31.
20. Zhou Y, Zhu J, Gurioli A, Yuan D, Luo J, Li Z, et al. Randomized study of ureteral catheter vs double-J stent in tubeless minimally invasive percutaneous nephrolithotomy patients. J Endourol. 2017;31(3):278–82.
21. Li Q, Gao L, Li J, Zhang Y, Jiang Q. Total tubeless versus standard percutaneous nephrolithotomy: a

meta-analysis. Minim Invasive Ther Allied Technol. 2019:1–9.
22. Lee JY, Jeh SU, Kim MD, Kang DH, Kwon JK, Ham WS, et al. Intraoperative and postoperative feasibility and safety of total tubeless, tubeless, small-bore tube, and standard percutaneous nephrolithotomy: a systematic review and network meta-analysis of 16 randomized controlled trials. BMC Urol. 2017;17(1):48.
23. Choi M, Brusky J, Weaver J, Amantia M, Bellman GC. Randomized trial comparing modified tubeless percutaneous nephrolithotomy with tailed stent with percutaneous nephrostomy with small-bore tube. J Endourol. 2006;20(10):766–70.
24. Shpall AI, Parekh AR, Bellman GC. Tubeless percutaneous nephrolithotomy with antegrade stent tether: clinical experience. J Endourol. 2007;21(9):973–6.
25. Mishra S, Sabnis RB, Kurien A, Ganpule A, Muthu V, Desai M. Questioning the wisdom of tubeless percutaneous nephrolithotomy (PCNL): a prospective randomized controlled study of early tube removal vs tubeless PCNL. BJU Int. 2010;106(7):1045–8; discussion 8–9.
26. Karami H, Gholamrezaie HR. Totally tubeless percutaneous nephrolithotomy in selected patients. J Endourol. 2004;18(5):475–6.
27. Husch T, Reiter M, Mager R, Steiner E, Herrmann TR, Haferkamp A, et al. The management of the access tract after percutaneous nephrolithotomy. World J Urol. 2015;33(12):1921–8.
28. Kara C, Resorlu B, Bayindir M, Unsal A. A randomized comparison of totally tubeless and standard percutaneous nephrolithotomy in elderly patients. Urology. 2010;76(2):289–93.
29. Akin Y, Basara I, Yucel S, Gulmez H, Ates M, Bozkurt A, et al. Is tubeless percutaneous nephrolithotomy really less injurious than standard in the midterm? J Endourol. 2013;27(10):1192–6.
30. Bhat S, Lal J, Paul F. A randomized controlled study comparing the standard, tubeless, and totally tubeless percutaneous nephrolithotomy procedures for renal stones from a tertiary care hospital. Indian J Urol. 2017;33(4):310–4.
31. Resorlu B, Kara C, Sahin E, Unsal A. Comparison of nephrostomy drainage types following percutaneous nephrolithotomy requiring multiple tracts: single tube versus multiple tubes versus tubeless. Urol Int. 2011;87(1):23–7.
32. Agrawal MS, Agrawal M. Are multiple nephrostomy tubes necessary after multitract percutaneous nephrolithotomy? A randomized comparison of single versus multiple nephrostomy tubes. J Endourol. 2009;23(11):1831–4.
33. Aghamir SMK, Mohseni MG, Hosseini SR, Salavati A, Ganjali H, Fallah MA, et al. Totally tubeless percutaneous nephrolithotomy is feasible in morbidly obese patients. Turk J Urol. 2017;43(2):162–4.
34. Kuntz NJ, Neisius A, Astroza GM, Tsivian M, Iqbal MW, Youssef R, et al. Does body mass index impact the outcomes of tubeless percutaneous nephrolithotomy? BJU Int. 2014;114(3):404–11.
35. Jackman SV, Hedican SP, Peters CA, Docimo SG. Percutaneous nephrolithotomy in infants and preschool age children: experience with a new technique. Urology. 1998;52(4):697–701.
36. Nouralizadeh A, Simforoosh N, Shemshaki H, Soltani MH, Sotoudeh M, Ramezani MH, et al. Tubeless versus standard percutaneous nephrolithotomy in pediatric patients: a systematic review and meta-analysis. Urologia. 2018;85(1):3–9.
37. Samad L, Zaidi Z. Tubed vs tubeless PCNL in children. J Pak Med Assoc. 2012;62(9):892–6.
38. Aghamir SM, Salavati A, Aloosh M, Farahmand H, Meysamie A, Pourmand G. Feasibility of totally tubeless percutaneous nephrolithotomy under the age of 14 years: a randomized clinical trial. J Endourol. 2012;26(6):621–4.
39. Song G, Guo X, Niu G, Wang Y. Advantages of tubeless mini-percutaneous nephrolithotomy in the treatment of preschool children under 3 years old. J Pediatr Surg. 2015;50(4):655–8.
40. Ozturk A, Guven S, Kilinc M, Topbas E, Piskin M, Arslan M. Totally tubeless percutaneous nephrolithotomy: is it safe and effective in preschool children? J Endourol. 2010;24(12):1935–9.
41. Keshavamurthy R, Kumar S, Karthikeyan VS, Mallya A, Nelivigi GG. Tubeless pediatric percutaneous nephrolithotomy: assessment of feasibility and safety. J Indian Assoc Pediatr Surg. 2018;23(1):16–21.
42. Iqbal N, Assad S, Hussain I, Hassan Y, Khan H, Farooq MA, et al. Comparison of outcomes of tubed versus tubeless percutaneous nephrolithotomy in children: a single center study. Turk J Urol. 2018;44(1):56–61.
43. Shoma AM, Elshal AM. Nephrostomy tube placement after percutaneous nephrolithotomy: critical evaluation through a prospective randomized study. Urology. 2012;79(4):771–6.
44. Jun-Ou J, Lojanapiwat B. Supracostal access: does it affect tubeless percutaneous nephrolithotomy efficacy and safety? Int Braz J Urol. 2010;36(2):171–6.
45. Yan MY, Lin J, Chiang HC, Chen YL, Chen PH. Supra-costal tubeless percutaneous nephrolithotomy is not associated with increased complication rate: a prospective study of safety and efficacy of supra-costal versus sub-costal access. BMC Urol. 2018;18(1):112.
46. Gonen M, Cicek T, Ozkardes H. Tubeless and stentless percutaneous nephrolithotomy in patients requiring supracostal access. Urol Int. 2009;82(4):440–3.
47. Shah HN, Hegde SS, Shah JN, Bansal MB. Safety and efficacy of supracostal access in tubeless percutaneous nephrolithotomy. J Endourol. 2006;20(12):1016–21.
48. Altschuler J, Jain R, Ganesan V, Monga M. Supracostal upper pole endoscopic-guided prone tubeless "maxi-percutaneous nephrolithotomy": a contemporary evaluation of complications. J Endourol. 2019;33(4):274–8.

49. Sourial MW, Francois N, Box GN, Knudsen BE. Supracostal access tubeless percutaneous nephrolithotomy: minimizing complications. World J Urol. 2019;37(7):1429–33.
50. Yu C, Xu Z, Long W, Longfei L, Feng Z, Lin Q, et al. Hemostatic agents used for nephrostomy tract closure after tubeless PCNL: a systematic review and meta-analysis. Urolithiasis. 2014;42(5):445–53.
51. Wang J, Zhang C, Tan G, Yang B, Chen W, Tan D. The use of adjunctive hemostatic agents in tubeless percutaneous nephrolithotomy: a meta-analysis. Urolithiasis. 2014;42(6):509–17.
52. Kim JJ, Suh YS, Han DH. Urolithiasis. 2019. https://doi.org/10.1007/s00240-019-01126-0.

Complications Related with PCNL and Their Management

12

Iliya Saltirov and Kremena Petkova

12.1 Introduction

Percutaneous nephrolithotomy (PCNL) is a standard procedure for the management of large and/or complex renal calculi [1]. Despite the advancements in endoscopic technologies and the refinements of PCNL surgical technique and training, the procedure is still associated with complications, which can occur during the intervention or in the early or late postoperative period. Therefore, detailed knowledge on PCNL complications and their diagnosis and management is essential to reduce procedure-related morbidity and improve patient outcomes.

12.2 Classification of PCNL Complications

Standardization of reporting and grading of surgical complications is important to compare outcomes between studies and improve patient care. The Modified Clavien-Dindo Classification of surgical complications, validated in many surgical procedures, is increasingly used for grading of complications in PCNL [2–5]. Recently, the CROES PCNL Group validated the modified Clavien-Dindo classification for PCNL and assigned Clavien scores to specific PCNL complications in order to improve reporting [4]. Although the complication rate reported in the CROES PCNL database was 20.5%, most complications were low grade and classified as Clavien score I, II and IIIa [5].

12.3 Preoperative Factors for Complications

The selection of patients indicated for PCNL and preoperative assessment of risk factors for complications are important steps when planning a PCNL procedure in order to reduce postoperative morbidity. Multiple studies have investigated the impact of different patient and stone-related factors and surgeon experience on the occurrence of intra- and postoperative adverse events.

12.3.1 Patient's Age and Comorbidities

With the worldwide increase in life expectancy and incidence of urolithiasis, advanced age is becoming a concern for perioperative morbidity. In a study of 3310 patients from the CROES PCNL study database, Okeke et al. compared PCNL outcomes between elderly (>70 years)

I. Saltirov (✉) · K. Petkova
Department of Urology and Nephrology, Military Medical Academy, Sofia, Bulgaria
e-mail: saltirov@vma.bg

G. Zeng, K. Sarica (eds.), *Percutaneous Nephrolithotomy*,
https://doi.org/10.1007/978-981-15-0575-1_12

and younger (18–70 years) patients [6]. In this study elderly patients had a significantly higher incidence of comorbidities, such as diabetes and cardiovascular disease, and were more likely to have preoperative anticoagulation therapy. Furthermore, in the matched analysis, elderly patients had a statistically significantly higher rate and grade of complications and longer hospital stay [6]. In another study, Unsal et al. analysed the correlation between Charlson Comorbidity Index (CCI), a validated classification of comorbid conditions, as a predictor for perioperative morbidity in PCNL [7]. In their series, higher CCI score and increased patient age correlated with increased complications rate following PCNL.

12.3.2 Obesity

Obesity has been linked to increased incidence of renal stones and other comorbidities, such as diabetes and cardiovascular disease [8, 9]. Obese patients have longer skin-to-stone distance, which may pose some technical challenges when performing PCNL. Furthermore, the prone position in obese patients may lead to decreased lung capacity and reduced venous return [10]. However, despite the increased preoperative and anaesthesiologic risk in obesity, several studies have found no adverse impact on PCNL morbidity [11–13]. In the CROES Global PCNL Study, obese patients had higher rate of comorbidities, preoperative anesthesiologic risk and increased incidence of preoperative anticoagulation therapy, but postoperative complication rates were comparable to normal weight patients [11]. However, high-grade complications were more common in morbidly obese patients [11].

12.3.3 Preoperative Anticoagulation Therapy

Patients on antiplatelet and anticoagulation therapy are an important concern for the endourologist when performing PCNL. The risk of intra- and postoperative bleeding and perioperative thromboembolic complications should be considered when discussing indications for surgery and choosing therapeutic procedure. Alternative treatment approaches, such as retrograde ureterorenoscopy, are reasonable in high-risk patients. A thorough preoperative evaluation, including history of coagulopathy or ongoing anticoagulation or antiplatelet therapy, is important. Anticoagulation medication should be discontinued before PCNL and patients should be monitored in the postoperative period [1]. It is advisable to stop antiplatelet agents for 5–7 days prior to the procedure except for patients at very high risk of thrombosis [14]. An interdisciplinary approach is necessary in order to guarantee patient safety and optimal discontinuation and reinitiation of anticoagulation and antiplatelet therapies [15].

12.3.4 Preoperative Urinary Tract Infection

Preoperative urinary tract infection (UTI) is a recognised risk factor for postoperative infectious complications in PCNL and should be diagnosed and treated before surgery [1, 16–18]. Multiple studies have found that positive preoperative midstream, pelvic urine and stone culture are associated with higher risk of infectious complications following PCNL [18, 19].

12.3.5 Renal Anomalies

Treatment of urolithiasis in abnormal kidneys may be challenging due to variable vascular and pyelocalyceal anatomy and renal position, which make percutaneous puncture and tract dilation more difficult. Available data from the literature has found that PCNL in patients with abnormal renal anatomy is safe when performed in experienced centres [20–22]. In the CROES Global PCNL study, patients with anomalous and normal kidneys had comparable results in terms of stone-free rates and overall complications [22]. However, operating times were longer and rate of failed percutaneous access was higher in patients with renal anomalies (87 min vs. 75 min, $p = 0.037$ and 5% vs. 1.7%, $p = 0.001$, respectively) [22].

12.3.6 Stone Type and Burden

Stone type and burden are important considerations when planning a PCNL procedure. Several preoperative systems for grading stone complexity have been developed as tools to predict stone-free rates and complications associated with PCNL, such as the Guy's Stone Score (GSS), the S.T.O.N.E. Nephrolithometry and the CROES nomogram [23–25]. These scoring systems take into account multiple factors: number, location, size and complexity of the stone, presence of renal anomalies, and skin-to-stone distance, which have been validated in several studies [23–27]. Therefore, they may be used preoperatively for patient counselling and planning of PCNL procedure as well as for the comparison of outcomes between studies.

12.3.7 Surgeon Experience and Learning Curve

PCNL is a complex procedure, and surgeon experience and case volume are important factors related to PCNL outcomes. Negrete-Pulido et al. and Quirke et al. observed a learning curve from 40 to 100 cases in order to reduce operating and fluoroscopy times, complication rates and increase stone-free rates [28, 29]. The CROES PCNL group found increased efficacy, lower perioperative morbidity and bleeding complications, and shorter hospital stay in high-volume centres and surgeons performing PCNL [30].

12.4 Intraoperative Complications and Their Management

12.4.1 Complications Related to Patient Positioning

Since the introduction of PCNL in clinical practice, the prone position has been considered the standard patient position for PCNL. Valdivia-Uria et al. introduced the supine position for PCNL and described its advantages over the prone position [31]. Since then, several modifications of the supine and flank positions have been proposed in order to overcome some of the disadvantages of the prone position [32–34]. However, comparative studies failed to show any differences in stone-free and complication rates [35, 36].

Complications specific to the prone position have been studied in orthopaedic and neurosurgery. Several studies demonstrated decreased venous return and cardiac index due to compression of the vena cava in the prone position [37, 38]. Other specific complications, such as postoperative ischaemic optic neuropathy, injuries to the cervical spine or peripheral nerves, have also been observed in spinal and orthopaedic surgery performed in prone position and have been associated with longer operating times [39–41]. In PCNL, the duration of surgery has also been linked to increased risk of nerve injuries associated with the prone position [42, 43].

12.4.2 Intraoperative Bleeding

Intraoperative bleeding of variable degree is commonly observed during PCNL. It may arise from the renal parenchyma or from injury of arterial or venous vessels. Technical aspects to reduce the risk of bleeding include papillary puncture of the targeted calyx, less angulation of the Amplatz sheath and the nephroscope, and fluoroscopic monitoring of the tract dilation [44]. Venous bleeding is usually self-limiting and resolves by tamponade of the renal parenchyma with the Amplatz sheath. In cases with significant bleeding and low endoscopic visibility, it is recommended to stop the procedure and clamp the nephrostomy tube [45]. Another option to tamponade the nephrostomy tract in cases with severe bleeding is to use a Kaye balloon catheter [46]. The cases with arterial bleeding are usually managed by renal angiography and selective embolisation of the bleeding vessel [47, 48].

12.4.3 Organ Injury

Injury of the neighbouring organs (lung, pleura, spleen, liver, colon) is rarely encountered during

PCNL. Pleural and/or lung injury is more likely during supracostal puncture above the 12th rib and may result in hydrothorax, pneumothorax, haemothorax, lung injury or nephropleural fistula [44]. The rate of intrathoracic complications reported in the literature, ranges from 0 to 11% in the modern series according to renal puncture location [44, 49, 50]. Hydrothorax occurs by extravasation of the irrigation fluid or urine along the nephrostomy tract during or after the procedure. Pneumothorax is caused by lung injury and penetration of air into the pleura. Haemothorax may result from renal parenchymal bleeding or injury of subcostal vessels. Nephropleural fistula is usually diagnosed after the extraction of the nephrostomy tube and extravasation of urine into the pleural space. Successful management of these complications relies on early diagnosis. Patients with small hydro- or pneumothorax and no respiratory distress may be managed conservatively. In cases of larger hydrothorax and nephropleural fistula, the kidney and pleural cavity should be drained separately by a nephrostomy tube or stent, and a chest tube.

Colon injuries following PCNL are uncommon, occurring in <1% of the cases [51]. Identified risk factors include presence of retrorenal colon, puncture located laterally to the posterior axillary line, prone position for PCNL, female patients with low body mass index and horseshoe kidney [52–54]. A preoperative computed tomography (CT) can identify the presence of a retrorenal colon, and ultrasound-guided puncture is recommended to avoid colon damage. Colonic perforation may be suspected by contrast medium extravasation into the bowel during the procedure. Postoperatively, colonic injury is diagnosed by the presence of diarrhoea, faecaluria through the nephrostomy tube or signs of peritonitis. Extraperitoneal perforations can be managed successfully with separate drainage of the kidney with ureteral stent and retraction of the nephrostomy tube into the bowel as a colostomy. Cases with intraperitoneal colon injuries and signs of peritonitis should be managed by immediate surgery.

Splenic and liver injuries are uncommon and are more likely in patients with hepato- and splenomegaly and supracostal punctures. Treatment options reported in the literature range from conservative measures to splenectomy, according to the timing of diagnosis and haemodynamic status of the patient [55, 56]. Hepatic injuries may be managed conservatively with local haemostatic agents and gradual retraction of the nephrostomy tube or with surgery in instable patients [57].

12.4.4 Collecting System Perforation

Perforation of the collecting system of the kidney may occur during nephrostomy tract dilation, nephroscopy and lithotripsy and may lead to extravasation of irrigation fluid and urine or migration of stone fragments outside of the kidney (Figs. 12.1 and 12.2). Risk factors include high irrigation pressure, forceful manipulation with the dilators, lithotripsy probe or other working instruments or excessive angulation of the nephroscope. Drainage of the kidney with nephrostomy tube and/or ureteral stent is the treatment of choice, and the majority of perforations close within 24–48 h [58]. In cases with stone

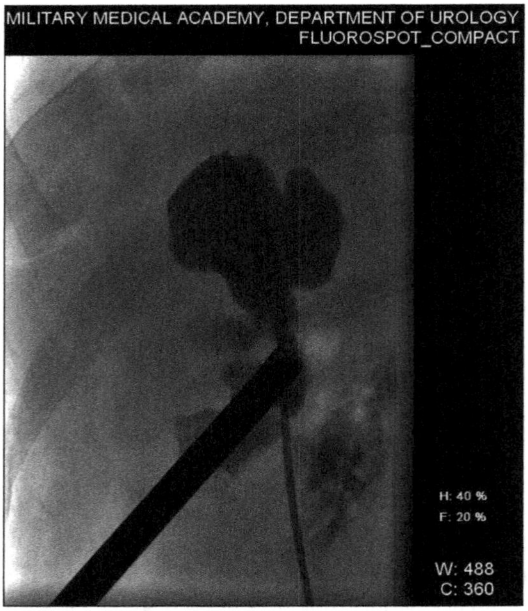

Fig. 12.1 Contrast extravasation through collecting system perforation during PCNL

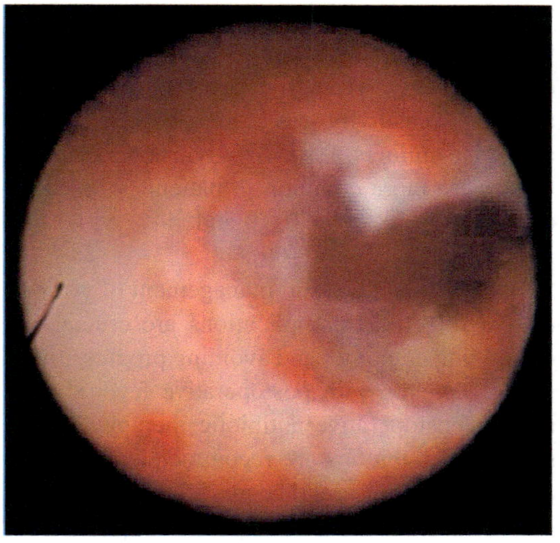

Fig. 12.2 Renal pelvis perforation due to overadvancement of the Amplatz dilator

fragments outside of the collecting system, efforts to extract them are not recommended because of the risk of further damage to the collecting system.

12.4.5 Loss of the Nephrostomy Tract

Loss of the nephrostomy tract may occur at any moment during PCNL and is caused by slipping of the guidewire or Amplatz sheath outside of the collecting system. The use of suitable guidewire and its placement in the ureter or through-and-through help prevent this complication. The presence of a safety guidewire ensures regaining of the access. In cases with no safety guidewire in place, injection of methylene blue mixed with contrast and visual inspection are useful to find the tract. If the nephrostomy access cannot be found, a new puncture or termination of the procedure may be considered.

12.4.6 Absorption of Irrigation Fluid

Absorption of irrigation fluid has been observed in transurethral prostate resection, but it has also been described in percutaneous stone surgery through the renal parenchymal vessels or from fluid extravasation [59, 60]. Kukreja et al. studied fluid absorption during PCNL in 148 patients [61]. Absorption of irrigation fluid was present in all cases and the amount absorbed increased with surgery duration, irrigation fluid volume, perforation of the collecting system and bleeding. In contrast, low-pressure irrigation and staged procedure were found to reduce the risk of this complication [61]. More recently, Guzelburc et al. compared the amount of absorbed fluid during retrograde intrarenal surgery and percutaneous nephrolithotomy for kidney stones >2 cm [62]. Fluid absorption was observed in all cases; however, no patients developed postoperative electrolyte imbalance. The volume of absorbed fluid increased significantly with duration of PCNL surgery.

12.5 Postoperative Complications and Their Management

12.5.1 Postoperative Fever and Sepsis

Postoperative infection is a common complication of PCNL and ranges from transient postoperative fever to sepsis. Despite the recommended use of antibiotic prophylaxis, from 10.5 to 39.8% of patients will develop postoperative fever [16, 44, 63]. Sepsis following PCNL has been reported in 0.3–1% of the cases but has a high mortality rate of 66–80% [44, 64, 65]. Therefore, preoperative microbiological evaluation of patients and assessment of pre- and intraoperative risk factors are crucial for prevention of postoperative fever and sepsis (Fig. 12.3).

The risk factors for postoperative fever and urinary tract infection have been studied extensively in the literature. Rivera et al. observed postoperative urinary tract infection rate of 5%, systemic inflammatory response syndrome (SIRS) in 9% and sepsis in 0.9% in a group of 227 patients [17]. In their study, the presence of struvite stone, positive stone culture and staghorn calculus correlated with higher rate of infectious complications. More recently, the CROES PCNL group analysed factors related with postoperative

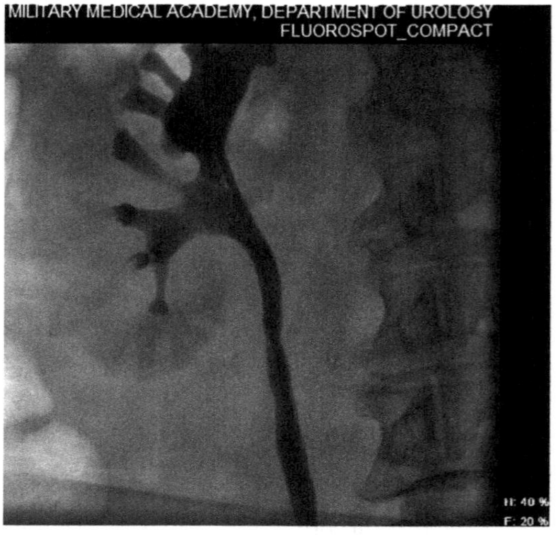

Fig. 12.3 Pyelotubular reflux during retrograde pyelography at the beginning of PCNL procedure. Patient developed postoperative fever

fever [16]. Overall postoperative fever rate was 10.4%. Increased duration of surgery, positive preoperative urine culture, presence of staghorn stone, residual stones, preoperative nephrostomy and diabetes were found to be independent predictors for postoperative fever [16].

Preoperative urinary tract infection increases the risk of postoperative infectious complications in PCNL. Therefore, preoperative urine culture and perioperative antibiotic prophylaxis are recommended [1]. However, postoperative infectious complications are observed even in cases with negative preoperative midstream urine culture [16]. Mariappan et al. investigated bladder, renal pelvic and stone cultures as predictors of postoperative sepsis following PCNL in a series of 54 patients [19]. Midstream bladder urine culture was positive in 11.1%, pelvic urine culture in 20.4% and stone culture in 35.2% [19]. The same microorganism was found in pelvic and stone cultures in 85.7% of cases, but none of the patients had the same type of microorganism between bladder and upper urinary tract. The risk of urosepsis was found to be four times higher with positive pelvic and stone cultures. More recently, Korets et al. analysed the correlation of bladder, pelvic and stone cultures and postoperative systemic inflammatory response syndrome (SIRS) following PCNL in 198 patients [66]. Thirty-three percent of patients with positive pelvic culture had negative midstream urine and the concordance between type of microorganism and antibiotic sensitivity was highest between pelvic and stone cultures. Positive pelvic and stone cultures were more common in patients with SIRS (26% vs. 10%, $p = 0.03$ and 44% vs. 17%, $p = 0.01$, respectively) [66].

Timely diagnosis and management of postoperative infectious complications are crucial for optimizing outcomes and avoiding progression to sepsis. Patients with postoperative fever should receive postoperative antibiotic therapy. Broad-spectrum antibiotics are recommended until the antibiotic therapy could be modified according to culture results. Renal drainage with nephrostomy tube or stent prevents ureteral obstruction or urinary leakage, which may worsen infectious complications. Early recognition of symptoms of sepsis and the results from midstream, pelvic and stone cultures are essential for the choice of appropriate therapeutic regimen and prevention of life-threatening complications.

12.5.2 Postoperative Bleeding

Postoperative bleeding is commonly observed in PCNL. In most cases there is some degree of haematuria following PCNL, which is usually minor and resolves within 24–48 h. Venous bleeding is usually not significant and resolves with clamping of the nephrostomy tube to create clot tamponade of the collecting system. Arterial bleeding arises from arterial laceration, arterio-venous fistula or pseudoaneurysm and may be observed at any time during the postoperative period (Fig. 12.4). It is usually significant and may present with macroscopic haematuria and perirenal haematoma leading to haemorrhagic shock (Fig. 12.5). In some cases bleeding may be managed by fluid resuscitation and haemotransfusion. However, in patients with persistent bleeding, renal angiography and selective embolization of the bleeding source are indicated (Fig. 12.6).

The reported in the literature incidence of haemotransfusion following PCNL ranges between 0.6 and 23.8% with severe haemorrhage requiring angioembolisation, observed in

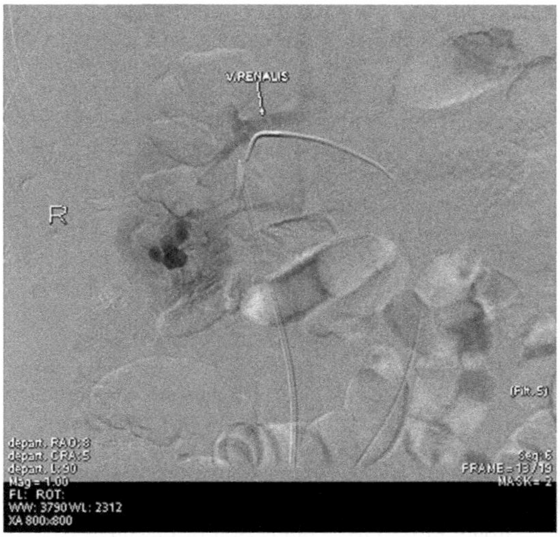

Fig. 12.4 Renal angiography of arterio-venous fistula following PCNL

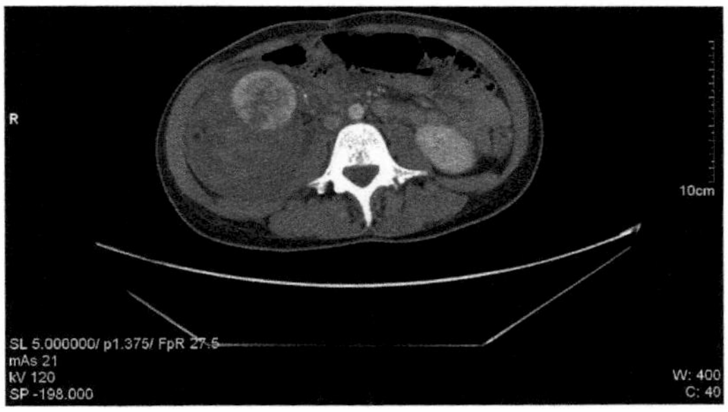

Fig. 12.5 Postoperative perirenal haematoma due to arterial laceration following miniaturised PCNL. Patient underwent renovasography with selective embolisation

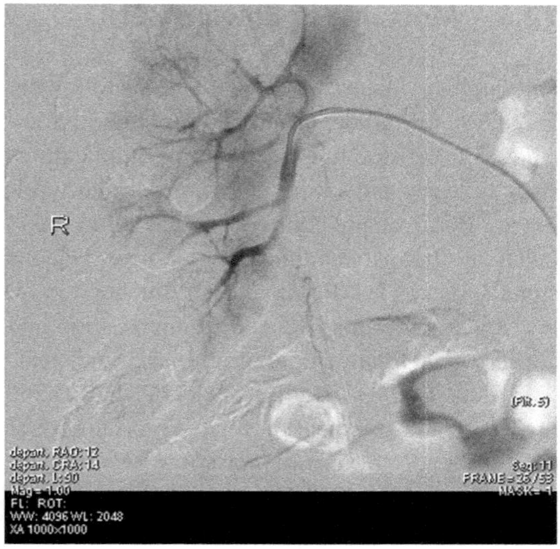

Fig. 12.6 Selective embolisation of arterio-venous fistula following PCNL

0.3–1.5% of the cases [47, 67–69]. Multiple studies have evaluated the predictors for haemotransfusion and haemorrhagic complications following PCNL. Kukreja et al. analysed risk factors for bleeding in 236 patients [68]. Multivariate analysis identified duration of surgery, method of tract dilation, size of tract, multiple tracts, renal parenchymal thickness and presence of diabetes as significant predictors for bleeding following PCNL. In another study, Turna et al. found that the presence of staghorn stones, Amplatz dilation, multiple tracts, diabetes and stone size is associated with blood loss in PCNL [69]. The CROES PCNL Group reported significant bleeding and haemotransfusion in 7.8% and 5.7%, respectively [70]. Balloon dilation was associated with increased incidence of bleeding and transfusion compared to telescopic/serial dilation [71]. However, other studies failed to demonstrate statistically significant differences in postoperative haemoglobin drop and haemotransfusion rate when comparing different methods for tract dilation in PCNL [72–74].

12.5.3 Postoperative Nephrocutaneous Fistula

Nephrocutaneous fistula is rare following PCNL and is usually caused by obstruction from mucosal oedema, stone fragment or clot. It is managed successfully by postoperative stent placement and relief of obstruction.

12.5.4 Late Complications

Late postoperative complications following PCNL include postoperative ureteropelvic junction stenosis and infundibular stenosis. These complications are rare and may result from intraoperative injury or ischaemia caused by impacted stones. Postoperative strictures can be managed endoscopically by laser incision and stent placement.

12.6 Mortality Following PCNL

Although the majority of complications following PCNL are low grade, the procedure can be associated with serious life-threatening complications such as sepsis and severe bleeding. Mortality following PCNL is not common, occurring in 0.03–0.2% of the patients undergoing percutaneous stone surgery [7, 70]. Recently, Whitehurst et al. investigated mortality related to intervention and conservative treatment of urolithiasis and analysed data from 34 studies [75]. PCNL had the highest rate of intervention-related mortality (507 patients, 85.3% of overall mortality). Main causes of death following PCNL were postoperative sepsis and haemorrhage; however, in the majority of patients the cause of death was not specified. Multiple comorbidities, spinal cord injury, high stone burden and obesity were identified as significant risk factors for mortality in all types of interventions. The authors' recommendations to prevent life-threatening complications were to decrease operating times, treat urinary tract infection preoperatively and use antibiotic prophylaxis, avoid multiple tracts and ensure adequate patient preparation in high-risk patients [75].

12.7 Conclusions

PCNL is standard treatment of renal stones and is a safe procedure with predominantly low grade of complications. However, despite improvements of endoscopes and surgical technique, PCNL is still associated with specific complications, which may result in life-threatening conditions. Detailed knowledge on PCNL complications and the risk factors for their occurrence is essential for their early diagnosis and successful management in order to reduce procedure-related morbidity without compromising patient outcomes.

References

1. Türk C, Skolarikos A, Neisius A, Petřík A, Seitz C, Thomas K, et al.; Members of the European Association of Urology (EAU) Guidelines Office. Guidelines on urolithiasis. 2019. https://uroweb.org/guideline/urolithiasis/. Accessed 1 May 2019.
2. Clavien PA, Sanabria JR, Strasberg SM. Proposed classification of complications of surgery with examples of utility in cholecystectomy. Surgery. 1992;111:518–26.
3. Dindo D, Demartines N, Clavien PA. Classification of surgical complications: a new proposal with evaluation in a cohort of 6336 patients and results of a survey. Ann Surg. 2004;240:205–13.
4. de la Rosette JJ, Opondo D, Daels FP, Giusti G, Serrano A, Kandasami SV, et al.; CROES PCNL Study Group. Categorisation of complications and validation of the Clavien score for percutaneous nephrolithotomy. Eur Urol. 2012;62(2):246–55.
5. Labate G, Modi P, Timoney A, Cormio L, Zhang X, Louie M, et al. The percutaneous nephrolithotomy global study: classification of complications. J Endourol. 2011;25(8):1275–80.
6. Okeke Z, Smith AD, Labate G, D'Addessi A, Venkatesh R, Assimos D, et al.; CROES PCNL Study Group. Prospective comparison of outcomes of percutaneous nephrolithotomy in elderly patients versus younger patients. J Endourol. 2012;26(8):996–1001.
7. Unsal A, Resorlu B, Atmaca AF, Diri A, Goktug HN, Can CE, et al. Prediction of morbidity and mortality after percutaneous nephrolithotomy by using the Charlson Comorbidity Index. Urology. 2012;79(1):55–60.
8. Wollin DA, Skolarikos A, Preminger GM. Obesity and metabolic stone disease. Curr Opin Urol. 2017;27(5):422–7.
9. Apovian CM. Obesity: definition, comorbidities, causes, and burden. Am J Manag Care. 2016;22(7 Suppl):s176–85.
10. Brodsky JB, Oldroyd M, Winfield HN, Kozlowski PM. Morbid obesity and the prone position: a case report. J Clin Anesth. 2001;13(2):138–40.
11. Fuller A, Razvi H, Denstedt JD, Nott L, Pearle M, Cauda F, et al.; CROES PCNL Study Group. The CROES percutaneous nephrolithotomy global study: the influence of body mass index on outcome. J Urol. 2012;188(1):138–144.
12. El-Assmy AM, Shokeir AA, El-Nahas AR, Shoma AM, Eraky I, El-Kenawy MR, et al. Outcome of percutaneous nephrolithotomy: effect of body mass index. Eur Urol. 2007;52(1):199–204.
13. Tomaszewski JJ, Smaldone MC, Schuster T, Jackman SV, Averch TD. Outcomes of percutaneous nephrolithotomy stratified by body mass index. J Endourol. 2010;24(4):547–50.
14. Tikkinen KAO, Cartwright R, Gould R, Naspro R, Novara G, Sandset PM, et al.; Members of the European Association of Urology (EAU) Guidelines Office. EAU guidelines on thromboprophylaxis in urological surgery. 2019. https://uroweb.org/guideline/thromboprophylaxis/. Accessed 2 May 2019.
15. Gross AJ, Bach T. Preoperative percutaneous stone surgery in patients receiving anticoagulant therapy. J Endourol. 2009;23(10):1563–5.
16. Gutierrez J, Smith A, Geavlete P, Shah H, Kural AR, de Sio M, et al.; CROES PCNL Study Group. Urinary tract infections and post-operative fever

in percutaneous nephrolithotomy. World J Urol. 2013;31(5):1135–40.
17. Rivera M, Viers B, Cockerill P, Agarwal D, Mehta R, Krambeck A. Pre- and postoperative predictors of infection-related complications in patients undergoing percutaneous nephrolithotomy. J Endourol. 2016;30(9):982–6.
18. Lai WS, Assimos D. Factors associated with postoperative infection after percutaneous nephrolithotomy. Rev Urol. 2018;20(1):7–11.
19. Mariappan P, Smith G, Bariol SV, Moussa SA, Tolley DA. Stone and pelvic urine culture and sensitivity are better than bladder urine as predictors of urosepsis following percutaneous nephrolithotomy: a prospective clinical study. J Urol. 2005;173(5):1610–4.
20. Mosavi-Bahar SH, Amirzargar MA, Rahnavardi M, Moghaddam SM, Babbolhavaeji H, Amirhasani S. Percutaneous nephrolithotomy in patients with kidney malformations. J Endourol. 2007;21(5):520–4.
21. Ozden E, Bilen CY, Mercimek MN, Tan B, Sarikaya S, Sahin A. Horseshoe kidney: does it really have any negative impact on surgical outcomes of percutaneous nephrolithotomy? Urology. 2010;75(5):1049–52.
22. Osther PJ, Razvi H, Liatsikos E, Averch T, Crisci A, Garcia JL, et al.; Croes PCNL Study Group. Percutaneous nephrolithotomy among patients with renal anomalies: patient characteristics and outcomes; a subgroup analysis of the clinical research office of the endourological society global percutaneous nephrolithotomy study. J Endourol. 2011;25(10):1627–1632.
23. Thomas K, Smith NC, Hegarty N, Glass JM. The Guy's stone score—grading the complexity of percutaneous nephrolithotomy procedures. Urology. 2011;78:277–81.
24. Smith A, Averch TD, Shahrour K, Opondo D, Daels FP, Labate G, et al. A nephrolithometric nomogram to predict treatment success of percutaneous nephrolithotomy. J Urol. 2013;190:149–56.
25. Okhunov Z, Friedlander JI, George AK, Duty BD, Moreira DM, Srinivasan AK, et al. S.T.O.N.E. nephrolithometry: novel surgical classification system for kidney calculi. Urology. 2013;81:1154–9.
26. Kumar S, Sreenivas J, Karthikeyan VS, Mallya A, Keshavamurthy R. Evaluation of CROES nephrolithometry nomogram as a preoperative predictive system for percutaneous nephrolithotomy outcomes. J Endourol. 2016;30(10):1079–83.
27. Vicentini FC, Serzedello FR, Thomas K, Marchini GS, Torricelli FCM, Srougi M, et al. What is the quickest scoring system to predict percutaneous nephrolithotomy outcomes? A comparative study among S.T.O.N.E score, Guy's stone score and CROES nomogram. Int Braz J Urol. 2017;43(6):1102–9.
28. Negrete-Pulido O, Molina-Torres M, Castaño-Tostado E, Loske AM, Gutiérrez-Aceves J. Percutaneous renal access: the learning curve of a simplified approach. J Endourol. 2010;24(3):457–60.
29. Quirke K, Aydin A, Brunckhorst O, Bultitude M, Khan MS, Dasgupta P, et al. Learning curves in urolithiasis surgery: a systematic review. J Endourol. 2018;32(11):1008–20.
30. Opondo D, Tefekli A, Esen T, Labate G, Sangam K, De Lisa A, et al. Impact of case volumes on the outcomes of percutaneous nephrolithotomy. Eur Urol. 2012;62(6):1181–7.
31. Valdivia Uria JG, Valle Gerhold J, Lopez Lopez JA, Villarroya Rodriguez S, Ambroj Navarro C, Ramirez Fabián M, et al. Technique and complications of percutaneous nephroscopy: experience with 557 patients in the supine position. J Urol. 1998;160(6):1975–8.
32. Kerbl K, Clayman RV, Chandhoke PS, Urban DA, De Leo BC, Carbone JM. Percutaneous stone removal with the patient in a flank position. J Urol. 1994;151(3):686–8.
33. Ibarluzea G, Scoffone CM, Cracco CM, Poggio M, Porpiglia F, Terrone C, et al. Supine Valdivia and modified lithotomy position for simultaneous anterograde and retrograde endourological access. BJU Int. 2007;100(5):233–6.
34. Bach C, Goyal A, Kumar P, Kachrilas S, Papatsoris AG, Buchholz N, Masood J. The Barts 'flank-free' modified supine position for percutaneous nephrolithotomy. Urol Int. 2012;89(3):365–8.
35. Shoma AM, Eraky I, El-Kenawy MR, El-Kappany HA. Percutaneous nephrolithotomy in the supine position: technical aspects and functional outcome compared with the prone technique. Urology. 2002;60(3):388–92.
36. DeSio M, Autorino R, Quarto G, Calabrò F, Damiano R, Giugliano F, et al. Modified supine versus prone position in percutaneous nephrolithotomy for renal stones treatable with a single percutaneous access: a prospective randomized trial. Eur Urol. 2008;54:196–203.
37. Yokoyama M, Ueda W, Hirakawa M, Yamamoto H. Hemodynamic effect of the prone position during anesthesia. Acta Anaesthesiol Scand. 1991;35:741–4.
38. Poon KS, Wu KC, Chen CC, Fung ST, Lau AW, Huang CC, Wu RS. Hemodynamic changes during spinal surgery in the prone position. Acta Anaesthesiol Taiwanica. 2008;46(2):57–60.
39. Lee LA, Roth S, Posner KL, Cheney FW, Caplan RA, Newman NJ, et al. The American Society of Anesthesiologists Postoperative Visual Loss Registry: analysis of 93 spine surgery cases with postoperative visual loss. Anesthesiology. 2006;105:652–9.
40. Ho VT, Newman NJ, Song S, Ksiazek S, Roth S. Ischemic optic neuropathy following spine surgery. J Neurosurg Anesthesiol. 2005;17:38–44.
41. Epstein NE. Perioperative visual loss following prone spinal surgery: a review. Surg Neurol Int. 2016;7(Suppl 13):S347–60.
42. Nasseh H, Pourreza F, Saberi A, Kazemnejad E, Kalantari BB, Falahatkar S. Focal neuropathies following percutaneous nephrolithotomy (PCNL)—preliminary study. Ger Med Sci. 2013;11:Doc07.
43. Agah M, Ghasemi M, Roodneshin F, Radpay B, Moradian S. Prone position in percutaneous nephrolithotomy and postoperative visual loss. Urol J. 2011;8(3):191–6.
44. Michel MS, Trojan L, Rassweiler JJ. Complications in percutaneous nephrolithotomy. Eur Urol. 2007;51:899–906.

45. Gallucci M, Fortunato P, Schettini M, Vincenzoni A. Management of hemorrhage after percutaneous renal surgery. J Endourol. 1998;12:509–12.
46. Kaye KW, Clayman RV. Tamponade nephrostomy catheter for percutaneous nephrostolithotomy. Urology. 1986;27:441–5.
47. Srivastava A, Singh KJ, Suri A, Dubey D, Kumar A, Kapoor R, et al. Vascular complications after percutaneous nephrolithotomy: are there any predictive factors? Urology. 2005;66(1):38–40.
48. Rastinehad AR, Andonian S, Smith AD, Siefel DN. Management of hemorrhagic complications associated with percutaneous nephrolithotomy. J Endourol. 2009;23(10):1763–7.
49. Gupta R, Kumar A, Kapoor R, Srivastava A, Mandhani A. Prospective evaluation of safety and efficacy of the supracostal approach for percutaneous nephrolithotomy. BJU Int. 2002;90(9):809–13.
50. Radecka E, Brehmer M, Holmgren K, Magnusson A. Complications associated with percutaneous nephrolithotripsy: supra- versus subcostal access. A retrospective study. Acta Radiol. 2003;44(4):447–51.
51. Öztürk H. Gastrointestinal system complications in percutaneous nephrolithotomy: a systematic review. J Endourol. 2014;28(11):1256–67.
52. Morse RM, Spirnak JP, Resnick MI. Iatrogenic colon and rectal injuries associated with urological intervention: report of 14 patients. J Urol. 1988;140(1):101–3.
53. Neustein P, Barbaric ZL, Kaufman JJ. Nephrocolic fistula: a complication of percutaneous nephrostolithotomy. J Urol. 1986;135(3):571–3.
54. Vallancien G, Capdeville R, Veillon B, Charton M, Brisset JM. Colonic perforation during percutaneous nephrolithotomy. J Urol. 1985;134:1185–7.
55. Desai AC, Jain S, Benway BM, Grubb RL 3rd, Picus D, Figenshau RS. Splenic injury during percutaneous nephrolithotomy: a case report with novel management technique. J Endourol. 2010;24(4):541–5.
56. Shah HN, Hegde SS, Mahajan AP, Sodha H, Shah R, Bansal M. Splenic injury: rare complication of percutaneous nephrolithotomy: report of two cases with review of literature. J Endourol. 2007;21:919–22.
57. Seitz C, Desai M, Häcker A, Hakenberg OW, Liatsikos E, Nagele U, Tolley D. Incidence, prevention, and management of complications following percutaneous nephrolitholapaxy. Eur Urol. 2012;61(1):146–58.
58. Kyriazis I, Panagopoulos V, Kallidonis P, Özsoy M, Vasilas M, Liatsikos E. Complications in percutaneous nephrolithotomy. World J Urol. 2015;33(8):1069–77.
59. Rao PN. Fluid absorption during urological endoscopy. Br J Urol. 1987;60(2):93–9.
60. Hahn RG. Fluid absorption in endoscopic surgery. Br J Anaesth. 2006;96(1):8–20.
61. Kukreja RA, Desai MR, Sabnis RB, Patel SH. Fluid absorption during percutaneous nephrolithotomy: does it matter? J Endourol. 2002;16(4):221–4.
62. Guzelburc V, Balasar M, Colakogullari M, Guven S, Kandemir A, Ozturk A, et al. Comparison of absorbed irrigation fluid volumes during retrograde intrarenal surgery and percutaneous nephrolithotomy for the treatment of kidney stones larger than 2 cm. Springerplus. 2016;5(1):1707.
63. Draga RO, Kok ET, Sorel MR, Bosch RJ, Lock TM. Percutaneous nephrolithotomy: factors associated with fever after the first postoperative day and systemic inflammatory response syndrome. J Endourol. 2009;23(6):921–7.
64. O'Keeffe NK, Mortimer AJ, Sambrook PA, Rao PN. Severe sepsis following percutaneous or endoscopic procedures for urinary tract stones. Br J Urol. 1993;72:277–83.
65. Negrete-Pulido O, Gutierrez-Aceves J. Management of infectious complications in percutaneous nephrolithotomy. J Endourol. 2009;23(10):1757–62.
66. Korets R, Graversen JA, Kates M, Mues AC, Gupta M. Post-percutaneous nephrolithotomy systemic inflammatory response: a prospective analysis of preoperative urine, renal pelvic urine and stone cultures. J Urol. 2011;186(5):1899–903.
67. Stoller ML, Wolf JS Jr, St Lezin MA. Estimated blood loss and transfusion rates associated with percutaneous nephrolithotomy. J Urol. 1994;152(6 Pt 1):1977–81.
68. Kukreja R, Desai M, Patel S, Bapat S, Desai M. Factors affecting blood loss during percutaneous nephrolithotomy: prospective study. J Endourol. 2004;18(8):715–22.
69. Turna B, Nazli O, Demiryoguran S, Mammadov R, Cal C. Percutaneous nephrolithotomy: variables that influence hemorrhage. Urology. 2007;69(4):603–7.
70. de la Rosette J, Assimos D, Desai M, Gutierrez J, Lingeman J, Scarpa R, et al.; CROES PCNL Study Group. The Clinical Research Office of the Endourological Society Percutaneous Nephrolithotomy Global Study: indications, complications, and outcomes in 5803 patients. J Endourol. 2011;25(1):11–7.
71. Yamaguchi A, Skolarikos A, Buchholz NP, Chomón GB, Grasso M, Saba P, et al.; CROES PCNL Study Group. Operating times and bleeding complications in percutaneous nephrolithotomy: a comparison of tract dilation methods in 5,537 patients in the Clinical Research Office of the Endourological Society Percutaneous Nephrolithotomy Global Study. J Endourol. 2011;25(6):933–9.
72. Srivastava A, Singh S, Dhayal IR, Rai P. A prospective randomized study comparing the four tract dilation methods of percutaneous nephrolithotomy. World J Urol. 2017;35(5):803–7.
73. Gönen M, Istanbulluoglu OM, Cicek T, Ozturk B, Ozkardes H. Balloon dilatation versus Amplatz dilatation for nephrostomy tract dilatation. J Endourol. 2008;22:901–4.
74. Amjadi M, Zolfaghari A, Elahian A, Tavoosi A. Percutaneous nephrolithotomy in patients with previous open nephrolithotomy: one-shot versus telescopic technique for tract dilatation. J Endourol. 2008;22:423–5.
75. Whitehurst L, Jones P, Somani BK. Mortality from kidney stone disease (KSD) as reported in the literature over the last two decades: a systematic review. World J Urol. 2019;37(5):759–76.

13 Microperc

Stefano Paolo Zanetti, Matteo Fontana, and Emanuele Montanari

13.1 Introduction

Microperc is defined [1] as a modified percutaneous nephrolithotomy (PCNL) in which the percutaneous access to the pyelocalyceal system and the subsequent nephroscopy are performed in a single step using a dedicated 4.85 ch. instrument, the "all-seeing needle." This device was first presented in 2010 at the annual meeting of the American Urological Association in San Francisco as an innovative approach through which a vision-guided calyceal puncture could be achieved. The optical and technical specifications of the device were assessed, and the feasibility of the technique was demonstrated in a small cohort of patients [2]: the device allowed the visualization of the entire percutaneous tract during the puncture and could be used by the urologist to directly verify the access to the designated calyx, to assess its quality prior to dilation, and to position a guidewire under vision. In this series, the obtained tract was subsequently dilated and the percutaneous procedure performed as a traditional PCNL.

Shortly afterwards, this concept was extended and the possibility of performing the entire PCNL procedure using this miniaturized device was explored as the employment of this system allowed the surgeon to avoid many maneuvers related to two key stages of PCNL: tract dilation and stabilization. These steps, in addition to being time consuming and requiring fluoroscopic control, can be associated with inadvertent complications such as tract bleeding, calyceal infundibular tearing and pelvic perforation. Using a dedicated connector to vehiculate a 200 μm laser fiber and to allow pressurized irrigation, the safety and feasibility of this technique for the percutaneous treatment of kidney stones were confirmed by Mahesh Desai, and microperc was born. In his original series [1], 10 patients with a mean stone size of 14.3 mm were treated, and although no significant complications were recorded, a single conversion to miniPCNL was necessary for stone clearance. A stone-free rate of 88.9% at the 1 month follow-up was achieved.

These promising results compelled other groups to explore the possibilities and the indications for this peculiar technique, both in adult and pediatric patients. Since then, microperc has been used to treat small to medium-size stones, and despite being heavily criticized due to its inherent limitations, it has reached considerable diffusion, being performed in 28% of centers according to a recent survey by the European Association of Urology Section of Urolithiasis (EULIS) [3].

The objective of this chapter is to summarize the available evidence regarding the use of micro-percutaneous surgery for the treatment of renal stones, reviewing the core concepts, armamentarium, surgical technique, outcomes in

S. P. Zanetti · M. Fontana · E. Montanari (✉)
Fondazione IRCCS Ca' Granda Ospedale Maggiore Policlinico, Department of Urology, Università degli Studi di Milano, Milan, Italy

G. Zeng, K. Sarica (eds.), *Percutaneous Nephrolithotomy*,
https://doi.org/10.1007/978-981-15-0575-1_13

terms of safety and efficacy in comparison with other techniques, and the advantages and limitations of this approach, in order to identify its role in the current landscape of endourological treatments for urolithiasis.

13.2 The Microperc Concept

13.2.1 PCNL Pathophysiology and Tract Miniaturization

The assumption that reducing the caliber of the percutaneous access fosters less tissue damage and scarring, although still controversial, represents the core premise for PCNL miniaturization. Minimizing the breach in the renal parenchyma, and the related trauma caused by the dilation and the stabilization of the percutaneous tract, is advocated to reduce the risk of bleeding, certainly one of the main setbacks of PCNL. Indeed, as reported in the literature, a hemorrhagic complication requiring blood transfusion occurs in around 7% (range 0–20%) of patients who undergo percutaneous surgery for stones [4, 5]. Although many factors have been advocated to influence the risk of bleeding in PCNL, tract size appears to be primarily responsible for this type of complication, and small-tract PCNL techniques are associated with a lower hemoglobin drop and transfusion rate [6], maintaining comparable stone-free rates.

The miniaturization of the percutaneous tract caliber affects the pathophysiology of PCNL in various ways [6, 7], including:

- Decreased risk of inadvertent damage to the pyelocalyceal system with easier access to smaller calyces, both during tract dilation and nephroscopy
- Reduced tract bleeding, often resulting in unclouded vision during nephroscopy
- Longer operation times due to the need for a fine laser lithotripsy, since fragment retrieval is not feasible through the downsized percutaneous sheath, and the choice of lithotripsy probes is restricted by the small operative channel of the scope
- Generally higher pressure in the renal pelvis during the procedure due to the limited irrigation fluid outflow
- Reduced need for prolonged postoperative urinary drainage and a higher rate of tubeless procedures, with possible lower postoperative patient discomfort and reduced need for analgesics
- Shorter hospitalization likely owing to fewer bleeding complications, reduced pain and shorter urinary drainage periods
- Better functional outcomes due to minimized parenchymal loss and tissue scarring even though further studies are warranted to demonstrate this point

13.2.2 Core Concepts

With this background, the creators of microperc have asked themselves whether they could eliminate the morbidity related to the percutaneous access by reducing its size to a minimum and by limiting the steps necessary for its establishment [1]. Microperc, which is performed through a very small tract with a one-step access by means of the puncture needle, incarnates this notion. For these reasons, the technique conceptually differs from other miniaturized PCNL techniques that duplicate standard PCNL but with the use of smaller instruments. It is important to point out that the term microperc not only illustrates the extremely reduced size of the access sheath but also refers to a specific set of operative concepts, techniques and instrumentation.

13.2.2.1 Advantages

In microperc, the concepts that have led to the birth of miniaturized PCNL are taken to extremes. The tract diameter is reduced to a minimum to cause the least trauma possible to the renal parenchyma. We know from studies regarding kidney needle biopsies that reducing the needle size by more than 16 gauge, which corresponds to the 4.85 ch of the all-seeing needle, produces no advantages in terms of blood loss [8, 9]. Although it has not been demonstrated, it is reasonable to assume that its effect on parenchymal loss is minimal when compared to large-caliber PCNL, particularly when multiple tracts are needed or when patients are submitted to repeated procedures over time. Moreover, the all-seeing needle, being so compact, minimizes the traumatic impact of nephroscopic exploration on the renal cavities, especially in pediatric patients and in cases of peculiar anatomical variations, narrow calyceal infundibula, or calyceal diverticula.

Through the microperc system, nephroscopic access to the renal cavities is achieved in a single step, avoiding the stages that are necessary in standard PCNL for the dilation and stabilization of the tract through the placement of a percutaneous sheath. These steps include many maneuvers, each of which is time-consuming, lengthens fluoroscopic time, increases tract bleeding and can be responsible for damage to the pyelocalyceal system, such as perforation or infundibular tearing. Moreover, the all-seeing needle allows the optical visualization of the entire percutaneous tract and could help to avoid inadvertent puncture of the surrounding organs. It can be used to directly confirm the access in the chosen calyx and to immediately assess its quality, enabling the urologist to correct it or to puncture a more appropriate site.

The technique avoids the retrograde transureteral route employed in the ureteroscopic approach for the treatment of renal stones, eliminating the risk of producing injuries to the ureter, that, although generally self-limiting, can be catastrophic and result in long-term consequences.

Since a tubeless procedure can be safely performed in the majority of cases and the need for a prolonged urinary drainage is minimal, patient discomfort is reduced and postoperative hospitalization is shorter than standard PCNL, with a length of stay of generally 24–48 h. Moreover, the need for a postoperative double-J stent is low [10], limiting the associated costs and morbidity.

13.2.2.2 Drawbacks

Nevertheless, this technique has many pitfalls that need to be addressed. Firstly, microperc optics, although acceptable, have limited resolutions compared to those of bigger nephroscopes or modern ureteroscopes, especially those with digital optical systems.

Due to the minimal caliber of the instrument's working channel, lithotripsy can only be performed through the energy vehiculated by a 200 μm laser fiber. Since the lapaxy of the stone fragments is not possible through the 4.85 ch sheath, fine stone fragmentation or complete dusting should be achieved through protracted laser lithotripsy, which is sometimes necessary to pause due to the cloudiness of the irrigation medium caused by the scarce irrigation. These limitations entail that prolonged operative time is one of the main drawbacks of this technique, limiting its application to small to medium-size stones only, as lithotripsy can be exceedingly time consuming for bigger stones.

Furthermore, the small caliber of the all-seeing needle implies a restriction in its movements during nephroscopy as the instrument can be easily bent and eventually broken. It must also be considered that flexible scopes cannot be employed during this procedure to explore the renal cavities and reach stones or scattered fragments in contrast to standard and miniPCNL. These limitations demand a careful planning and a precise realization of the tract in order to ensure easy access to the stone and limit the chances of its displacement during lithotripsy, potentially rendering the access ineffective. The conversion rate to miniPCNL due to the impossibility to visualize or reach the stone during the procedure, although generally lower than 10%, must be taken into consideration [10].

Finally, lacking a urinary drainage other than the ureteral catheter, it has been demonstrated that renal pelvic pressure during the procedure frequently exceeds the threshold that is considered safe for the risk of infectious complications, even though no clinical consequences have been observed [11].

13.3 Indications

The role of microperc in the panorama of stone treatment is not clearly defined by the European Association of Urology (EAU) Guidelines. In order to obtain the best results from this peculiar technique and to outline its possible indications, it is mandatory to optimize patient selection according to the available scientific evidence. The pioneer center for this technique, after analyzing the impact of various factors on the outcomes of the procedure, defined microperc as a promising treatment method for solitary renal stones with volume <1000 mm^3 and with low density (HU), regardless of stone location [12].

Considering the previously reported limitations of the technique, the stone size is an important variable to be taken into account while indicating and planning the procedure. Although even larger stones could technically be treated with microperc, it seems there is some consensus posing and adequate limit on 1.5–2 cm stones. Indeed, the attempt to treat bigger and harder stones would likely result in a longer, less meticulous lithotripsy, possibly leading to significant residual fragments. In case of softer stones, when a satisfactory dusting can be efficiently achieved, the size limit could be slightly exceeded without excessively prolonging the operation time. However, no evidence is available on this specific topic.

Once established the adequate stone size and density range, the specific cases in which microperc could be indicated have to be identified.

Given that only limited stone burden can be approached with this technique, microperc cannot be considered as an alternative to standard PCNL but could compete with ESWL or RIRS.

In all cases of ESWL or RIRS failure, when a percutaneous surgery would be advised, microperc is a safe and minimally invasive option: as mentioned before, since the miniaturization of the tract caliber is associated with less bleeding, it appears logic to use a micro-access when the stone burden permits it.

As a primary indication, microperc can be used when RIRS and ESWL are not feasible for unfavorable anatomical conditions, such as in case of stones in lower calyces with steep infundibular-pelvic angles or with infundibular stenosis, or when the retrograde approach is difficult or non-viable (i.e. ureteric stenosis, kinking, reimplantation or other congenital or acquired abnormalities of the urinary tract).

Furthermore, considering its minimally invasive profile, microperc is a suitable option in pediatric patients who require a percutaneous surgery for stones up to 15–20 mm.

One more possible role of microperc is its use as an ancillary procedure. When treating staghorn or complex stones, the creation of multiple tracts can help achieving a higher success rate, albeit at the cost of more frequent access-related complications. The association of a standard- or mini-access with one or more complementary micropercutaneous tracts could limit morbidity while maintaining a high success rate [13].

Another interesting possible application is the combination of microperc and RIRS in the micro-endoscopic combined intrarenal surgery (micro-ECIRS): although very scarce evidence is available on this topic, this procedure can be performed in selected cases [14].

Finally, going further the typical indication for kidney stones, some authors described the anecdotal use of the microperc set in other peculiar settings. A recent study reported the intraoperative postperfusion micro-nephrolithotomic treatment of a stone in a kidney allograft [15]. Another group assessed the feasibility of using the microperc set for the treatment of distal ureteral stones in women (micro-ureteroscopy, or mURS) [16]. Lastly, the creators of microperc described the use of the all-seeing needle to treat ureteric, bladder and urethral stones and even non-calculus diseases such as posterior urethral valves and vesicoureteric reflux [17].

To resume, microperc can be indicated:

- To treat stones smaller than 2 cm when a percutaneous approach is required due to previous ESWL or RIRS failure or because there are factors contraindicating these techniques
- To perform an ancillary access during other endourological procedures for stones such as RIRS, standard- or miniPCNL
- To perform a minimally invasive percutaneous treatment of kidney stones in pediatric patients
- To treat different conditions of the urinary tract taking advantage of the all-seeing needle

13.4 Microperc Armamentarium

The microperc set is manufactured by *PolyDiagnost* (Pfaffenhofen, Germany) and it is composed of a specific puncture needle, a microfiber optical system and a three-way connector [2].

The puncture needle comprises a needle shaft, a puncture stylet, an inner stylet and a Y-connector:

- The needle shaft, used as a working sheath during the procedure, has an outer diameter of 1.6 mm (4.85 ch/16 gauge), an inner diameter of 1.4 mm and a working length of 200 mm.
- The beveled-tip puncture stylet, having an outer diameter of 1.3 mm (3.9 ch/18 gauge) and an inner diameter of 1.05 mm, is inserted in the needle shaft and hosts the microfiber optic during the puncture, allowing the urologist to perform the maneuver under vision.
- The inner stylet, being radiopaque, can be used for fluoroscopic-guided puncture if necessary.
- The Y-connector can be used to maintain irrigation during access to the pyelocalyceal system.

The highly flexible microfiber optic has a nitinol outer cover and an integrated illumination bundle composed of 200 optic fibers. It has a diameter of 0.9 mm and a length of 275 mm, and it is characterized by a resolution of 10.000 pixels and a field of view of 120° in air and 105° in water. It can be inserted in both the puncture stylet and the shaft of the puncture needle, and its length can be adjusted inside the needle sheath via a slide adapter.

The three-way connector is attached at the proximal end of the needle shaft following the puncture (Fig. 13.1), allowing for the introduction of the microfiber optical system through its central port and a 200 μm laser fiber through one of the side ports. The remaining port is connected to an irrigation line that can either be attached to an irrigation pump or to a manually operated 20 mL syringe.

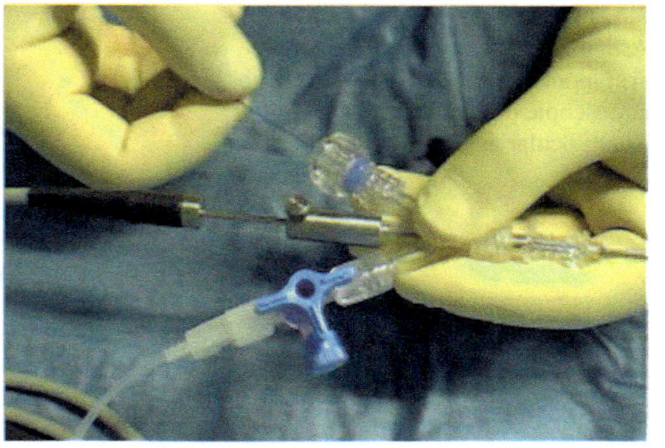

Fig. 13.1 The three-way connector with the microfiber optic and the laser fiber inserted, and the irrigation line connected

The optical fiber is connected via a zoom ocular and a light adapter to a standard endoscopic camera system and a xenon light source with a power of at least 100 W. The camera and light cables are held and suspended by an articulated multi-joint arm, which can be mounted laterally to the surgical table or on the endoscopic column (Fig. 13.2). This arm allows for easy positioning of the nonsterile components and relieves the surgeon of the weight of the optical and light cables.

A specifically designed 8 ch. sheath can be employed to perform the so-called mini-microperc [18]: this sheath enables an easier navigation during nephroscopy without bending the instrument and allows for the introduction of a 1.6 mm ultrasonic or ballistic probe, as well as fine forceps for fragments retrieval, in order to obtain a faster clearance of the stones. A 14 G angiocath has been alternatively used as a microsheath to stabilize the tract and to allow for the extraction of the all-seeing needle during the procedure [19]: this system can be useful in order to clean the optics and to balance the intrarenal pressure by draining the renal cavities. This method, however, other than being limited to pediatric patients due to the limited tract length

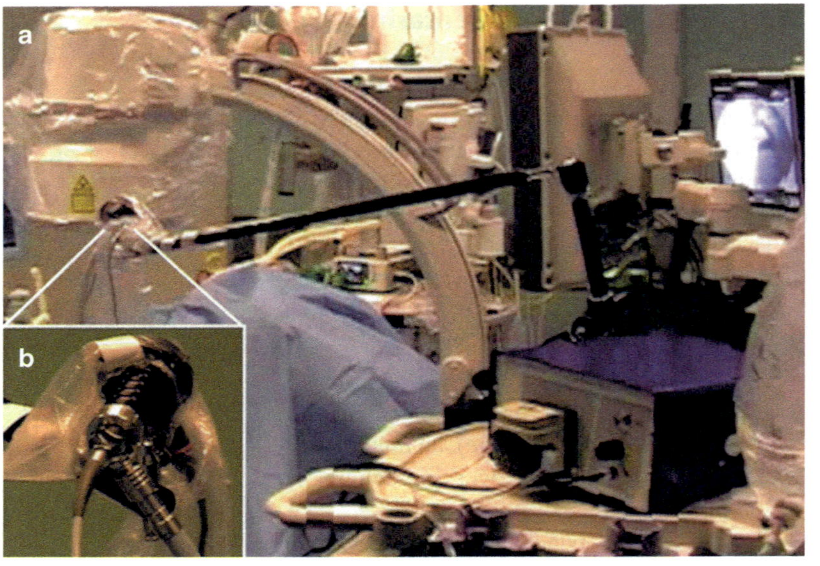

Fig. 13.2 (**a**) Articulated multi-joint arm mounted on the endoscopic column. (**b**) Zoom ocular and light adapter

that can be obtained with the angiocath partially contradicts the concept of the microperc.

13.5 Surgical Technique

Microperc, similarly to other percutaneous procedures for stones, is generally performed under general anesthesia although spinal anesthesia has been reported to be feasible: indeed, a retrospective comparative study of 116 patients conducted by Katarag and colleagues showed that the procedure has similar outcomes with both types of anesthesia [20].

Regarding patient positioning, the majority of surgeons perform the procedure in the prone position, even though, as demonstrated by a few reports [21–23] either the prone or supine positions can be chosen according to the surgeon's preference.

The procedure begins with the retrograde positioning of a 5–8 ch ureteral catheter in the renal pelvis, which is essential to drain the renal cavities during the procedure as no irrigation fluid can be evacuated through the miniaturized percutaneous sheath. Moreover, it can be used to assist the puncture by means of the distension of the pyelocalyceal system and the injection of contrast medium.

Afterwards, the carefully selected calyx is punctured with the assembled all-seeing needle. This allows for the optical visualization of the entire percutaneous tract and can assist in the evaluation of the quality of the access to the pyelocalyceal system. The puncture can be performed under ultrasonographic or fluoroscopic guidance, or using both control modalities in conjunction.

Subsequently, the beveled-tip puncture stylet is removed together with the microfiber optic, and the three-way connector is attached to the proximal end of the 4.85 ch. needle shaft, acting as a percutaneous sheath. The miniaturized optic is then introduced through the central port, and its length adjusted through the slide adapter. The irrigation line is connected to one of the lateral ports, and, as soon as the target stone is identified, a 200 μm laser fiber is inserted through the remaining lateral port of the connector as previously described (Fig. 13.3). Laser lithotripsy is performed, possibly using a dusting setting (i.e. high frequency, low energy, long pulse length), in order to obtain maximal stone pulverization and leave only very small fragments that can be spontaneously passed, since they cannot be extracted through the microperc sheath. Alternatively the 8 ch. sheath can be assembled in the mini-microperc configuration, as discussed, in order to enhance lithotripsy and enable litholapaxy to quicken the procedure.

Although a holmium:yttrium-aluminum-garnet (Ho:YAG) laser source is generally used, an initial report has been published in which the Thulium SuperPulse Fiber Laser (TSPFL) was utilized during microperc [24]: being able to reach very high frequencies, it could be employed as a more time-efficient way to dust larger stones and to limit fragment scattering.

Depending on the available laser, stone characteristics and the anatomy of the excretory system, complete pulverization can sometimes be difficult or impossible to obtain. In these cases, it is appropriate to reduce the caliber of the fragments as much as possible by performing a meticulous lithotripsy in an attempt to avoid conversion to mini- or standard PCNL.

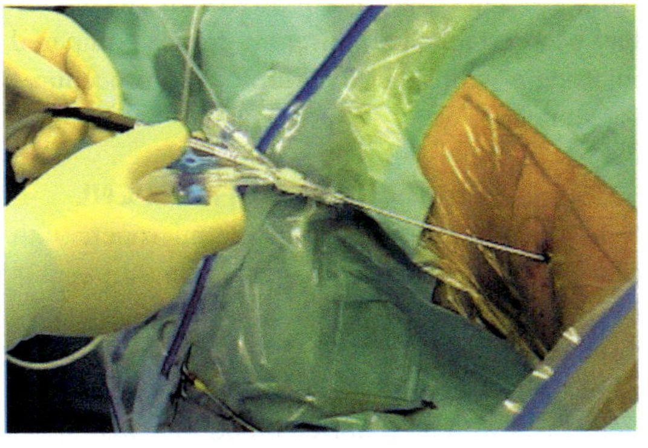

Fig. 13.3 The all-seeing needle with the three-way connector in the operative setting

Occasionally, stone fragments can migrate to sites that are not safe to reach from the percutaneous access without running the risk of bending and breaking the instrument as the small-caliber all-seeing needle requires very precise and delicate movements. In these cases, stone migration may require conversion to a larger caliber PCNL or performing a retrograde access (RIRS): once again, to avoid this possible complication, it is essential to perform lithotripsy methodically and to maintain adequate vision during the entire procedure. The vision provided by the microfiber optic is not comparable to the quality offered by standard or miniPCNL optics due to technical limitations, but it is sufficient, in standard situations, to comfortably and safely perform the procedure (Fig. 13.4).

It is also important to periodically check the emission of irrigation fluid through the ureteral catheter in order to maintain low intrarenal pressures, this being the only drainage route for the renal cavities. Once lithotripsy is completed, the all-seeing needle is removed, leaving a millimetric skin incision.

The placement of a nephrostomy tube is generally not necessary; postoperatively, the ureteral catheter, usually kept in place for 24 h, assures drainage. Optionally, considering the patient's

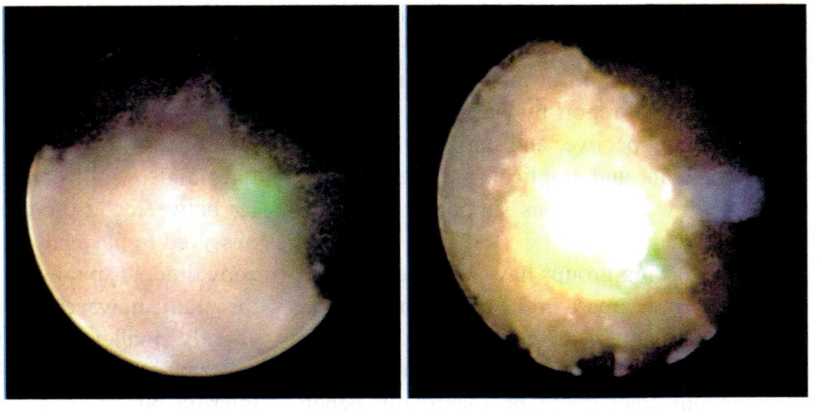

Fig. 13.4 Endoscopic vision during microperc

characteristics and in all the cases in which a satisfactory dusting is not obtainable, a double-J ureteral stent should be placed at the end of the procedure to prevent a possible postoperative renal colic and the related complications.

13.6 Reported Outcomes

13.6.1 Microperc Series

In the original microperc series published by M. Desai and colleagues in 2011 [1], 10 patients with a mean stone diameter of 14.3 mm were treated without any recorded blood transfusion or postoperative complication and with a mean (±SD) hospital stay of 2.3 (±1.2) days. In a single case, conversion to miniPCNL was necessary due to intraoperative bleeding and subsequent poor vision. In the remaining nine patients, the authors reported a stone-free rate of 88.9% 1 month after the procedure.

Since then, many other microperc series have been published by different groups (Table 13.1) [10, 12, 25–28]. The mean stone size of the patients treated in these studies was inferior to 20 mm, with a reported mean operative time of approximately 60 min and a mean hospital stay of 1–2 days. The obtained stone-free rates ranged from 82 to 96% with complication rates varying from 6 to 17% although most of the reported complications were low grade (Clavien ≤2). The need for a blood transfusion was generally low and the conversion rate to mini- or standard PCNL ranged from 4 to 22%. Although these results are seemingly optimal, all of the cited studies, apart from the original report by Desai and colleagues [1], were retrospective, and both the number of treated patients and implicated centers are too small to draw conclusions supported by a high level of evidence.

Other working groups have analyzed the possible role of microperc in the treatment of stones smaller than 20 mm in the pediatric population (Table 13.2) in which the miniaturization of the percutaneous tract could be maximally beneficial [23, 29–32]. In these studies the reported outcomes were similar to the adult series. In particular, the mean operation time ranged from 51 to 75 min and the mean hospital stay from 2 to 4 days. Complication rates varied from 6 to 30% with a high predominance of low-grade complications (Clavien ≤2); the hemoglobin drop was minimal with no reported transfusions in any of the studies. The stone-free rates ranged from 80 to 100% and the conversion rate to other techniques varied from 5 to 20%. Once again, these results appear to be promising but, because they include only small series, can't support unquestionable conclusions.

13.6.2 Comparison with Other Techniques

Once the safety and feasibility of the technique had been established, different groups compared microperc with other endourological procedures for stones.

13.6.2.1 Comparison with miniPCNL

Some researchers have compared microperc with miniPCNL. A retrospective study on 98 patients by Tok and colleagues [33] compared these techniques in patients with 10–20 mm lower calyceal stones, showing similar stone-free and complications rates with no reported blood transfusions in both groups. However, microperc was associated with less blood loss, shorter operation and fluoroscopy times, shorter hospital stays and higher tubeless rates.

Similar results have been described in pediatric populations. A retrospective study of 119 pediatric patients from three referral centers [34] compared microperc and miniPCNL for 10–20 mm stones: operation times, success rates and overall complication rates were similar between the procedures, but microperc was observed to have advantages in terms of fluoroscopy time, hospital stay and hemoglobin drop. In this study, however, microperc was employed for slightly smaller stones than miniPCNL. Another paper by Dundar et al. [35], comparing mini- and microPCNL in pediatric patients with stones smaller than 20 mm, confirmed similar success rates for the two techniques with advantages in

Table 13.1 Published series of microperc

Authors	Treated renal units, *n*.	Stone size, mean ± SD (range)	Anatomic abnormalities	Operative time (min), mean ± SD (range)	Fluoroscopy time (s), mean ± SD (range)	Conversion to mini/ standardPCNL *n*. (%)	Peroperative DJ stent placement, *n*. (%)	Hospital stay, mean ± SD (range)	Hb drop (mg/dL), mean ± SD (range)	Transfusions, *n*. (%)	Postoperative complications, *n*. (%) and details (Clavien score)	Postoperative DJ placement for colic, *n*. (%)	Stone clearance, *n*. (%)
Desai, 2011 [1]	10	14.3 ± 6.3 mm	1 ectopic kidney	Not reported	Not reported	1 (10)	4 (40)	2.3 ± 1.2 days	1.4 ± 1	0 (0)	0 (0)	0 (0)	Complete in 8/9 (88.9) completed with microperc; CIRF in 1/9 (11.1); completed with microperc
Piskin, 2012 [25]	9	12.8 mm (7–18)	Not reported	108 (60–130)	Not reported	2 (22.2)	4 (44.4)	2.6 days (1–3)	Not reported	Not reported	1 (14.3): 1 RC treated conservatively (I)	0 (0)	Complete in 6/7 (85.7); completed with microperc; 4 mm residual fragment in 1/7 (14.3)
Tepeler, 2013 [26]	21	17.8 ± 5.9 mm (9–29)	Not reported	62.8 ± 25.2 (30–100)	150.5 ± 92.8 (20–320)	1 (4.8)	Not reported	37.5 ± 14.4 h (14–76)	0.8 ± 0.6 (0.1–2.3)	0 (0)	2 (9.5): 1 UTI (II), 1 RC with DJ placement (IIIa)	1 (4.7)	Complete in 18 (85.7); CIRF in 1 (4.8)
Armagan, 2013 [27]	30	17.9 ± 5 mm (10–30)	1 horseshoe kidney; 1 pelvic kidney, 1 Kyphoscoliosis	63.5 ± 36.8 (20–200)	150.5 ± 90.4 (45–360)	3 (10)	Not reported	35.5 ± 18.6 h (14–96)	1.1 ± 0.8 (0–2.8)	0 (0)	5 (16.6): 2 RC treated conservatively (I), 2 steinstrasse with DJ placement (IIIa), 1 extravasation with drain placement (IIIB)	2 (6.7)	Complete in 25 (83); CIRF in 3 (10)
Hatipoglu, 2014 [10]	140	15.1 ± 5.15 mm (6–32)	1 horseshoe kidney; 1 pelvic kidney, 1 Kyphoscoliosis	55.76 ± 30.83 (20–200)	107.4 ± 79.07 (0–360)	12 (8.57)	9 (6.43)	1.76 ± 0.65 days (1–4)	0.87 ± 0.84 (0–4.1)	1 (0.7)	20 (14.28): 7 RC treated conservatively (I), 3 UTI (II), 1 BT (II), 1 RC with DJ placement (IIIa), 2 steinstrasse with DJ placement (IIIa), 3 steinstrasse with DJ placement in pediatric pts. (IIIb), 3 extravasation with drain placement (IIIb)	6 (4.3)	Complete in 115 (82.14); CIRF in 17 (12.14)
Katarag, 2015 [28]	70	122 ± 83 mm^2 (27–450)	Not reported	40.6 ± 23.8 (10–150)	108.4 ± 72.6 (30–300)	Not reported	Not reported	27.5 ± 12.4 h (15–60)	0.95 ± 0.7 (0.1–1.5)	0 (0)	4 (5.7): 1 UTI (I), 3 RC with DJ placement (IIIa)	3 (4.3)	Complete in 67 (95.7)
Ganpule, 2016 [12]	139	1095 ± 1035 mm^3 (105–6650)	2 duplex systems, 1 pelvic kidney, 1 horseshoe kidney	50.15 ± 9.8 (35–85)	Not reported	9 (6.47)	Not reported	2.36 ± 0.85 (2–5)	0.63 ± 0.84 (0–3.7)	1 (0)	15 (11.53): 8 RC treated conservatively (I), 3 UTI (II), 4 RC with DJ placement (IIIa)	4 (3.1)	Complete in 119 (91.53)

CIRF clinically insignificant residual fragments, *RC* renal colic, *UTI* urinary tract infection

Table 13.2 Published series of microperc in the pediatric population

Authors	Treated renal units, *n*.	Stone size (mm), mean ± SD (range)	Anatomic abnormalities	Operative time (min), mean ± SD (range)	Fluoroscopy time, mean ± SD (range)	Conversion rate, *n*. (%)	Peroperative DJ stent placement, *n*. (%)	Hospital stay, mean ± SD (range)	Hb drop (mg/dL), mean ± SD (range)	Transfusions, *n*. (%)	Postoperative complications, *n*. (%) and details (Clavien score)	Postoperative DJ placement for colic, *n*. (%)	Stone clearance, *n*. (%)
Silay, 2013 [29]	19	14.8 ± 6.8 (7–32)	1 pelvic kidney	72.5	2.3 min	2 (10.5) converted to miniPCNL	4 (21)	1.8 ± 0.8 days (1–3)	0.1 ± 0.3 (0–1.1)	0 (0)	3 (15.7): 2 RC treated conservatively (I), 1 extravasation with drain placement (IIIb)	0 (0)	Complete in 17 (89.5), CIRF in 2 (10.5)
Caione, 2014 [23]	5	15.0 (±2.5)	0	56 ± 23	Not reported	1 (20) converted to RIRS	1 (20)	2.4 ± 0.6 days	0.44	0 (0)	1 (10): 1 UTI (II)	0 (0)	Complete in 5 (100)
Bodakçi, 2015 [30]	25	13.45 ± 3.11 (10–20)	Not reported	51.45 ± 30.69 (20–120)	45.2 s (20–90)	Not reported	3 (12)	3.18 ± 1.77 (2–7)	0.46 ± 0.63	0 (0)	3 (6): 1 bleeding managed conservatively (I), 2 fever (I)	0 (0)	Complete in 23 (92)
Daggulli, 2016 [31]	40	16.5 (10–36)	0	75 (20–110)	3.7 min (1.2–7.9)	2 (5) converted to miniPCNL	11 (27.5)	3.8 ± 1.2 days (1–10)	0.7 ± 0.3 (0–1.7)	0 (0)	12 (30): 7 Clavien I, 3 Clavien II, 1 Clavien IIIa, 1 Clavien IIIb	0 (0)	Complete in 20 (80), CIRF in 3 (5)
Dede, 2016 [32]	24	13.5 ± 3.84	0	53.7 ± 10.35	1.4 ± 0.9 min	Not reported	4 (16.7)	2.5 ± 0.8	0.51 ± 0.34	0 (0)	6 (25): 4 RC treated conservatively (I), 2 fever (I)	0 (0)	Complete in 32 (83.3); CIRF in 2 (12.5)

CIRF clinically insignificant residual fragments, *RC* renal colic, *UTI* urinary tract infection favor of microperc concerning operation time, hospital stay, hemoglobin drop and transfusions rates.

Conversely, a recent survey paper by the European Association of Urology Section of Urolithiasis (EULIS) group, comparing all of the available endoscopic techniques for the treatment of kidney stones, reported lower stone-free rates and longer operative times for microperc than for all of the other techniques. However, this study confirmed the satisfactory safety profile and the low hemoglobin drop guaranteed by this procedure [36].

Considering the limitations of microperc in terms of stone burden, it appears more reasonable to compare it to retrograde intrarenal surgery (RIRS) or external shockwave lithotripsy (ESWL) rather than to other percutaneous procedures.

13.6.2.2 Comparison with RIRS

Sabnis and colleagues [37], in a prospective randomized study including 35 patients submitted to microperc and 35 patients submitted to RIRS, compared the two techniques for stones smaller than 15 mm. The stone clearance rate, operation time and hospital stay duration were similar in the two groups, but microperc was associated with a greater hemoglobin drop, more pain and higher analgesic requirement; conversely RIRS was associated with a higher rate of intraoperative double-J stenting and greater surgeon discomfort score. A prospective study by Cepeda et al. [38], comparing 17 RIRS and 18 microperc, obtained similar results in terms of success rate and hospital stay, which did not differ between the two groups with a significantly greater hemoglobin drop and longer operative time for microperc. Both procedures were confirmed to be safe, reporting only Clavien ≤ 2 complications for both techniques.

Other groups have compared microperc and RIRS focusing on lower calyceal kidney stones. Armagan and colleagues [39], in their study of a total of 127 procedures (59 RIRS, 68 microperc) for lower pole stones smaller than 20 mm, showed better results for microperc, which was associated with a higher stone-free rate, shorter operative time and lower complication rate than RIRS. However, RIRS was associated with a smaller hemoglobin drop and shorter fluoroscopy time and hospital stay. In a similar study including lower pole stones up to 15 mm, Kandemir et al. [40] did not describe any statistically significant differences between RIRS and microperc in terms of operative times, hemoglobin drops, stone-free and postoperative complications rates, but microperc was associated with longer fluoroscopy times and hospital stays. Another recent study [41] investigated this topic randomizing a total of 116 patients into two equal groups, submitted to microperc and flexible ureteroscopy (fURS). No significant differences between the groups were observed concerning hemoglobin drop, hospital stay or stone-free and complications rates, but fURS was associated with a slightly longer operative time.

Other researchers have compared microperc and RIRS in pediatric patients with stones smaller than 20 mm without observing any significant differences in terms of operative times, success rates and complication rates. They did, however, report longer fluoroscopy times for microperc [42, 43]. In one of these studies RIRS was associated with a shorter hospital stay and a higher rate of intraoperative double-J stenting [42].

13.6.2.3 Comparison with ESWL

Concerning ESWL, Hatipoglu and colleagues [44] retrospectively compared 37 microperc and 103 ESWL in a population of pediatric patients with radiopaque single kidney stones. The mean stone size was 11.32 mm in the SWL group and 14.78 mm in the microperc group ($P < 0.001$). Patients submitted to ESWL needed more retreatments to obtain satisfactory results, but experienced shorter hospital stays and a lower radiation times than patients who had undergone microperc. The complication rates were comparable between the two groups.

13.6.2.4 Key Messages

Microperc appears to be a good alternative to RIRS, ESWL and miniPCNL for stones smaller than 15–20 mm. This technique is characterized by satisfactory stone clearance rates, and lower bleeding and transfusion rates than miniPCNL. It seems to be associated with greater hemoglobin drops than RIRS without implicating a higher rate of blood transfusions: indeed, the absence of transfusions in many published studies is worth mentioning, this being a percutaneous technique.

It is important to emphasize the minimally invasive profile of microperc. As discussed, the complication rate is low in all of the published series. One of the most frequent postoperative complications is renal colic, which is managed by medical treatment or ureteral catheterization. This complication is likely a result of the low rate of double-J catheter placement at the end of the procedure and the possible presence of residual fragments following lithotripsy.

Despite the elevated intrapyelic pressures, urinary tract infections and fever rates were not relevant in any of the published series. Some authors have reported irrigation fluid extravasation, leading to the need for percutaneous drainage [10, 27, 29]: this complication could be due to the rise in pressure in cases of prolonged surgery or impacted stones. Although the rate of this complication is minimal, it is advisable to prevent intrapyelic hyperpressure by always placing a ureteral catheter, periodically checking its functionality, and limiting operative times.

As already stressed, we must take into account that the reported series have been published by just a few centers with extensive experience with this technique and high-quality evidence in still lacking.

More prospective randomized controlled comparative studies are required to be able to properly define the role of microperc in the current panorama of stone treatment.

However, the versatility of this system and its applicability in many different situations make it very attractive for the skilled endourologist.

References

1. Desai MR, Sharma R, Mishra S, Sabnis RB, Stief C, Bader M. Single-step percutaneous nephrolithotomy (microperc): the initial clinical report. J Urol. 2011;186:140–5.
2. Bader MJ, Gratzke C, Seitz M, Sharma R, Stief CG, Desai M. The "all-seeing needle": initial results of an optical puncture system confirming access in percutaneous nephrolithotomy. Eur Urol. 2011;59:1054–9.
3. Zanetti SP, Boeri L, Catellani M, Gallioli A, Trinchieri A, Sarica K, Montanari E. Retrograde intrarenal surgery (RIRS), regular and small sized percutaneous nephrolithotomy (PCNL) in daily practice: European Association of Urology Section of Urolithiasis (EULIS) Survey. Arch Ital di Urol e Androl. 2016;88:212.
4. de la Rosette JJMCH, Assimos D, Desai M, Gutierrez J, Lingeman J, Scarpa R, Tefekli A. The Clinical Research Office of the Endourological Society Percutaneous Nephrolithotomy Global Study: indications, complications, and outcomes in 5803 patients. J Endourol. 2011;25:11–7.
5. Seitz C, Desai M, Häcker A, Hakenberg OW, Liatsikos E, Nagele U, Tolley D. Incidence, prevention, and management of complications following percutaneous nephrolitholapaxy. Eur Urol. 2012;61:146–58.
6. Ruhayel Y, Tepeler A, Dabestani S, et al. Tract sizes in miniaturized percutaneous nephrolithotomy: a systematic review from the European Association of Urology Urolithiasis Guidelines Panel [figure presented]. Eur Urol. 2017;72:220–35.
7. Heinze A, Gozen AS, Rassweiler J. Tract sizes in percutaneous nephrolithotomy. Curr Opin Urol. 2019;29:118–23.
8. Gazelle GS, Haaga JR, Rowland DY. Effect of needle gauge, level of anticoagulation, and target organ on bleeding associated with aspiration biopsy. Radiology. 1992;183:509–13.
9. Mai J, Yong J, Dixson H, Makris A, Aravindan A, Suranyi MG, Wong J. Is bigger better? A retrospective analysis of native renal biopsies with 16 gauge versus 18 gauge automatic needles. Nephrology. 2013;18:525–30.
10. Hatipoglu NK, Tepeler A, Buldu I, et al. Initial experience of micro-percutaneous nephrolithotomy in the treatment of renal calculi in 140 renal units. Urolithiasis. 2014;42:159–64.
11. Tepeler A, Akman T, Silay MS, Akcay M, Ersoz C, Kalkan S, Armagan A, Sarica K. Comparison of intrarenal pelvic pressure during micro-percutaneous nephrolithotomy and conventional percutaneous nephrolithotomy. Urolithiasis. 2014;42:275–9.
12. Ganpule A, Chhabra JS, Kore V, Mishra S, Sabnis R, Desai M. Factors predicting outcomes of micropercutaneous nephrolithotomy: results from a large single-centre experience. BJU Int. 2016;117:478–83.
13. Buldu İ, Tepeler A, Karatağ T, İnan R, Armağan A, İstanbulluoğlu O. Combined micro-and standard percutaneous nephrolithotomy for complex renal calculi. Turk Urol Derg. 2016;42:150–4.
14. Cossu M, Poggio M, Fiori C, Serra N, Manfredi M, Cattaneo G, Bertolo R, Porpiglia P. Micro-ECIRS (Endoscopic Combined Intrarenal Surgery) for kidney stones: our initial experience. Eur Urol Suppl. 2014;13:eV3.

15. Favi E, Raison N, Zanetti S, Sampogna G, Montanari E, Ferraresso M. Intra-operative postperfusion micronephrolithotomy for renal allograft lithiasis: a case report. Transplant Proc. 2018;50:3950–3.
16. Caballero-Romeu J-P, Galán-Llopis J-A, Pérez-Fentes D, Budia-Alba A, Cepeda-Delgado M, Palmero-Marti J-L, Cansino-Alcaide J-R, Caballero-Pérez P, Ibarluzea-Gonzalez G. Assessment of the effectiveness, safety, and reproducibility of micro-ureteroscopy in the treatment of distal ureteral stones in women: a multicenter prospective study. J Endourol. 2016;30:1185–93.
17. Ganpule A, Chhabra JS, Sudharsan SB, Jairath A, Vijaykumar M, Sabnis R, Desai MR. Extending indications of micropercutaneous nephrolithotomy: it is not just about cracking stones. Arab J Urol. 2017;15:17–23.
18. Sabnis RB, Ganesamoni R, Ganpule AP, Mishra S, Jagtap J, Desai M, Vyas J. Current role of microperc in the management of small renal calculi. Indian J Urol. 2013;29:214.
19. Penbegul N, Bodakci MN, Hatipoglu NK, Sancaktutar AA, Atar M, Cakmakci S, Yildirim K. Microsheath for microperc: 14-gauge angiocath. J Endourol. 2013;27:835–9.
20. Karatag T, Tepeler A, Buldu I, Akcay M, Tosun M, Istanbulluoglu MO, Armagan A. Is micro-percutaneous nephrolithotomy surgery technically feasible and efficient under spinal anesthesia? Urolithiasis. 2015;43:249–54.
21. Pérez-Fentes D, Blanco-Gómez B, García-Freire C. Nefrolitotomía micropercutánea: una nueva opción terapéutica para la litiasis renal pediátrica. Actas Urol Esp. 2014;38:483–7.
22. Ramón de Fata F, García-Tello A, Andrés G, Redondo C, Meilán E, Gimbernat H, Angulo JC. Comparative study of retrograde intrarenal surgery and micropercutaneous nephrolithotomy in the treatment of intermediate-sized kidney stones. Actas Urol Esp. 2014;38:576–83.
23. Caione P, De Dominicis M, Collura G, Matarazzo E, Nappo SG, Capozza N. Microperc for pediatric nephrolithiasis: technique in Valdivia-modified position. Eur J Pediatr Surg. 2014;25:94–9.
24. Martov AG, Andronov A, Dutov S, Traxer O. Thulium SuperPulse Fiber Laser (TSPFL) for micro-PCNL. Eur Urol Suppl. 2019;18:e2251.
25. Piskin MM, Guven S, Kilinc M, Arslan M, Goger E, Ozturk A. Preliminary, favorable experience with microperc in kidney and bladder stones. J Endourol. 2012;26:1443–7.
26. Tepeler A, Armagan A, Sancaktutar AA, Silay MS, Penbegul N, Akman T, Hatipoglu NK, Ersoz C, Erdem MR, Akcay M. The role of microperc in the treatment of symptomatic lower pole renal calculi. J Endourol. 2013;27:13–8.
27. Armagan A, Tepeler A, Silay MS, Ersoz C, Akcay M, Akman T, Erdem MR, Onol SY. Micropercutaneous nephrolithotomy in the treatment of moderate-size renal calculi. J Endourol. 2013;27:177–81.
28. Karatag T, Buldu I, Inan R, Istanbulluoglu MO. Is micropercutaneous nephrolithotomy technique really efficacicous for the treatment of moderate size renal calculi? Yes. Urol Int. 2015;95:9–14.
29. Silay MS, Tepeler A, Atis G, Sancaktutar AA, Piskin M, Gurbuz C, Penbegul N, Ozturk A, Caskurlu T, Armagan A. Initial report of microperc in the treatment of pediatric nephrolithiasis. J Pediatr Surg. 2013;48:1578–83.
30. Bodakçi MN, Penbegul N, Dağgülli M, Dede O, Utangaç MM, Hatipoglu NK, Sancaktutar AA. Ultrasound-guided micropercutaneous nephrolithotomy in pediatric patients with kidney stones. Int J Urol. 2015;22:773–7.
31. Dağgülli M, Utanğaç MM, Dede O, Bodakçi MN, Penbegül N, Hatipoğlu NK, Atar M, Bozkurt Y, Sancaktutar AA. Micro-percutaneous nephrolithotomy in the treatment of pediatric nephrolithiasis: a single-center experience. J Pediatr Surg. 2016;51:626–9.
32. Dede O, Sancaktutar AA, Baş O, et al. Micro-percutaneous nephrolithotomy in infants: a single-center experience. Urolithiasis. 2016;44:173–7.
33. Tok A, Akbulut F, Buldu I, Karatag T, Kucuktopcu O, Gurbuz G, Istanbulluoglu O, Armagan A, Tepeler A, Tasci AI. Comparison of microperc and mini-percutaneous nephrolithotomy for medium-sized lower calyx stones. Urolithiasis. 2016;44:155–9.
34. Karatag T, Tepeler A, Silay MS, Bodakci MN, Buldu I, Daggulli M, Hatipoglu NK, Istanbulluoglu MO, Armagan A. A comparison of 2 percutaneous nephrolithotomy techniques for the treatment of pediatric kidney stones of sizes 10-20 mm: microperc vs miniperc. Urology. 2015;85:1015–8.
35. Dundar G, Gokce G, Gokcen K, Korgali E, Asdemir A, Kaygusuz K. Microperc versus miniperc for treatment of renal stones smaller than 2 cm in pediatric patients. Urol J. 2016;13:2829–32.
36. Zanetti SP, Talso M, Palmisano F, et al. Comparison among the available stone treatment techniques from the first European Association of Urology Section of Urolithiasis (EULIS) Survey: do we have a queen? PLoS One. 2018;13:e0205159.
37. Sabnis RB, Ganesamoni R, Doshi A, Ganpule AP, Jagtap J, Desai MR. Micropercutaneous nephrolithotomy (microperc) vs retrograde intrarenal surgery for the management of small renal calculi: a randomized controlled trial. BJU Int. 2013;112:355–61.
38. Cepeda M, Amón JH, Mainez JA, De La Cruz B, Rodríguez V, Poza M, Alonso D, Martínez-Sagarra JM. Retrograde intrarenal surgery and micro-percutaneous nephrolithotomy for renal lithiasis smaller than 2 cm. Eur Urol Suppl. 2017;16:e737.
39. Armagan A, Karatag T, Buldu I, Tosun M, Basibuyuk I, Istanbulluoglu MO, Tepeler A. Comparison of flexible ureterorenoscopy and micropercutane-

ous nephrolithotomy in the treatment for moderately size lower-pole stones. World J Urol. 2015;33: 1827–31.
40. Kandemir A, Guven S, Balasar M, Sonmez MG, Taskapu H, Gurbuz R. A prospective randomized comparison of micropercutaneous nephrolithotomy (microperc) and retrograde intrarenal surgery (RIRS) for the management of lower pole kidney stones. World J Urol. 2017;35:1771–6.
41. Jiang K, Chen H, Yu X, Chen Z, Ye Z, Yuan H. The "all-seeing needle" micro-PCNL versus flexible ureterorenoscopy for lower calyceal stones of ≤ 2 cm. Urolithiasis. 2019;47(2):201–6.
42. Baş O, Dede O, Aydogmus Y, Utangaç M, Yikilmaz TN, Damar E, Nalbant İ, Bozkurt ÖF. Comparison of retrograde intrarenal surgery and micro-percutaneous nephrolithotomy in moderately sized pediatric kidney stones. J Endourol. 2016;30:765–70.
43. Sen H, Seckiner I, Bayrak O, Dogan K, Erturhan S. A comparison of micro-PERC and retrograde intrarenal surgery results in pediatric patients with renal stones. J Pediatr Urol. 2017;13:619.e1–5.
44. Hatipoglu NK, Sancaktutar AA, Tepeler A, et al. Comparison of shockwave lithotripsy and microperc for treatment of kidney stones in children. J Endourol. 2013;27:1141–6.

Ultra-Mini PCNL (UMP) 14

Janak D. Desai

The urological surgeon has been performing PCNL for stone removal for the last four decades. In the early days, the instruments were of large caliber and stone-disintegrating devices were not very advanced. Several advances in medical instruments like endoscopes, endo-vision cameras and stone-breaking devices happened in late 1970s and early 1980s, and the endoscopic stone removal techniques became more standardized. These key hole surgeries were hugely dependent on advances in fiberoptics and imaging equipment like fluoroscopy and high-resolution sonography. Lasers as stone-breaking energy paved the way for flexible instrumentation that are now used not only for diagnosis but for stone disintegration also. Miniaturized techniques of mini-PCNL and UMP could be developed because very thin laser fibers could be passed through this extremely small caliber instruments (Fig. 14.1).

PCNL is efficacious for stone removal but is associated with morbidity in some situations. The most common problem of bleeding is directly proportional to track size [1]. The question asked was "How can we make PCNL safer?" The natural fall out was to make instruments that needed a much smaller track size and, thereby, reduce the most common complication of bleeding. In 2010, Janak Desai and investigators in India developed what they called ultra-mini-PCNL (UMP). The first articles on UMP were published in 2013 [2, 3]. UMP consists of a telescope of 1 mm size and a sheath size of either 11 Fr or 13 Fr. The sheath's design is special that enables to create a vortex of fluid in the pelvicalyceal system and that removes fragments that are already created by laser disintegration. This moves the stone fragments from high pressure in the PC system to the low pressure area which is the lumen of the sheath [2].

Whilst doing standard PCNL we observed that there was minimal bleeding when we used the initial Teflon dilators—upto 14–16 Fr; the bleeding was seen when the dilation was stepped up and when a 18 Fr dilator was exchanged for the next 20 Fr dilator, we saw a sudden gush of blood in some situations. Therefore we concluded that the renal parenchyma could withstand a dilation upto about 14 Fr because of tissue elasticity; however, if the dilation was increased the possibility of lateral tear increased and that lead to bleeding. Therefore UMP has been designed to keep the largest instrument with a 13 Fr outer diameter. The telescope is 1 mm thick and has a resolution of 17,000 pixels. The inner sheath allows a laser fiber up to 365 μm and also irrigation of saline. The stones are disintegrated into very small particles, and they are pulled out by creating a vortex of fluid by injecting saline

Electronic Supplementary Material The online version of this chapter (https://doi.org/10.1007/978-981-15-0575-1_14) contains supplementary material, which is available to authorized users.

J. D. Desai (✉)
Samved Hospital, Ahmedabad, India

G. Zeng, K. Sarica (eds.), *Percutaneous Nephrolithotomy*,
https://doi.org/10.1007/978-981-15-0575-1_14

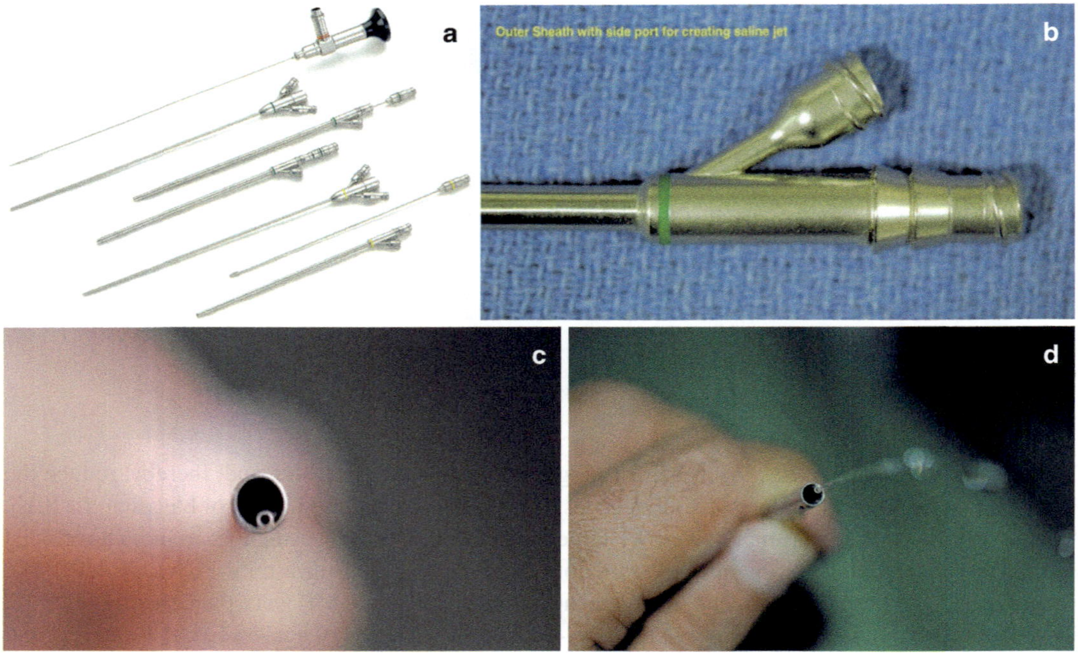

Fig. 14.1 UMP instruments. (**a**) Full ultra-mini-PCNL set consisting of 11 and 13 F shafts and dilatators as well as a miniaturized nephroscope. (**b**) Outer sheath with a side-port connecting to the waterjet tube inside. (**c**) View of waterjet tube inside the sheath. (**d**) Demonstration of the "waterjet" function. (Reproduced with permission of Schoelly Fiberoptics GmbH, Denzlingen, Germany & Dr. Janak Desai)

through the specially designed small tube, running parallel to the outer sheath (tube). There is no need of suction; however, if you want to pull out a clot, suction can be done by a 20 cc syringe (see Video 14.1).

The whirlpool can also be created by pushing saline from the previously placed ureteric catheter. The fluid will move from the high-pressure zone of the renal pelvicalyceal system to the outer sheath and will carry the fragments along with it. This vortex effect carrying the fragments towards the outer sheath can be seen in Video 14.2. In this video the endoscopic view is picked up by a flexible ureteroscope. UMP operation can be used for small and midsize stones up to 20 mm in size. It can also be used as a second puncture surgery when a small stone is in another calyx and we want to avoid a second large puncture (Table 14.1).

UMP is less expensive than RIRS because the use of consumables is limited and it can be finished in lesser time than RIRS.

RIRS and UMP are compared in Table 14.2 [4]. These statistics are only from a few users of UMP and need to be confirmed by other centers of the world.

Table 14.1 Transfusion rates in relation to sheath size in percutaneous nephrolithotomy [1]

Sheath size	No. of patients	Blood transfusion (*n* (%))
Small (18 Fr and below)	271	3 (1.1%)
Medium (24 Fr and 26 Fr)	1039	50 (4.8%)
Large (27 Fr, 28 Fr, and 30 Fr)	3533	208 (5.9%)
Largest (32 Fr, 33 Fr, and 34 Fr)	371	45 (12.1%)

14.1 Synopsis

UMP is a rather delicate technique and needs high level of surgeon experience before undertaking it. With the development of miniaturized PCNL, there is a revival of PCNL and investigators are trying to study the stone-free rates and complication rates of UMP and RIRS. We still need results from high-quality studies but initial data points out that UMP gives better stone free rates compared to RIRS, and the complication rates of UMP are lesser than standard PCNL.

The common complication of bleeding, which worries the surgeons doing standard PCNL, is reduced to a great extent. The need for placing a nephrostomy is also reduced to a great extent. This in turn reduces the post-operative pain and the patient can be discharged within 24 h [5, 6]. Larger access sheaths produce more bleeding and sometimes because of impaired vision the procedure needs to be terminated also [6, 7]. Investigators have already looked into the possibility of reduced bleeding if the track size is reduced [7].

For a large stone, the main bulk can be removed by standard PCNL, and the stone in an otherwise inaccessible calyx can be removed by UMP. This can help the surgeon prevent a second large puncture. Familiarity with the full spectrum of different endoscopic techniques facilitates a minimally invasive approach to the entire urinary tract.

As the instrumentation of treatment modalities available to the urologist has been increased, new debates regarding the indications for these options have developed. Currently, urologists face the challenge of selecting the optimal treatment modality on the basis of the patient's and the stone's characteristics. The choice also depends on the availability of instruments (and thereby experience) in the hospital (Tables 14.3 and 14.4).

Recent technological advances in PCNL might initiate safer and more efficient management of renal stones. A lack of prospective ran-

Table 14.2 Comparison between ultra-mini-percutaneous nephrolithotomy and retrograde intrarenal surgery [4]

	RIRS	UMP
Total cases	20	32
Operation time (min)	98	46
Hospitalization (h)	32	24
Cost of disposables (euros)	484	80
Complication rate	8%	6%
Stone-free rate	80%	88%
Auxiliary procedure	100%	1%
Fever (percentage of patients)	20%	12.5%

UMP ultra-mini-percutaneous nephrolithotomy, *RIRS* retrograde intrarenal surgery

Table 14.4 Comparison between miniaturized percutaneous nephrolithotomy instruments [8]

	Mini-PCNL	UMP	Micro-perc
Size of sheath	18–22 Fr	11.0 Fr and 13 Fr	4.85 Fr
Stone removal	Forceps and ultrasonic disintegration with suction	Creating a fluid vortex	Leave for natural expulsion
Telescope size	3 mm	1 mm	0.9 mm
Resolution of telescope	30,000 pixels	17,000 pixels	10,000 pixels

Table 14.3 Observational comparison among minimally invasive treatment modalities for kidney stones [8]

	Mini-PCNL	UMP	RIRS	Micro-perc
Learning curve	Puncture skill required	Puncture skill required	Relatively easy	Puncture skill required
Cost of equipment	Moderate	Moderate	High	Moderate
Stone-free rate	Good; even for large stone	Good, up to 2.0 cm	Good, up to 1.5 cm	Good up to 1.0 cm
Auxiliary procedure	Almost nil	Almost nil	Stent removal; pre-procedure stenting sometimes	Steinstrasse removal sometimes
Hospitalization	48–72 h	24 h	24 h	24 h

domized trials comparing treatment modalities coupled with the vast disparity in the access to resources worldwide continues to individualize rather than standardize stone treatment in patients. Also, when treating a patient with a renal calculus, the urologist must ask: "Is single session ESWL possible in this patient or other treatment options should be deployed?" It is not surprising that the urologist will choose an endoscopic treatment for his/her patient whilst he may choose ESWL for himself or his family member.

References

1. Yamaguchi A, Skolarikos A, Buchholz NP, et al. Operating times and bleeding complications in percutaneous nephrolithotomy: a comparison of tract dilation methods in 5537 patients in the Clinical Research Office of the Endourological Society Percutaneous Nephrolithotomy Global Study. J Endourol. 2011;25:933–9.
2. Desai J, Solanki R. Ultra-mini percutaneous nephrolithotomy (UMP): one more armamentarium. BJU Int. 2013;112:1046–9.
3. Janak D, Solanki R. Ultra-mini percutaneous nephrolithotripsy. J Endourol Videourol. 2013.
4. Desai J, Solanki R. E93 comparison of UMP v/s RIRS for lower calyx stone. Eur Urol Suppl. 2013;12(3):62.
5. Akman T, Binbay M, Yuruk E, et al. Tubeless procedure is most important factor in reducing length of hospitalization after percutaneous nephrolithotomy: results of univariable and multivariable models. Urology. 2011;77:299–304.
6. Wells H, Rukin N, Wright A, et al. Outcome-based comparison of percutaneous procedures for urinary lithiasis with calibre of instrumentation less than 12Fr. Curr Urol Rep. 2015;16:53.
7. Kukreja R, Desai M, Patel S, et al. Factors affecting blood loss during percutaneous nephrolithotomy: prospective study. J Endourol. 2004;18:715–22.
8. Smith AD, Preminger GM, Kavoussi LR, Badlani GH, Rastinehad AR, editors. Smith's Textbook of Endourology. 4th ed: Wiley; 2018. ISBN: 9781119245193.

Super-Mini-PCNL (SMP) 15

Guohua Zeng and Wei Zhu

According to the updated European Association of Urology (EAU) guidelines, PCNL is recommended as the therapy of choice for large renal calculi (>20 mm) and also for smaller stones (10–20 mm) of the lower renal pole when unfavourable factors for SWL exist [1]. It offers high stone-free rates and is less invasive than open surgery. However, PCNL is still a challenging surgical technique and can be associated with significant complications that may compromise its efficacy. Bleeding and injury to the kidney and its adjacent structures are the most troublesome morbidities. PCNL complications tend to be associated with the accuracy of the nephrostomy tract placement and its size. A modification of the standard PCNL has been developed to reduce morbidity associated with larger instruments such as blood loss, postoperative pain, and potential renal damage. This is performed through a miniature endoscope via a small percutaneous tract (14–20 F) and has been known as minimally invasive PCNL or mini-PCNL or mini-Perc. In addition to mini-Perc, Desai et al. [2] have reported their ultra-mini-PCNL (UMP), and lastly micro-PCNL has been introduced for clinical use [3]. Reducing the size of nephrostomy tracts mandates the development of miniature endoscopes and access sheaths. Also, with smaller nephrostomy tracts the problem of a compromised visual field arises and increased difficulty in stone extraction. Increasing irrigation, using a pressure pump, could enhance the visualization and passive egress of stone fragments, but it would also boost the intra-luminal pressure.

The super-mini-PCNL (SMP) technique was developed to improve the critical limitations of miniaturised PCNLs [4, 5]. SMP is a recent addition to the options for miniaturized PCNL using an access sheath size of 10–14 F. Its design aims not only at preventing excessive intrarenal pressure but also at improving visualization and extraction of stone fragments.

15.1 Materials

The essential components of the SMP system include an 8.0 Fr miniaturized nephroscope and a newly designed irrigation-suction sheath [6].

15.1.1 Miniaturized Nephroscope

The nephroscope has an 8.0/7.5 F (outer diameter/inner diameter) dismountable sheath. The telescope consists of a fibre optic bundle of 1.4 mm (4.2 F) with a viewing angle of 120° and resolution of up to 40,000 pixels. When the telescope is

G. Zeng (✉) · W. Zhu
Department of Urology and Guangdong Key Laboratory of Urology, The First Affiliated Hospital of Guangzhou Medical University, Guangzhou, China

G. Zeng, K. Sarica (eds.), *Percutaneous Nephrolithotomy*,
https://doi.org/10.1007/978-981-15-0575-1_15

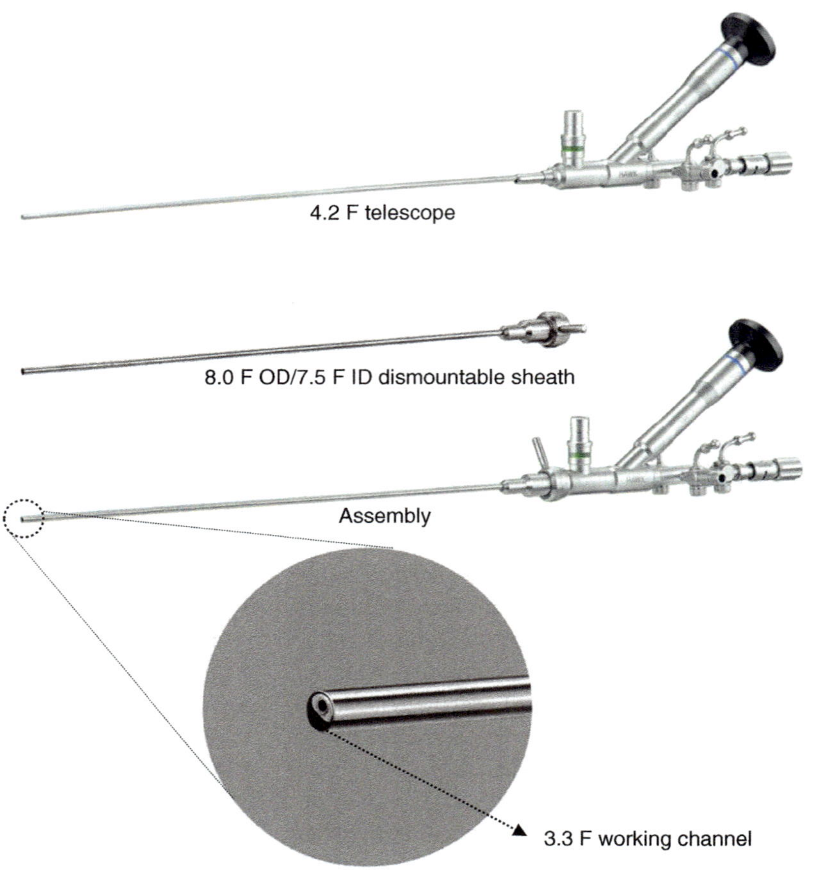

Fig. 15.1 Detailed structure of the miniaturized nephroscope. *OD* outer diameter, *ID* inner diameter

inserted into the sheath, a 3.3 F space remains in the lower half of the sheath to serve as the working channel (Fig. 15.1). A laser fibre up to 550 μm, a 0.8 mm pneumatic lithotripter probe, and a 3.0 F stone basket or forceps can be used in the working channel. The working length of the scope is 25.2 cm.

15.1.2 Irrigation-Suction Sheath

The irrigation-suction sheath was developed to provide an easy alternative to improve irrigation and stone clearance during SMP. The irrigation-suction sheath consists of a straight sheath and a 'handle'. The straight sheath is a metal structure of two layers available from 12 to 14 F. The sheath has 8 or 14 cm working length. The space between the sheath's two layers acts as a channel for irrigation, and the sheath's central lumen acts as a constant suction conduit. At the distal tip, the sheath has side holes that enable the irrigation egress through the irrigation channel.

The 'handle' consists of an irrigation port with an integral stopcock, a straight tube, and a 45 ° oblique bifurcated tube. The irrigation port is connected to an irrigation pump. The straight tube is adjacent to the suction conduit of the straight sheath and has a proximal end receptacle for a rubber cap. A continuous negative pressure aspirator is connected to the end of the oblique tube. The negative pressure of the aspiration can be adjusted by occluding or opening the pressure vent in the oblique tube axis (Fig. 15.2). To facili-

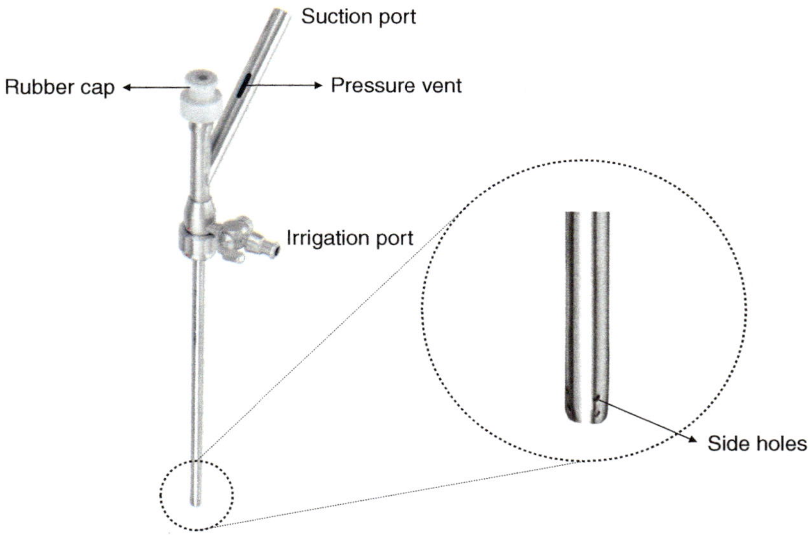

Fig. 15.2 Irrigation-suction sheath

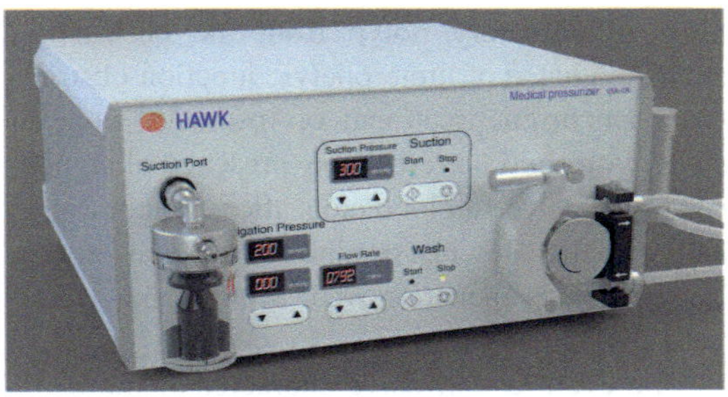

Fig. 15.3 A specially designed irrigation and aspiration device dedicated to SMP surgery

tate stone fragments collection, a sample collection container is added between the handle and the aspirator.

15.1.3 Irrigation and Aspiration Pump

The irrigation and aspiration pump includes an irrigation unit for conducting fluid under pressure to the irrigation port of the sheath, and an aspiration unit for simultaneous removal of fluid via the suction port of the sheath (Fig. 15.3). The optimum adjustment of pressure and flow parameters allows for efficient irrigation and effective aspiration of fluid during SMP procedures.

15.2 Indications and Contraindications

15.2.1 Indications

- Adult patients with stone size 1.5–3.0 cm, including previous failure of SWL or ureteroscopic lithotripsy, cystine calculi, and anatomic abnormalities precluding retrograde access or the distal passage of stones
- Patients not suitable for RIRS due to unfavourable anatomy (a narrow (<5 mm) or long (>30 mm) infundibulum)
- Paediatric patients with stone size <2.5 cm in whom SWL therapy failed

15.2.2 Contraindications

- Anticoagulant therapy must be discontinued before the procedure. Patients receiving aspirin, for example, should discontinue it 7 days before SMP while those on warfarin need to stop the drug 5 days before SMP
- Untreated urinary tract infections (UTIs), pregnancy, atypical interposition of visceral organs (bowel, spleen or liver), tumour in the probable access tract area, and potential malignant renal tumour

15.3 Technique

All routine preoperative biochemical testing and preparation is performed as for any of percutaneous surgery. The preoperative assessment involves a close study and analysis of the image including CT and IVU. This helps to determine the primary calyx of puncture by which the majority of the stone bulk is to be cleaned; stones located in distinct calyces are also recognized that are unlikely to be removed through the primary tract. In these calyces, the secondary tracts are generally established.

Traditionally, SMP has been performed in the prone position. This allows direct access to the posterior calyx. SMP can also be performed in supine with the benefits of combined antegrade and retrograde methods, making it simpler for patients with cardiac co-morbidities to switch from regional to general anaesthesia and useful. However, in the supine position, establishing multiple channels would be challenging and space is restricted.

Under general anaesthesia, a 5 F ureteral catheter is first inserted into the target kidney in a retrograde manner using ureteroscope. A Foley catheter is placed into the bladder to provide drainage during the procedure. Percutaneous access is achieved using an 18-gauge coaxial needle to puncture the desired calix under fluoroscopic or ultrasonic guidance. A 0.035″ flexible tip guidewire is inserted through the needle. The dilatation is performed with 10 F fascial dilators. An irrigation-suction straight sheath is then advanced over the guidewire and inserted into the pelvicalyceal system. Then remove the guidewire and connect the 'handle' to the straight sheath. The irrigation port of the irrigation-suction sheath is connected to the irrigation unit of the irrigation-aspiration pump. The sheath's oblique tube is connected to the collection bottle of samples and the bottle to the pump's aspirator unit. The irrigation pressure is set at 200–250 mmHg while the suction pressure is adjusted at 100–150 mmHg. The miniature endoscope is inserted into the sheath through the cap. The stone is visualized and lithotripsy is performed using either a holmium-yttrium-aluminium garnet (YAG) laser or pneumatic lithotripter. Laser lithotripsy is a preferred method. The pneumatic lithotripter could be used in the centres where laser lithotripters are not available. The small stone fragments would move through the space between the scope and the sheath with effective and constant suction, then exit through the oblique sluice. The negative pressure can be adjusted by either partially or completely occluding the pressure vent with the surgeon's thumb whilst holding the handle with the rest of the hand. If the stone fragments are too large to pass around the scope within the sheath, the scope can be slowly removed proximal to the bifurcation to create an unblocked channel for larger fragments to evacuate. For staghorn stones, multiple tracts are usually necessary and are created in the same session. At the end of the procedure, a single fluoroscopic image is obtained to assess the stone-free status. A double-J stent is placed only when there is the presence of a ureteric inflammatory polyp from the obstruction stone, evidence of ureteropelvic junction obstruction, concurrent treatment of ipsilateral ureteric stone with rigid ureteroscope, presence of significant pyelocalyceal blood clots after the lithotripsy, and in patients with significant residual stones. The sheath is then removed, sealing the wound with absorbable gelatin.

The even less invasive character of the SMP due to smaller access tracts makes the procedure feasible in a tubeless or totally tubeless manner, especially in uncomplicated cases when a stone-free status is achieved. Assumed advantages of a tubeless procedure are better patient comfort, less postoperative pain, shorter hospital stay, and quicker recovery.

Nephrostomy tube placement indications include significant residual stone fragments, which would require a second-look operation and significant pyelocalyceal blood clots or bleeding after the lithotripsy.

15.4 Advantages over Other Miniaturized PCNLs

1. *Active removal of stone fragments and maintaining low renal pelvic pressure (RPP)*
   Stone fragments are removed through negative pressure aspiration in SMP with the ultimate goal of making the patient completely stone

free at the end of the procedure. When using SMP, there are several benefits. Firstly, stone extraction is feasible; therefore, both stone fragmentation and dusting can be used. Secondly, stone fragments tend to aggregate at the opening of the sheath, making lithotripsy and stone fragments removal more effective. Thirdly, the visual field is clearer with the capacity to use constant irrigation despite being in a miniaturized system. This is because with such an irrigation system, 'dust storm' caused by stone pulverization is minimized. Bleeding caused by large PCNL tracts is minimized by using a miniaturized puncture system that further enhances the field of vision. Finally, the use of negative pressure aspiration promotes irrigation drainage while maintaining a low average RPP during the entire operation [7].

2. *Improved irrigation*
   In most of miniaturized PCNLs, the main irrigation is delivered through the same channel used for working instruments. This cause a dramatic reduction in irrigation efficiency once the laser fibre or pneumatic lithotripter probe was inserted. The irrigation-suction sheath in SMP system could improve the irrigation efficiency. The irrigation-suction sheath is a structure of two-layered metal. The space between the sheath's two layers is an independent irrigation channel. Using this SMP system, the irrigation is delivered through the sheath, thus freeing the nephroscope's working channel space that enables the use of larger instruments (as 550 μm laser fibre or 1.0 mm lithotripter) without decreasing irrigation efficiency.
3. *A more efficient hydrodynamic mechanism for retrieval of fragments*
   In irrigation systems used in other miniaturized PCNLs, both irrigation inflow and outflow take place within the same sheath lumen. As a consequence, the inflow partly offsets the outflow impact, eventually pushing back stone fragments into the collecting system, possibly leading to stone migration and increasing operation time. The irrigation-suction sheath in the SMP system enables the inflow and outflow to follow separate channels, establishing a one-way flow system. The inflow that enters the collecting system through the sheath's irrigation channel is then removed from the system via the sheath's suction conduit (Fig. 15.4). This system makes stone removal effective and reduces operating time.

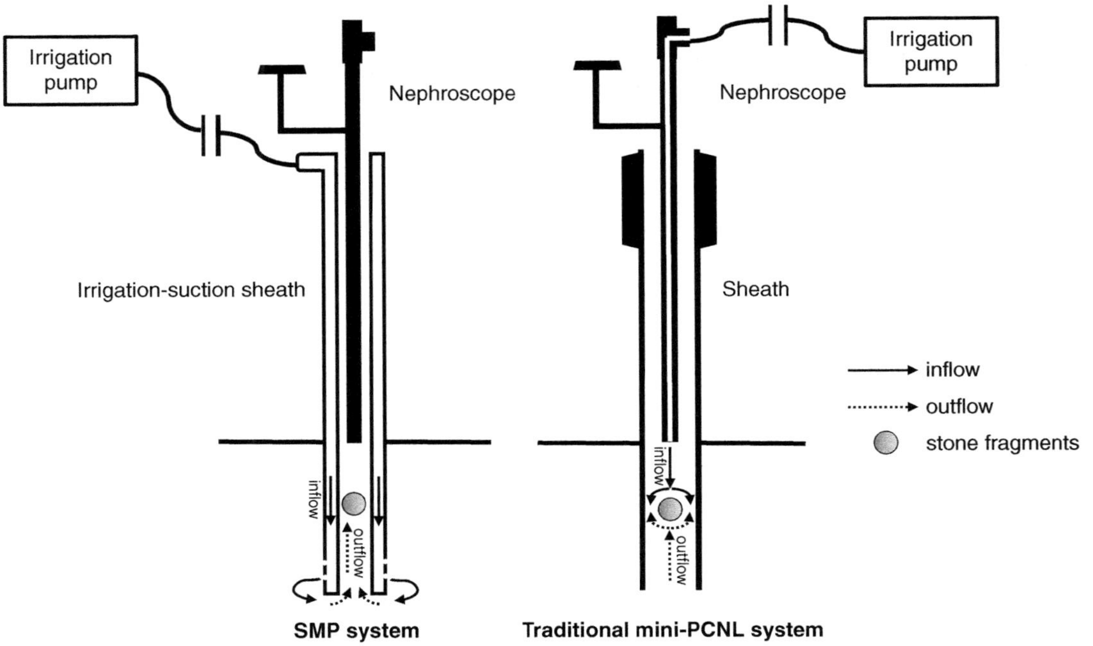

Fig. 15.4 The hydrodynamic mechanisms for retrieval fragments in SMP system and traditional mini-PCNL system

15.5 Comment

Despite being first described a few years ago, SMP technique has yet to gain widespread acceptance. The safety and effectiveness of the SMP in both adults and paediatric populations were explored [8, 9]. The results from a multicentre, prospective, randomized controlled trial showed that SMP was more effective than RIRS in treatment of lower calyceal calculi with a better stone-free rate and lesser auxiliary rate [10]. SMP appears to be a reasonable option for patients with small to medium stones and has been shown to be associated with a greater totally tubeless rate [8]. In some centres, it is most commonly used to manage moderate-sized renal calculus or in patients with multiple renal calculi. Although SMP can be used in the management of larger stones, the choice to use SMP should be prudent, and the operation should be performed by an experienced surgical team familiar with the equipment. Selection of patients is of paramount significance for successful treatment with SMP.

References

1. Professionals S-O. Urolithiasis. In: Uroweb. https://uroweb.org/guideline/urolithiasis/. Accessed 13 Apr 2019.
2. Desai J, Zeng G, Zhao Z, Zhong W, Chen W, Wu W. A novel technique of ultra-mini-percutaneous nephrolithotomy: introduction and an initial experience for treatment of upper urinary calculi less than 2 cm. Biomed Res Int. 2013;2013:490793.
3. Desai M, Mishra S. "Microperc" micro percutaneous nephrolithotomy: evidence to practice. Curr Opin Urol. 2012;22:134–8.
4. Zeng G, Wan S, Zhao Z, et al. Super-mini percutaneous nephrolithotomy (SMP): a new concept in technique and instrumentation. BJU Int. 2016;117:655–61.
5. Zeng G, Zhu W, Liu Y, Fan J, Zhao Z, Cai C. The new generation super-mini percutaneous nephrolithotomy (SMP) system: a step-by-step guide. BJU Int. 2017;120(5):735–8. https://doi.org/10.1111/bju.13955.
6. Zeng G, Zhu W, Lam W. Miniaturised percutaneous nephrolithotomy: its role in the treatment of urolithiasis and our experience. Asian J Urol. 2018;5:295–302.
7. Alsmadi J, Fan J, Zhu W, Wen Z, Zeng G. The influence of super-mini percutaneous nephrolithotomy on renal pelvic pressure in vivo. J Endourol. 2018;32:819–23.
8. Liu Y, AlSmadi J, Zhu W, Liu Y, Wu W, Fan J, Lan Y, Lam W, Zhong W, Zeng G. Comparison of super-mini PCNL (SMP) versus Miniperc for stones larger than 2 cm: a propensity score-matching study. World J Urol. 2018;36(6):955–61. https://doi.org/10.1007/s00345-018-2197-7.
9. Sarica K, Eryildirim B, Tuerxun A, Batuer A, Kavukoglu O, Buz A, Zeng G. Super-mini percutaneous nephrolithotomy for renal stone less than 25mm in pediatric patients: could it be an alternative to shockwave lithotripsy? Actas Urol Esp. 2018;42(6):406–13. https://doi.org/10.1016/j.acuro.2017.08.005.
10. Zeng G, Zhang T, Agrawal M, et al. Super-mini percutaneous nephrolithotomy (SMP) vs retrograde intrarenal surgery for the treatment of 1-2 cm lower-pole renal calculi: an international multicentre randomised controlled trial. BJU Int. 2018;122:1034–40.

Minimal-Invasive PCNL (Mini-PCNL)

16

Sven Lahme

16.1 Introduction

Over a long period of about 20 years, the so-called conventional PCNL was the surgical procedure of choice for the treatment of larger stones of the upper urinary tract. The advantage of the conventional PCNL was the very high stonefree rate compared to extracorporeal shockwave lithotripsy. Percutaneous treatment of large stones was superior to all other treatment alternatives (retrograde endoscopic treatment, extracorporeal shockwave lithotripsy), especially in the lower calyx. However, conventional PCNL was associated with a significant morbidity, e.g. the transfusion rate was approximately 10%. In solitary cases serious complications were observed, such as loss of kidney. In addition, the large instruments of a conventional PCNL can only be used with restrictions in the treatment of pediatric stones of the upper urinary tract. The difficulty to perform percutaneous stone removal in children led to a miniaturization of the conventional PCNL. Jackman described a miniaturized PCNL in children using a 13 F Amplatz sheath and showed that PCNL with miniaturized instruments is feasible. He reached a stonefree rate of 89% in nine pediatric patients. Transfusions were not needed [1].

Based on the good results of the miniaturization of PCNL in children, a miniaturization of the conventional PCNL in adults was evaluated in 1999. The aim was to combine the low mobility of extracorporeal shockwave lithotripsy with the good efficacy of the conventional PCNL in adult patients. In 2001 the first specially designed miniaturized nephroscope was published for the application of Mini-PCNL in adult patients [2] (Fig. 16.1).

Meanwhile, the Mini-PCNL has become widely accepted as the new standard of percutaneous nephrolithotomy. Numerous international publications confirm the minimal invasiveness and the excellent stonefree rate of Mini-PCNL [3–5]. Since about 8 years various modifications of the 2001 published original version of the Mini-PCNL had been published. These include the Micro-PCNL, the Ultra-Mini-PCNL (UMP) [6] and the Super-Mini-PCNL (SMP) [7].

S. Lahme (✉)
Department of Urology, Goldstadt Private Clinic, Pforzheim, Germany
e-mail: lahme@goldstadt-privatklinik.com

G. Zeng, K. Sarica (eds.), *Percutaneous Nephrolithotomy*,
https://doi.org/10.1007/978-981-15-0575-1_16

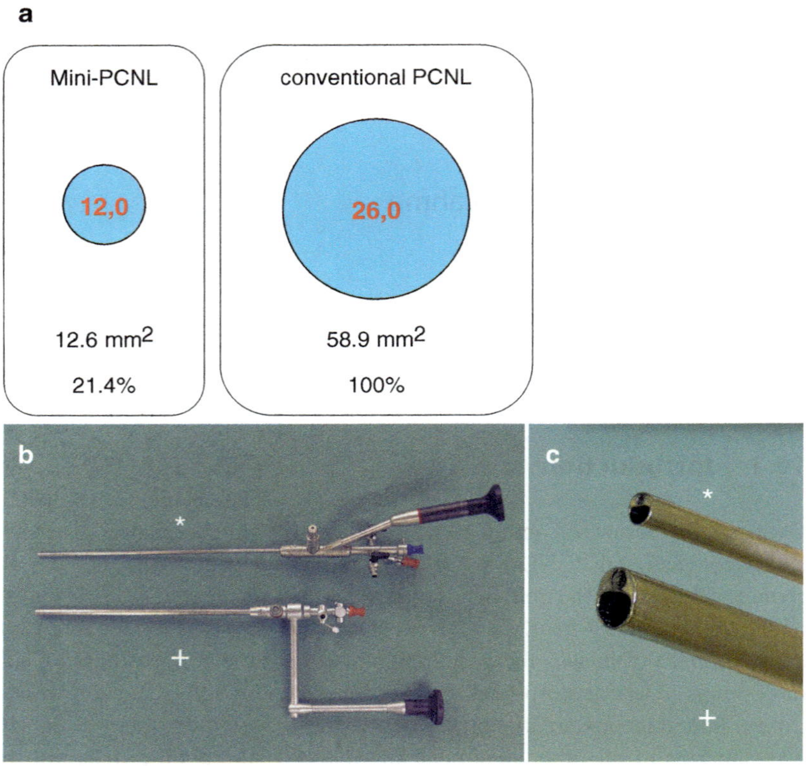

Fig. 16.1 Comparison of Mini-PCNL and conventional PCNL. (**a**) The Mini-nephroscope has only 21.4% of the cross section of the conventional nephroscope. (**b**) Comparison of Mini-nephroscope (∗) to conventional nephroscope (+). (**c**) Characteristics of the Mini-Perc procedure in comparison to a conventional PCNL

16.2 Indications for Mini-Perc

The European Association of Urology (EAU) recommends percutaneous treatment of stones from the upper urinary tract if the diameter of the urinary stone is more than 2 cm. For urinary stones with a diameter between 1 and 2 cm, percutaneous stone treatment is only a second-choice therapy. If the renal stone is less than 1 cm in diameter, percutaneous nephrolithotomy is only recommended as a third-line treatment [8]. In this context, it must be kept in mind, that these recommendations of the scientific societies are based on publications that are only dealing with conventional PCNL. In other words, this means that the indications for Mini-PCNL may differ from the general recommendations for performing conventional PCNL. At present there is still the difficulty that only a limited number of publications are available for the indication of Mini-PCNL and, therefore, so far no consideration was given in the guidelines. Based on the publications available so far, it can be assumed that Mini-PCNL can be recommended as a primary treatment option in urinary calculi of the upper urinary tract if the diameter is at least 1 cm [9]. However, it must again be emphasized that these indications cannot yet be based on the recommendations of the scientific societies. At present, this means that in the case of a Mini-PCNL of urinary stones with a diameter of less than 2 cm, appropriate information must be provided for the patient. The patient must always be informed about the treatment alternatives (extracorporeal shockwave lithotripsy and flexible ureterorenoscopy). Nevertheless the Mini PCNL is currently a minimally invasive procedure with low morbidity. However, so far it cannot be used on the basis of the current guidelines of the scientific societies [10].

16.3 Treatment Alternatives to Mini-PCNL

Depending on the size of the stone and the location of the stone, there are different treatment alternatives to the Mini-PCNL. In the case of stones of the upper urinary tract, the principal alternative treatment options are extracorporeal shockwave lithotripsy and flexible ureterorenoscopy. Shock wave lithotripsy offers a low morbidity; however, the stonefree is very low and the retreatment rate high. In addition, the treatment time of shockwave lithotripsy is very long.

In the case of retrograde flexible ureterorenoscopy as a minimally invasive treatment alternative, the stonefree rate is high and the morbidity of the procedure is also low. However, in the case of urinary stones larger than 1 cm in diameter, the operation time is significantly longer. For urinary calculi larger than 2–3 cm, retrograde flexible ureterorenoscopy cannot be recommended as the first-choice treatment [11, 12]. In contrast to Mini-PCNL, flexible ureterorenoscopy allows easier access to the ureter by using a ureteral access sheath. In addition, the instruments for flexible ureterorenoscopy are very expensive and fragile. In case of damage, high repair costs have to be expected (Fig. 16.2).

16.4 Equipment

The successful implementation of Mini-PCNL depends above all on the availability of appropriate instruments and suitable disposables.

In the first part of Mini-PCNL, a retrograde pyelography is performed using a special ureteral catheter (5 F). The use of contrast dye and methylene blue is required for dilatation, as well as for the radiographic and endoscopic identification of the renal calyceal system.

To perform a Mini-PCNL a 12 F nephroscope is needed. Furthermore, a so-called one-step dilator (15 F) and a reusable stainless steel Amplatz sheath are used. For lithotripsy, a holmium laser should be used. As a postoperative urinary diversion the insertion of a nephrostomy tube is advisable. As a treatment option, the antegrade use of a flexible endoscope through percutaneous access or the use of forceps and stone graspers may be necessary in solitary cases.

	Mini-PCNL	**flexible URS**
access	experience required	easy
stonefree rate	+++	++
hemostatic disorders	absolute contraindication	relative contraindication
prefered stone localization	lower pole	upper pole mid calix
cost effectiveness	+++	–
lithotripsy	Holmiumlaser	Holmiumlaser
transfusion rate	≈ 1%	< 1%

Fig. 16.2 Comparison of Mini-PCNL to flexible ureterorenoscopy

16.5 Surgical Procedure

The procedure of a Mini-PCNL consists of two steps [13]. The first step of the procedure is a retrograde pyelography. Preferably, a ureteral balloon catheter is used. The retrograde pyelography allows getting all information about the morphology of the ureter, such as strictures, kinkings or additional ureteral stones. The ureteral catheter is placed above the ureteropelvic junction and the balloon is inflated.

The next step is to reposition the patient. Mini-PCNL can be performed in the prone or supine position. Most Mini-PCNL procedures are done in the prone position. A percutaneous access to the renal calyceal system is established, the urinary stone disintegration is performed and the stone fragments are removed by means of the irrigation flow (Fig. 16.3a–f).

16.5.1 Retrograde Pyelography

First, a diagnostic endoscopy of the bladder is performed to exclude additional pathological findings of the lower urinary tract. Subsequently, a 5 F ureteral catheter is inserted through the ureteral orifice. The retrograde pyelography then shows any additional abnormalities of the ureter. In the case of a balloon ureteral catheter, it is blocked above the ureteral pelvic junction with approximately 0.5–1.0 mL of sterile saline. This is done under fluoroscopic control. In individual cases, the blockage of the ureteral balloon catheter can also be done in the proximal ureter under radiological guidance. This is always to be preferred if the urinary stone mass in the renal pelvis does not permit the position of the ureteral catheter in the renal pelvis due to limited space of the renal pelvis. Finally, after retrograde pyelography and the insertion of the ureteral catheter, the insertion of a transurethral catheter is performed (Fig. 16.3b).

16.5.2 Repositioning of the Patient

Upon completion of the ureteral catheter insertion, the patient is repositioned to perform the Mini-PCNL. This can be done either in the prone or supine position. The decision on the type of positioning primarily depends on the experience of the surgeon. In case of prone positioning, the kidney may be fixed by a cushion positioned under the abdomen. Alternatively, the pelvis and the thorax can be elevated by means of a cushion to have a mobile kidney to perform Mini-PCNL. Through the ureteral catheter a mixture of contrast dye and methylene blue is applied. This leads to a dilatation of the renal pelvis and facilitates the puncture of the renal calyceal system. In addition, the successful puncture of the renal calyceal system is easier to monitor after applying methylene blue through the ureteral catheter.

16.5.3 Puncture of the Calyceal System

The puncture of the renal pelvis can be done either under ultrasound control, under radiographic control or by a combination of both methods. After application of a mixture of contrast dye and methylene blue, the successful puncture of the renal calyceal system can be easily detected fluoroscopically and clinically. If the calyceal system had been punctured successfully, the next step is to insert a guidewire (Fig. 16.3c). Then the puncture needle is removed and a so-called single step dilator is inserted under radiological guidance. The next step is to insert a stainless steel Amplatz sheath, which exactly fits to the stainless steel dilator. Finally, the stainless steel dilator is removed (Fig. 16.3d). By means of the mini-nephroscope, an endoscopic evaluation of the renal calyceal system is performed. If the Amplatz sheath is placed properly and no further difficulties are detected by mini-nephroscopy, the guidewire can be removed. The removal of the guidewire in Mini-PCNL is always recommended as without the guidewire the so-called vacuum-cleaner effect is facilitated (see below).

16.5.4 Nephroscopy

The nephroscopy is performed with the mini-nephroscope, which has a diameter of 12 F. It can be inserted through the stainless steel Amplatz

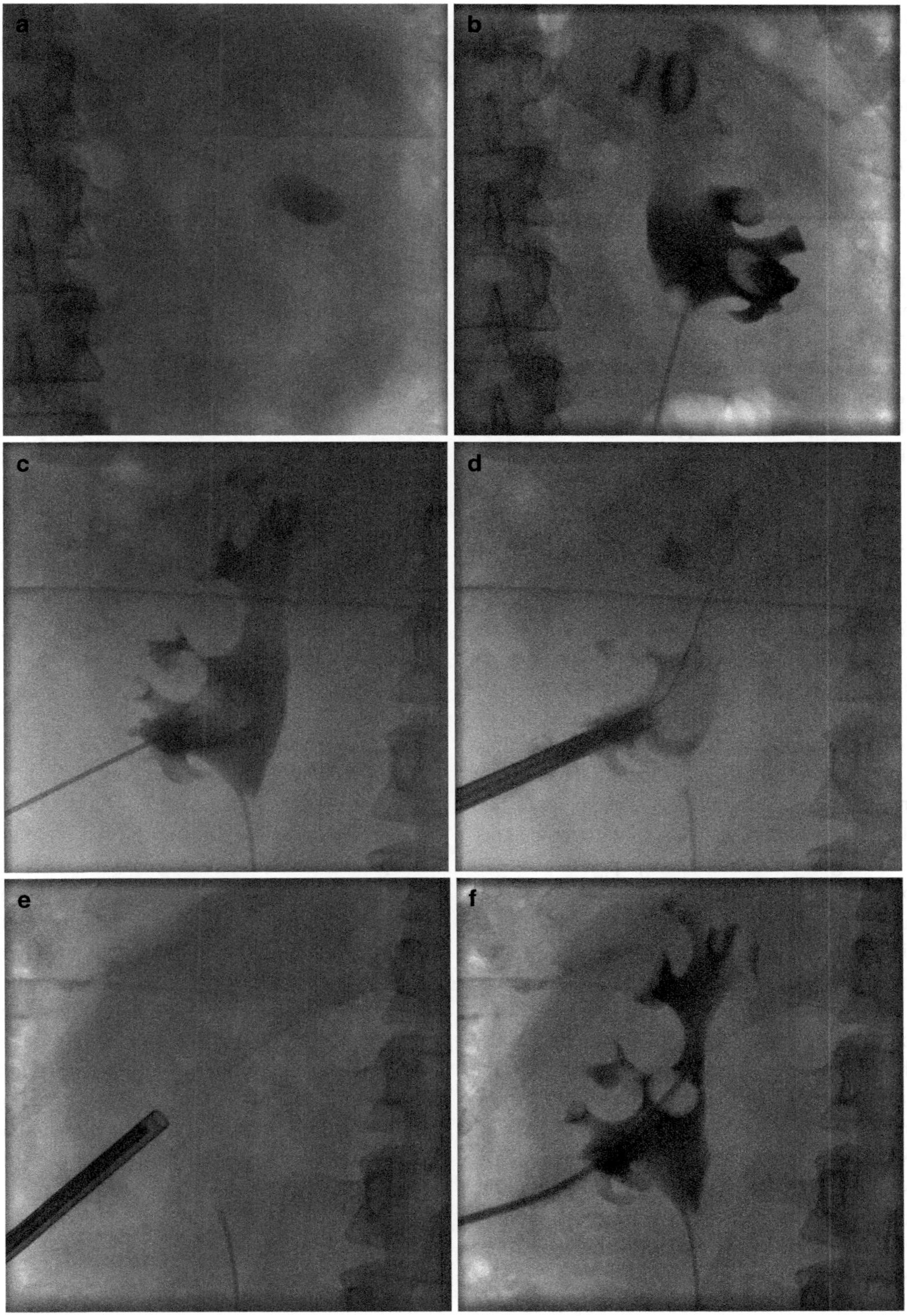

Fig. 16.3 Mini-Perc procedure. (**a**) 2 cm renal pelvic stone. (**b**) Retrograde pyelography and insertion of ureteral balloon catheter. (**c**) Puncture of the renal calyceal system. (**d**) Dilation of the tract and insertion of an Amplatz sheath. (**e**) Stonefree-status at the end of the procedure. (**f**) Insertion of nephrostomy tube

sheath. Once the correct position of the Amplatz sheath has been verified under nephroscopic vision, the still inserted guide wire can be removed. The aim of the removal of the guidewire is that the fragments later produced by holmium-laser lithotripsy can be more easily rinsed through the Amplatz sheath and the guidewire is not an obstruction, which stops the migration of stone fragments. For inspection of the renal calyceal system flexible endoscopes can also be used. Here, the indication is based on the morphology of the renal calyceal system. The orientation during nephroscopy is mainly done under endoscopic view. But it can be additionally facilitated by fluoroscopy and contrast dye application.

16.5.5 Stone Disintegration

The stone disintegration in Mini-PCNL should preferably be done by means of a holmium laser. The reason for this recommendation is that the cross-section of the holmium-laser fiber is very small and thus no decrease of the irrigation flow takes place. In addition, due to the different settings of a holmium laser, various different types of stone disintegration can be applied. According to the particular stone situation, disintegration into fragments, and disintegration into dust or a popcorn-effect can be performed. The goal in any Mini-PCNL case is to achieve such small stone fragments, which automatically can leave the renal calyceal system through the space between the mini-nephroscope and the Amplatz sheath. In holmium-laser lithotripsy, the laser fiber is brought close to the surface of the urinary stone. When applying the laser, the fragment size can be varied depending on the frequency and energy used. In the case of a Mini-PCNL, it is recommended to generate as small as possible fragments of the stone and to prevent the simultaneous formation of several larger fragments of the initial stone. If an ultrasound device is used for stone disintegration, it should be noted on the one hand that a reduction of the irrigation flow occurs due to the cross section of the ultrasound probe and, on the other hand, a collapse of the renal pelvis can occur due to the suction effect of the ultrasound probe. Therefore in Mini-PCNL a holmium-laser lithotripsy is most suitable.

16.5.6 Stone Extraction

In Mini-PCNL, the removal of disintegrated urinary stone fragments occurs only through the flushing stream of the irritation. In this respect, the use of forceps or baskets is not required. Due to the special ratio of the diameter and length of the Amplatz sheath a special suction effect occurs, which is known as the so-called vacuum-cleaner effect. This effect does not occur in the conventional PCNL and is considered to be the main difference of the Mini-PCNL to the conventional PCNL. If peripheral renal calculi are present in the renal calyceal system, the use of flexible endoscopes via the Mini-PCNL Amplatz sheath may be useful. The aim of the Mini-PCNL is in any case to treat the patient endoscopically and radiologically confirmed stonefree.

16.5.7 Postoperative Drainage of the Calyceal System

For the postoperative drainage of the renal calyceal system, the insertion of a 12 or 14 F nephrostomy tube is recommended. The insertion of a percutaneous nephrostomy tube reduces the risk of postoperative fever. In addition, the percutaneous access to the kidney is preserved so that, if necessary, a second procedure can be performed without a new puncture of the renal calyceal system. If one refrains from inserting a percutaneous nephrostomy and inserts a DJ stent instead, one speaks of a tubeless PCNL. If neither a percutaneous nephrostomy nor a DJ stent is inserted, this is called a totally tubeless PCNL (Fig. 16.3e, f) [14].

16.5.8 Particular Situations

In the case of very large masses of stone, it may be necessary to create multiple accesses to the

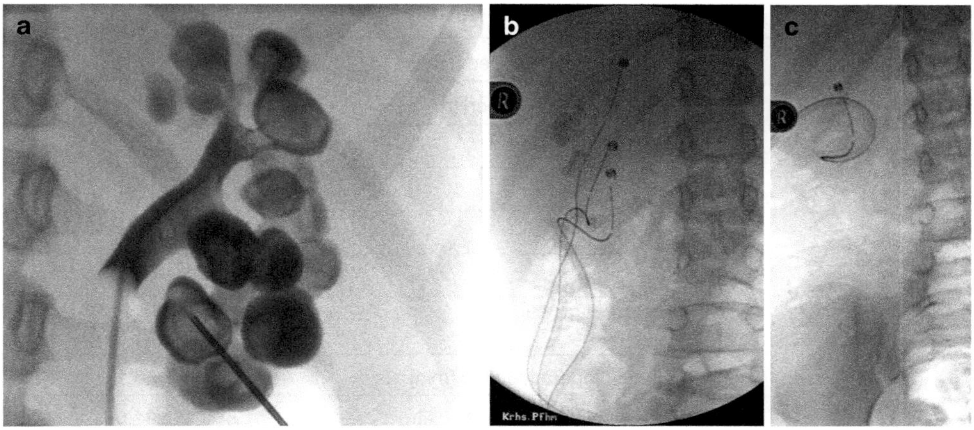

Fig. 16.4 In staghorn calculi, Mini-PCNL can be performed by multiple accesses. (**a**) Primary puncture of the lower calyx. (**b**) Multiple punctures due to peripheral stone mass. (**c**) Complete removal of all stones after seven sessions with no complications

kidney. In this case we are talking about a multitract Mini-PCNL (Fig. 16.4). If it is not possible to completely remove the stones in a Mini-PCNL, it is advisable to perform a second puncture [15].

In some cases a multiple tract PCNL can be expected before the procedure starts. In these cases it is recommended first to perform multiple punctures but not to perform any dilation. After multiple punctures had been done and guidewires in each access had been placed, the dilation of one tract can be started. Later one of the additional guidewires can be used for dilation and introducing an additional Amplatz sheath. According to the success of the procedure in some cases not all punctures are needed to insert an Amplatz sheath. At the end of the procedure any remaining guidewires can be removed without any difficulties.

In obese patients, using a longer Amplatz sheath may be helpful. However, in this case, the effect of the "vacuum-cleaner effect" is reduced.

16.6 Effectiveness of Mini-Perc

In experienced hands, the Mini PCNL is an effective and safe treatment modality for midsized stones of the renal calyceal system. The overall stonefree rate of the Mini PCNL is approximately 94%. The average operation time is approximately 65 min. If large urinary stones are treated, the operation time can be significantly longer. Interestingly the results of large upper urinary tract stones are comparable to the overall results. If an increase of the retreatment rate and a slight increase of the operating time are accepted, large stones can also be successfully treated by Mini-PCNL (Fig. 16.5) [16].

16.7 Complications

Basically complications of Mini-PCNL do not vary from complications of conventional PCNL—but frequency differs significantly. The main complications of Mini-PCNL are febrile urinary tract infections, perforation of the calyceal system, bleeding, strictures of the calyceal neck, fistulas and alterations of inner organs. Almost all perforations are treated with a prolonged insertion of a DJ-stent. No further difficulties remain in these cases. Major complications in Mini-PCNL are very rare. The transfusion rate is approximately 1% (Fig. 16.5) [17].

Fig. 16.5 Results of Mini-Perc in $n = 1048$ cases

		overall	> 5cm^2
stone burden [cm^2]		4.1	9.6
localisation [n]	calix	425	
	diverticulum	79	
	renal pelvis	353	
	part. staghorn	168	
	prox. ureter	18	
	horse shoe kidney	5	
operative time [min]		63.1	76.5
stonefree rate [%]		91.6	93.2
retreatment rate [%]		23.1	33.2
transfusion rate [%]		1.3	1.1
pyelonephritis [%]		7.0	7.7

16.8 Mini-PCNL in Particular Situations

Mini-PCNL is not only suitable in adult patients suffering from upper urinary tract calculi. Mini-PCNL can also be applied in particular situations which are challenging for endourological stone treatment.

16.8.1 Calyceal Diverticulum Stones

In calyceal diverticulum stones, the stones and the underlying morphological obstruction have to be treated simultaneously. There is almost no localization of calyceal diverticulum stones which cannot be reached by means of Mini-PCNL. This is a significant advantage in comparison to flexible ureterorenoscopy as in flexible ureterorenoscopy sometimes calyceal diverticula cannot be reached. In the case of Mini-PCNL, first the puncture is done. Then the calyceal diverticulum stone is disintegrated and removed. As the diverticulum is usually very narrow and there is only a limited space to place the nephroscope, Mini-PCNL is superior to conventional PCNL in this situation. Subsequently the diverticulum neck is passed by a guidewire by an antegrade way. Along the guidewire a holmium-laser incision of the diverticulum neck is done. Finally a nephrostomy tube is inserted and left in place for some days. There is scientific evidence that the percutaneous treatment of calyceal diverticulum stones is more effective than by means of flexible ureterorenoscopy (Fig. 16.6a–e).

16.8.2 Stone Removal in Transplanted Kidneys

Stones in transplanted kidneys can easily be reached by means of a Mini-PCNL. In contrast to pelvic kidneys, transplanted kidneys are located next to the abdominal wall with no interposition of the bowel. The ultrasound-guided puncture of the calyx of a transplanted kidney is often easy. Mini-PCNL also avoids any passage of the fragile ureteral anastomosis of the transplanted kidney. This means that Mini-PCNL in transplanted kidneys preserves the fragile anatomy of the transplanted ureter.

16.8.3 Pediatric Upper Urinary Tract Stones

The anatomy of the renal calyceal system in children is characterized by a limited space and a small diameter of the calyceal necks. Mini-PCNL with its limited diameter of the Amplatz sheath avoids any damage of the fragile infant calyceal system. Mini-PCNL is an ideal treatment option in upper urinary tract stones in childhood [1, 18]. Even in early born infants, Mini-PCNL can be applied. Remember that Mini-PCNL initially was designed for the treatment of upper urinary tract stones in children. A special chapter in this book deals with this topic (refer Chap. 19 by Dr. Kemal Sarica).

16.9 Recent Modifications of the Original Version of Mini-PCNL

From 2001 to 2011 Mini-PCNL has only been performed in its original version. Starting in 2011 several modifications of Mini-PCNL were presented. The main aim was to further minimize the risk of complications and to receive a comparable stonefree rate.

16.9.1 Micro-PCNL

Bader et al. published the Micro-PCNL technique in 2011. They developed a further minia-

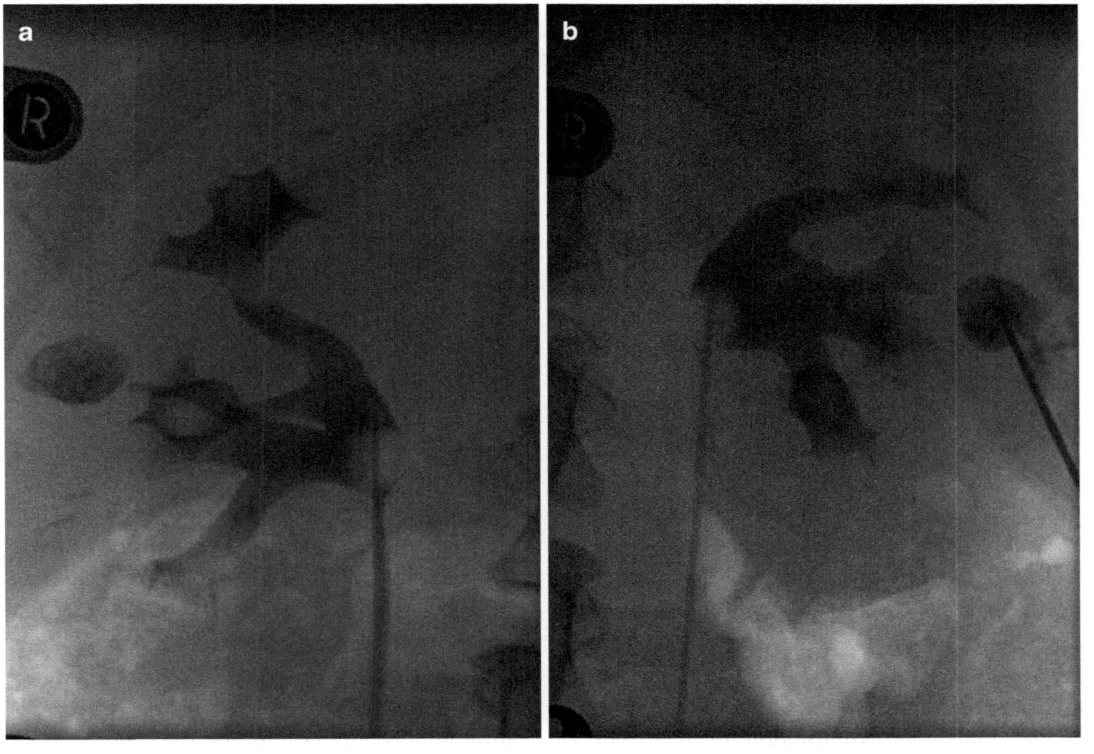

Fig. 16.6 (**a**) Calyceal diverticulum stone. (**b**) Retrograde pyelography in prone position. (**c**) Percutaneous puncture and removal of stone by Mini-PCNL. (**d**) Antegrade insertion of guidewire and holmium laser incision of the calyceal neck. (**e**) Insertion of nephrostomy tube

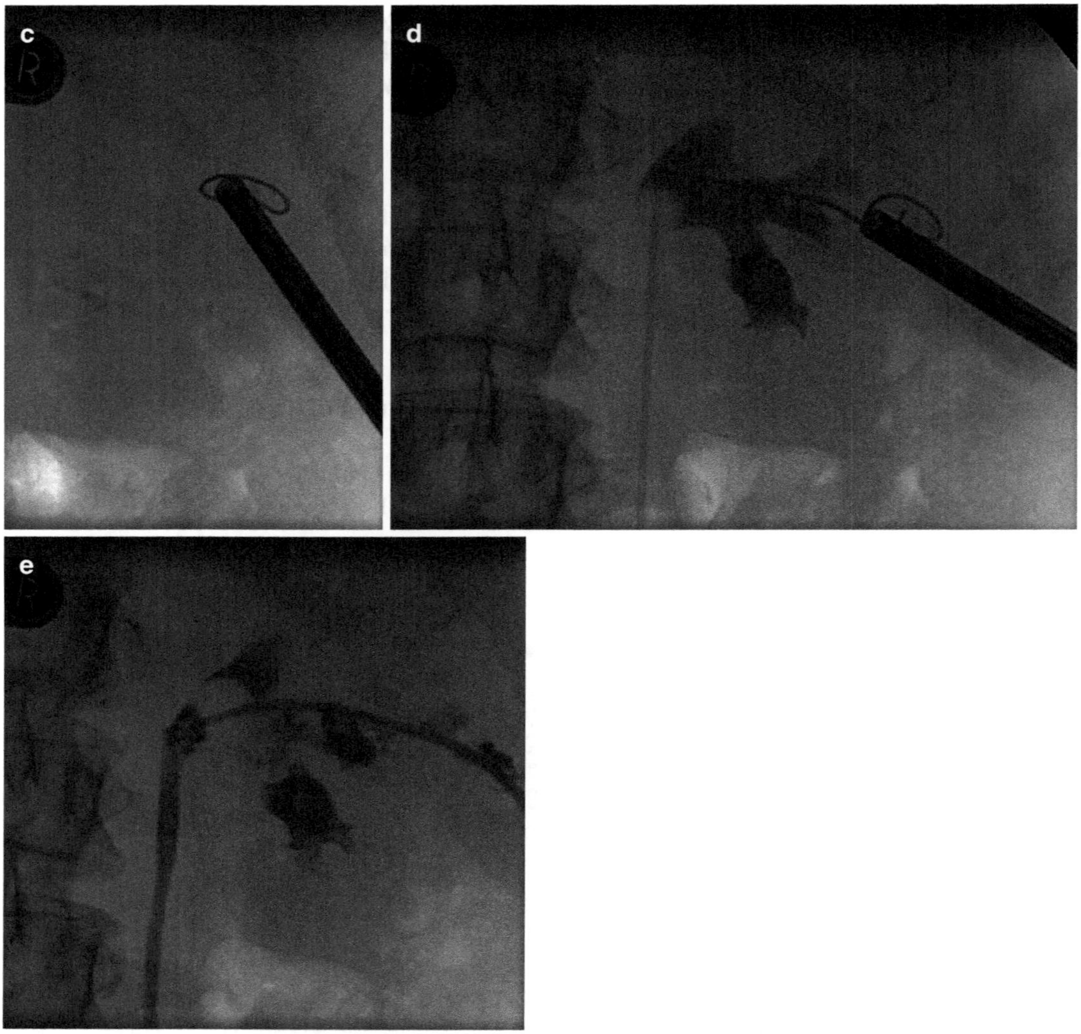

Fig. 16.6 (continued)

turized nephroscope which was inserted in a special puncture needle. As the nephroscope was used during the puncture, this particular needle was called the "all-seeing needle." The diameter of the needle is 5 F, and the puncture of the renal calyceal system is done under direct endoscopic vision and ultrasound and/or fluoroscopic guidance. No dilation of the tract is needed. The only type of stone disintegration that works with Micro-PCNL is the holmium-laser lithotripsy. Due to the limited diameter of the Micro-PCNL Amplatz sheath, no stone removal is possible. The aim is to produce stone dust. These very small dust particles have to pass the ureter. The Micro-PCNL technique leads to a disintegration of the renal stones but does not provide any immediate stonefree status after the procedure. Furthermore there is no low pressure in the renal calyceal system as the irrigation flow is applied through the scope, but no space is available to allow the irrigation water to come out of the calyceal system. This is the reason why most urologists performing Micro-PCNL prefer to insert a large ureteral catheter.

The missing percutaneous outflow of the irrigation flow also leads to an increase of the pressure of the renal calyceal system, which is also a significant disadvantage. The stonefree rate of Micro-PCNL is significant lower than in original Mini-PCNL, and the probability to convert to Mini-PCNL is up to 15% [19].

16.9.2 Ultra-Mini-PCNL (UMP)

An UMP is performed by means of a 6 F nephroscope and an 11 F Amplatz sheath. The underlying principle of UMP is the same as in the original Mini-PCNL. After puncturing the renal calyceal system, a dilation of the tract is performed. Lithotripsy is performed by means of a holmium laser. Small fragments can be washed out of the calyceal system by means of the irrigation flow. This means that the so-called vacuum-cleaner effect also occurs in UMP. Unfortunately the stone fragments have to be very small. Otherwise it is impossible to wash out the stone fragments. UMP provides a low morbidity and an acceptable stonefree rate. But the operative time is longer and UMP is not recommended in large stone burden. UMP usually is performed as a tubeless procedure, which means, that no nephrostomy tube is inserted after the procedure [6, 20].

16.9.3 Super Mini-PCNL (SMP)

SMP had been evaluated by Zeng et al. The puncture and the dilation are similar to the original Mini-PCNL. In contrast to the original Mini-PCNL in SMP, active irrigation and active suction are used. The SMP Amplatz sheath consists of a particular connection to apply suction. The result is that with active irrigation and active suction the stone fragments can be washed out quicker. Particular in larger stone burden, the SMP is an advantage. The disadvantage is that the equipment is more complex to install and more expensive.

16.9.4 Minimal Invasive PNL (MIP XS, S, M, L)

The MIP technique works similar to the original Mini-PCNL. After puncturing the calyceal system, a single-step dilation is performed. The particular instrument used is chosen according to the stone burden, e.g. MIP S in small stones, MIP L in staghorn stones. The size of the nephroscope corresponds to each size of the Amplatz sheath, which means that different Amplatz sheaths have different nephroscopes.

16.9.5 Perfect Perc (PP)

The PP was introduced in 2014. This technique is based on a variety of different Amplatz sheaths, which can be combined with the same further miniaturized nephroscope with a diameter of 4.5 F. The idea is to adjust the size of the Amplatz sheath to the size of the stone but always to use the same mini-nephroscope. Amplatz sheaths are available from 10 to 16 F. As the nephroscope is only used to have an endoscopic view of the stone and to apply the laser, a very small mini-nephroscope is suitable for all sizes of Amplatz sheaths. As the same mini-nephroscope fits to all sizes of Amplatz sheaths, the PP is a very cost-effective procedure. In addition not only the diameter of the Amplatz sheaths can be adjusted to the size of the stone but also the length of the Amplatz sheath. All different sizes of the Amplatz sheaths are available in different lengths from 120 to 180 mm according to the obesity of the patient. As the “vacuum-cleaner effect” depends on the diameter and length of the Amplatz sheath, the PP can provide the optimum combination of Amplatz sheath diameter and length at any time.

16.10 When to Choose Mini-PCNL

As already discussed numerous modifications of the original Mini-PCNL are available. Figure 16.7 gives an overview of which type of Mini-PCNL

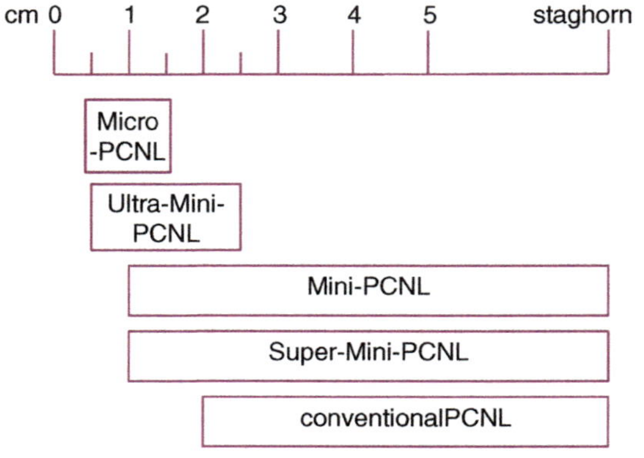

Fig. 16.7 Differential indications for PCNL according to stone sizes

to choose for which type of stones. Mini-PCNL can be recommended for stones exceeding a diameter of 1 cm. There is no limitation according to the stone size. The surgeon should always take into consideration that Mini-PCNL in stones from 1 to 2 cm is not yet covered by the guidelines. The type of PCNL used depends on the stone burden. According to the stone size, different types of PCNL can be recommended (Fig. 16.7) [21].

16.11 Conclusions

Mini-PCNL is a minimal-invasive modification of conventional PCNL. By means of a miniaturized instrument, a minimally invasive percutaneous procedure can be performed. Depending on stone size, location and composition, stonefree rate of 90% or more can be reached. As the puncture of the calyceal system is the most important step of the procedure, Mini-PCNL requires a lot of experience of the surgeon. Stone extraction, like in conventional PCNL, is not needed due to the effect by irrigation flow. It is expected that Mini-PCNL will be the percutaneous approach of choice and will be considered in the guidelines as soon as prospective trials are available to determine the effectiveness of Mini-PCNL even in smaller stone masses.

References

1. Jackman SV, Docimo SG, Cadeddu JA, Bishoff JT, Kavoussi LR, Jarrett TW. The "mini-perc" technique: a less invasive alternative to percutaneous nephrolithotomy. World J Urol. 1998;16(6):371–4.
2. Lahme S, Bichler KH, Strohmaier WL, Götz T. Minimally invasive PCNL in patients with renal pelvic and calyceal stones. Eur Urol. 2001;40(6):619–24.
3. Li X, He Z, Wu K, Li SK, Zeng G, Yuan J, He Y, Lei M. Chinese minimally invasive percutaneous nephrolithotomy: the Guangzhou experience. J Endourol. 2009;23(10):1693–7.
4. Nagele U, Schilling D, Anastasiadis AG, Walcher U, Sievert KD, Merseburger AS, Kuczyk M, Stenzl A. Minimally invasive percutaneous nephrolitholapaxy (MIP). Urologe A. 2008;47(9):1068–73.
5. Zhu W, Liu Y, Liu L, Lei M, Yuan J, Wan SP, Zeng G. Minimally invasive versus standard percutaneous nephrolithotomy: a meta-analysis. Urolithiasis. 2015;43(6):563–70.
6. Desai J, Solanki R. Ultra-mini percutaneous nephrolithotomy (UMP): one more armamentarium. BJU Int. 2013;112(7):1046–9.
7. Zeng G, Wan S, Zhao Z, Zhu J, Tuerxun A, Song C, Zhong L, Liu M, Xu K, Li H, Jiang Z, Khadgi S, Pal SK, Liu J, Zhang G, Liu Y, Wu W, Chen W, Sarica K. Super-mini percutaneous nephrolithotomy (SMP): a new concept in technique and instrumentation. BJU Int. 2016;117(4):655–61.
8. Turk C, Petrik A, Sarica K, Seitz C, Skolarikos A, Straub M, Knoll T. EAU guidelines on interventional treatment for urolithiasis. Eur Urol. 2016;69(3):475–82.
9. Zanetti SP, Talso M, Palmisano F, Longo F, Gallioli A, Fontana M, De Lorenzis E, Sampogna G, Boeri L, Albo G, Trinchieri A, Montanari E. Comparison among the available stone treatment techniques from the first European Association of Urology Section of Urolithiasis (EULIS) survey: do we have a Queen? PLoS One. 2018;13:e0205159.
10. Lahme S. Miniaturisation of PCNL. Urolithiasis. 2018;46(1):99–106.
11. Gao XS, Liao BH, Chen YT, Feng SJ, Gao R, Luo DY, Liu JM, Wang KJ. Different tract sizes of miniaturized percutaneous nephrolithotomy versus retrograde intrarenal surgery: a systematic review and meta-analysis. J Endourol. 2017;31(11):1101–10.
12. Hyams ES, Munver R, Bird VG, Uberoi J, Shah O. Flexible ureterorenoscopy and holmium laser lithotripsy for the management of renal stone burdens that measure 2 to 3 cm: a multi-institutional experience. J Endourol. 2010;24(10):1583–8.
13. Lahme S, Zimmermanns V, Hochmuth A, Janitzki V. Minimally invasive PCNL (mini-perc). Alternative treatment modality or replacement of conventional PCNL? Urologe A. 2008;47(5):563–8.

14. Schilling D, Winter B, Merseburger AS, Anastasiadis AG, Walcher U, Stenzl A, Nagele U. Use of a gelatine-thrombin matrix for closure of the access tract without a nephrostomy tube in minimally invasive percutaneous nephrolitholapaxy. Urologe A. 2008;47(5):601–7.
15. Zhong W, Zeng G, Wu W, Chen W, Wu K. Minimally invasive percutaneous nephrolithotomy with multiple mini tracts in a single session in treating staghorn calculi. Urol Res. 2011;39(2):117–22.
16. Abdelhafez MF, Bedke J, Amend B, Elganainy E, Aboulella H, Elakkad M, Nagele U, Stenzl A, Schilling D. Minimally invasive percutaneous nephrolitholapaxy (PCNL) as an effective and safe procedure for large renal stones. BJU Int. 2012;110(11 Pt C):E1022–6.
17. Jones P, Elmussareh M, Aboumarzouk OM, Mucksavage P, Somani BK. Role of minimally invasive (micro and ultra-mini) PCNL for adult urinary stone disease in the modern era: evidence from a systematic review. Curr Urol Rep. 2018;19(4):27.
18. Yan X, Al-Hayek S, Gan W, Zhu W, Li X, Guo H. Minimally invasive percutaneous nephrolithotomy in preschool age children with kidney calculi (including stones induced by melamine-contaminated milk powder). Pediatr Surg Int. 2012;28(10):1021–4.
19. Bader MJ, Grützke C, Seitz M, Sharma R, Stief CG, Desai M. The "all-seeing-needle": initial results of an optical puncture system confirming access in percutaneous nephrolithotomy. Eur Urol. 2011;59(6):1054–9.
20. Desai JD. Prospective outcomes of 11-13Ch. Ultra-mini percutaneous nephrolithotomy (UMP): a consecutive cohort study. Arch Esp Urol. 2017;70(1):202–10.
21. Hennessey DB, Kinnear NK, Troy A, Angus D, Bolton DM, Webb DR. Mini PCNL for renal calculi: does size matter? BJU Int. 2017;119(Suppl 5):39–46.

ECIRS (Endoscopic Combined IntraRenal Surgery): From Background Actor to Main Character of the Endourological Treatment of Urolithiasis

17

Cesare Marco Scoffone and Cecilia Maria Cracco

17.1 The Acronym ECIRS

ECIRS is an acronym standing for Endoscopic Combined IntraRenal Surgery, coined in 2008 [1], and duplicating the already existing acronym RIRS, standing for Retrograde IntraRenal Surgery.

For a long time our group has been the only one using it, both as an acronym and surgical approach for the treatment of large and/or complex urolithiasis [1, 2], but year after year ECIRS has come into the play. ECIRS has been included in the EAU (European Association of Urology) Guidelines on Urolithiasis since 2018 [3] and is nowadays used all over the world including Europe, South America and Asia in up to 30% of the percutaneous nephrolithotripsy (PNL) cases [4]. On the other hand, ECIRS is still not very popular in North America and Australia, although the interest seems to be somehow rising lately [5].

17.2 A Bit of History

PNL and retrograde flexible ureteroscopy (fURS) occasionally intersected within the same renal stone surgery during the 1980s, but retrograde fURS became an essential tool rather than a complementary step of PNL only in the 1990s thanks to the Spanish urologist Gaspar Ibarluzea, who regularly employed it along with a new modified supine position, later named Galdakao-modified supine Valdivia (GMSV) position [6]. His inheritance has been taken over by many urologists who experienced the advantages of the combined approach in terms of safety and efficacy although not all of them shifted from the prone to the supine/supine-modified positions [6–10].

17.3 Patient Positioning for ECIRS: From Prone to Supine and Supine-Modified Positions

Prone positioning of the patient for PNL was not a clinically reasoned choice but simply an inheritance from the radiologists, percutaneously draining hydronephrotic kidneys without passing through the renal parenchyma. When urologists developing the PNL technique took the renal puncture away from the radiologists' hands, establishing themselves the percutaneous renal access, they did not consider the possibility to modify the patient's position, which became the traditional one and remained such for decades [6].

In the past, only occasionally urologists tried alternative positions for PNL in selected and challenging cases like high-risk or obese patients,

C. M. Scoffone (✉) · C. M. Cracco
Department of Urology, Cottolengo Hospital of Torino, Torino, Italy

G. Zeng, K. Sarica (eds.), *Percutaneous Nephrolithotomy*,
https://doi.org/10.1007/978-981-15-0575-1_17

elderly or children, mainly because of the positive anaesthesiological effects.

During the late 1980s Josè Gabriel Valdivia Urìa from Spain started to regularly perform PNL in his supine-modified position with the operated flank elevated. Later on, another Spanish urologist, Gaspar Ibarluzea, proposed to add to the Valdivia supine position an asymmetric lithotomic arrangement of the lower limbs (Fig. 17.1), in order to associate the anaesthesiological advantages of the supine decubitus with an easy retrograde access to the collecting system. This position was named the Galdakao-modified supine Valdivia (GMSV) position, from the name of the hospital where Dr. Ibarluzea worked in Bilbao, and became our favourite one for ECIRS, optimally supporting this kind of approach [6].

Many urologists additionally described a variety of oblique, flank, complete supine and modified prone positions, allowing ECIRS and smooth anaesthesiological intraoperative management. Anaesthetists themselves confirmed the better cardiovascular and airway controls, the reduced risk of pressure damages and ischemia, the improved hemodynamic and pharmacokinetic conditions, the decreased risk of accidental extubation and kinking of the tracheal tube while turning the patient prone [5, 9, 10].

Urological and management benefits have been less evident for a long time, especially because the discussion remained blocked on the anaesthesiological issue, and the equivalent urological outcomes in terms of safety and efficacy clouded some obvious considerations [1, 2, 5, 6, 9]. Such benefits include the easy, safe and com-

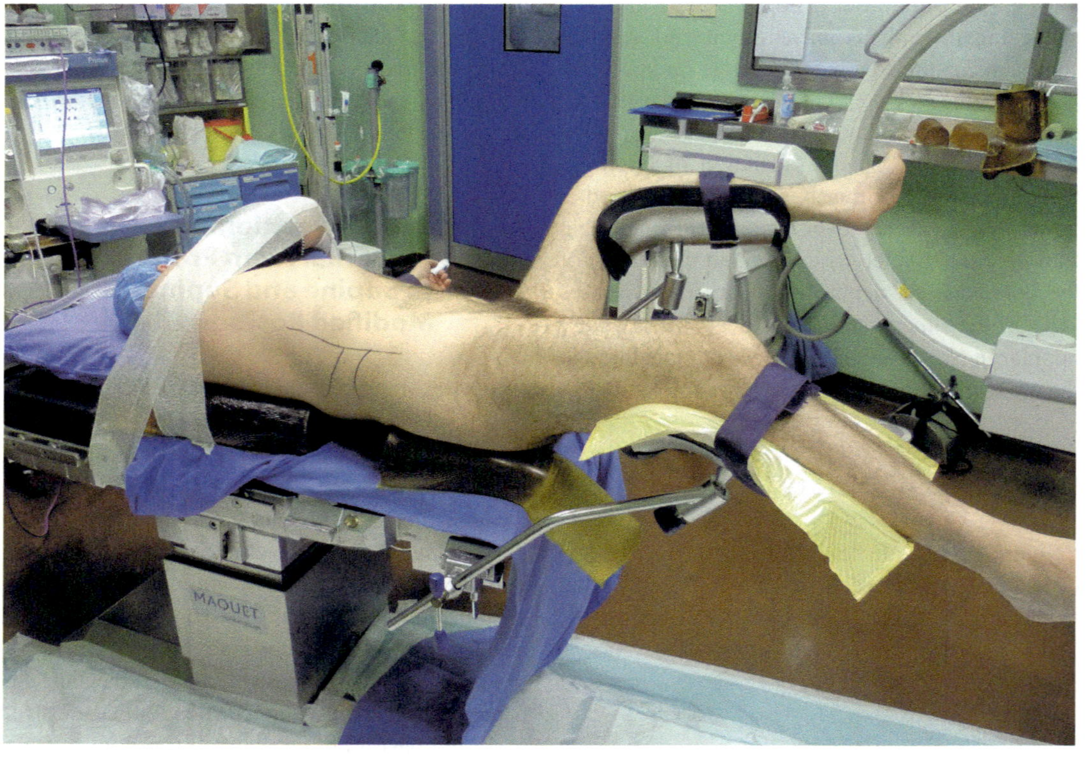

Fig. 17.1 The Galdakao-modified supine Valdivia (GMSV) position with the operated flank elevated by two jelly pillows and the legs arranged in a asymmetric lithotomic position with the ipsilateral leg slightly extended and the contralateral one well flexed and abducted

fortable supine patient positioning with no intraoperative changes, less need of nurses, diminished time and manipulation of the anaesthetized patient, decreased occupational risk related to shifting heavy loads, lowered risk of pressure damages, and no need for the sterile redraping of the patient (Fig. 17.2). The antegrade surgeon can work sitting down (Fig. 17.3) with the hands outside the fluoroscopic field; the colon moves away from the puncture area especially in the Valdivia supine and all the supine-modified positions because it drops down on the opposite side. The Amplatz sheath is horizontal or slightly inclined downwards (Fig. 17.4), favouring irrigation outflow and lowering intrarenal pressures with a reduced uroseptic risk as well as a better spontaneous drainage of stone fragments.

We have to underline also some disadvantages of the supine positions, mainly an increased mobility of the kidney, sometimes requiring an auxiliary help in order to stabilize the kidney (coordinated abdominal counterpressure, brief apnoea in maximal inspiration, through-and-through guidewire) and a restricted working space compared to the large working field of the prone position, even though the elevation of the flank helps enlarging the working space outlined by the reference lines (posterior axillary line, 12th rib and iliac crest) as well as patient positioning near the edge of the operating table (Fig. 17.5).

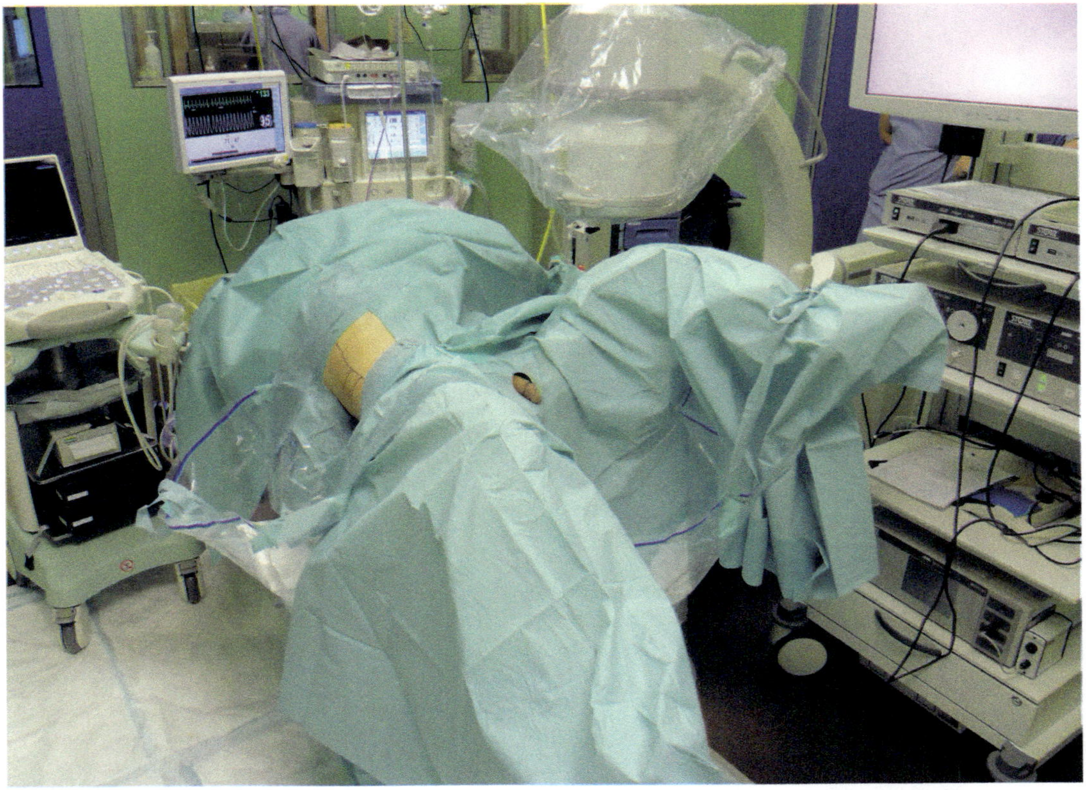

Fig. 17.2 The unique sterile draping of the patient for ECIRS with both antegrade and retrograde operating fields. Part of the organization of the operating room is also visible with the ultrasound device, the anaesthesiological armamentarium, the C-arm and the video tower

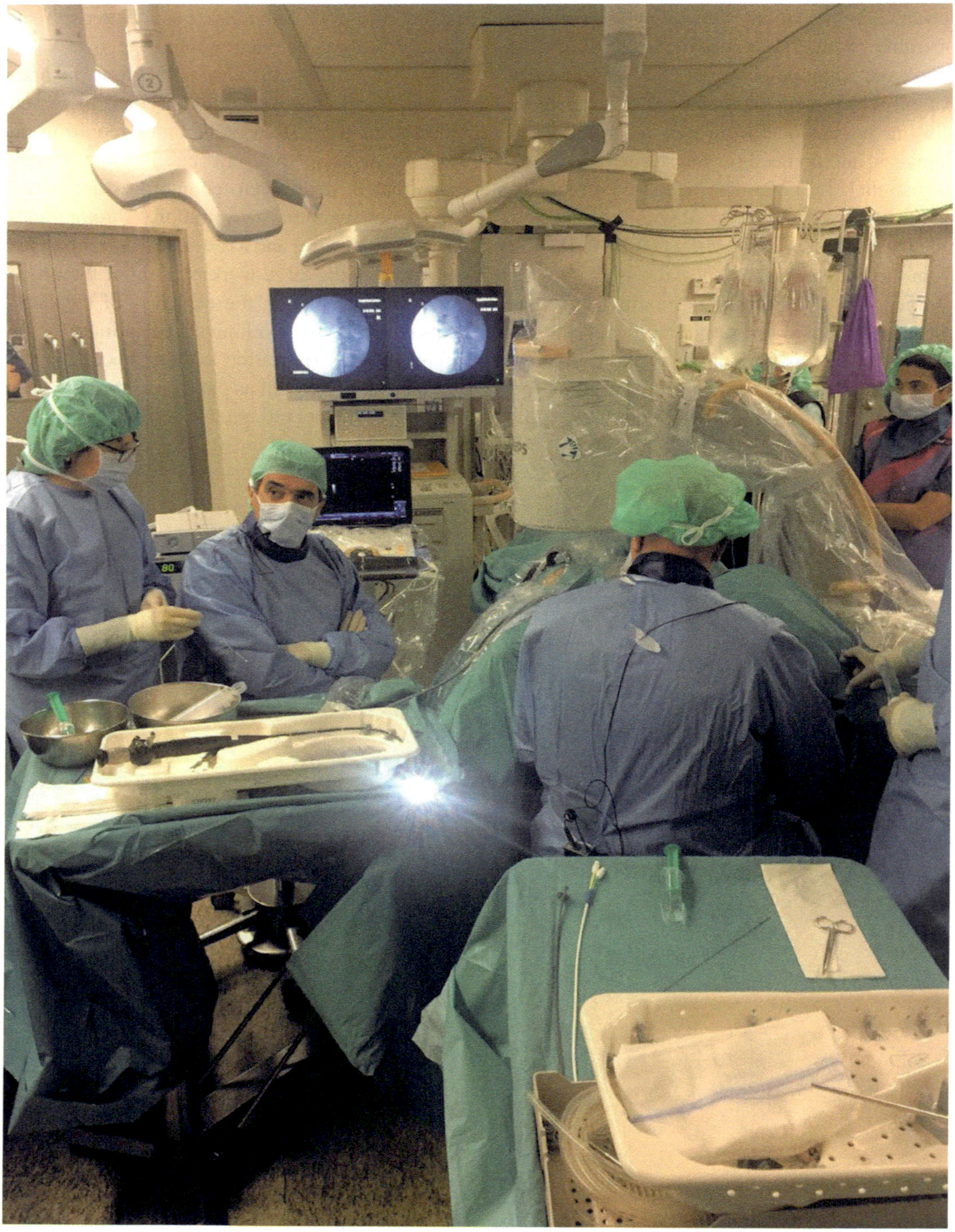

Fig. 17.3 The antegrade surgeon can work sitting down

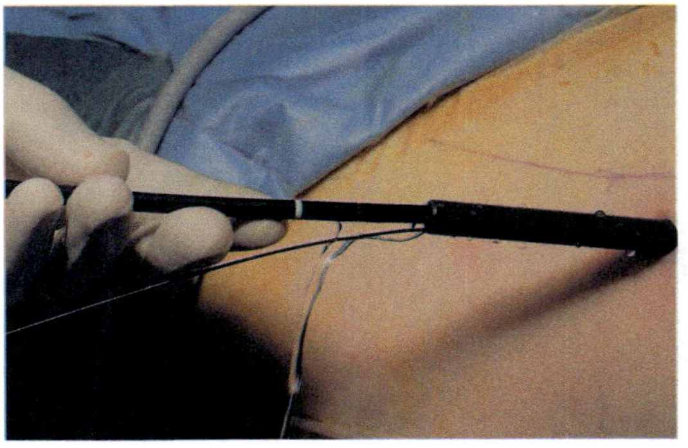

Fig. 17.4 During ECIRS in the GMSV position the direction of the Amplatz sheath is horizontal or slightly inclined downwards with optimal irrigation outflow and stone fragments' spontaneous drainage

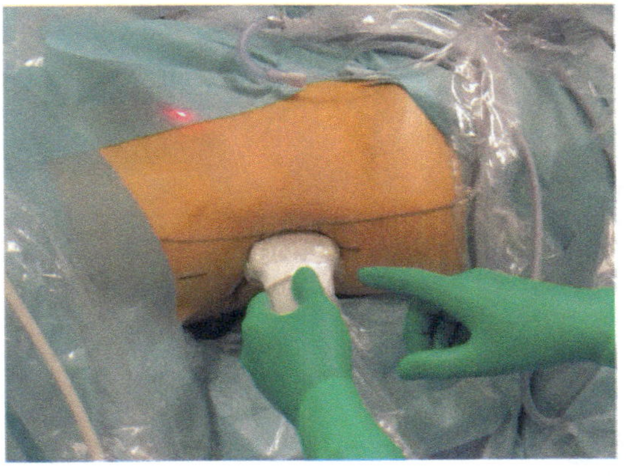

Fig. 17.5 The reference lines (posterior axillary line, 12th rib and iliac crest) are drawn on the skin of the operated side. Two small additional lines define the horizontal plane which can be followed straight forward to reach with the needle the lateral margin of the kidney, identified by means of ultrasound examination

17.4 Setup of the Operating Room and Preparation of Instruments/Devices/Accessories

In view of an ECIRS, a standardized organization of the operating room and a reasoned preparation of all instruments, devices and accessories are fundamental.

The operating table has to be radiolucent, with no interposed radiopaque bars, mobile in order to host the C-arm of the fluoroscope with the possibility to be arranged with the padded leg stirrups for the modified lithotomic position of the lower limbs. The floor underneath is usually covered by absorbent paddings in order to prevent fluid spilling although the sterile draping has pouches for both accesses.

During ECIRS the operating room is for sure very crowded; therefore, a thorough, standardized and coordinated preparation is required (Figs. 17.1, 17.2, and 17.3). The organization differs in case of right or left surgery. The result is a well-organized team work including urologists, anaesthetist and all nurses.

- Ultrasound and fluoroscopy screen are put on the side to be operated
- The anaesthetist and the needed equipment are located behind the head of the patient
- Lithotripsy devices (laser and ballistic/ultrasonic lithotripters) are placed behind the antegrade surgeon, sitting in front of the flank to be operated
- The C-arm of the fluoroscope with the radiology technician and video tower are positioned in front of the antegrade surgeon and on the side of the patient opposite to surgery
- Antegrade irrigation is near the C-arm and the head of the patient; retrograde irrigation is near the video tower and the legs of the patient
- The scrub nurse stands between the antegrade and the retrograde surgeons with the retrograde surgeon being between the lower limbs of the patient, the antegrade table behind the antegrade surgeon and the retrograde table behind the retrograde surgeon (Fig. 17.6).

The operation modes of all the devices must have been previously checked; all needed materials (like lead aprons, jelly pillows and paddings, or adhesive stripes) and accessories (like guidewires, ureteral catheters, nephrostomies, double-J stents, laser fibers, ballistic/ultrasound probes, needle for the renal puncture, progressive silicon dilators, Alken dilators and balloons of various sizes, Amplatz sheath, or ureteral access sheaths) must be prepared and ready in the operating room. All the operators must work without obsta-

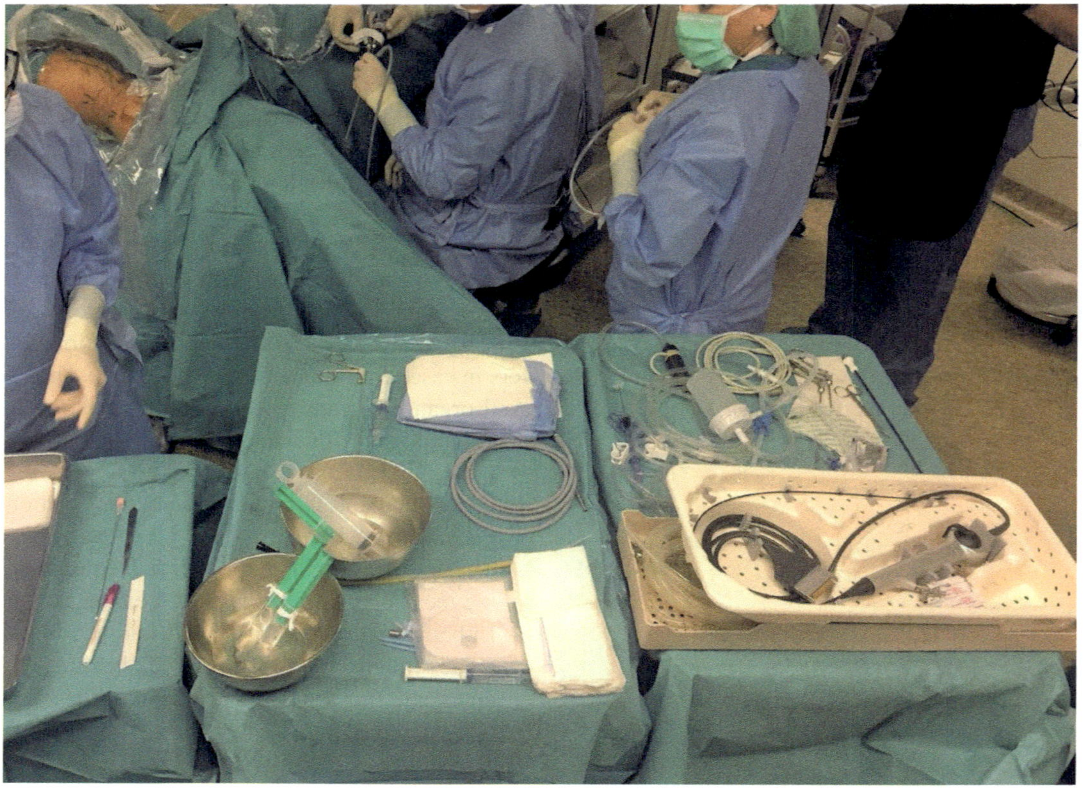

Fig. 17.6 The antegrade and retrograde scrub nurse tables

cles, having everything they need within arm's reach and comfortable.

17.5 The Rationale of ECIRS

ECIRS is an innovative interpretation of PNL because it introduces the standardized cooperation of retrograde flexible ureteroscopy (fURS) with the traditional antegrade percutaneous approach to the stone disease.

When we started to regularly employ retrograde fURS before and during PNL in 2003, we were very intrigued by the promises of the associated retrograde approach [1]. The very first and immediate addition was the possibility to perform the so-called Endovision percutaneous access, endoscopically checking the penetration of the needle through the tip of the papilla (Fig. 17.7),

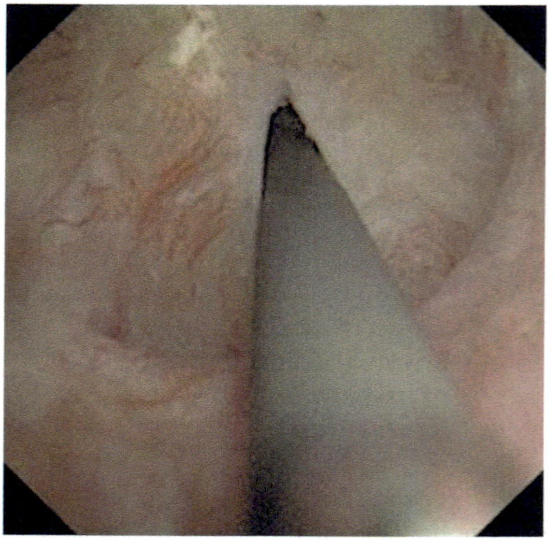

Fig. 17.7 The Endovision aspect of the hydrophilic guidewire inserted through the needle, papillary puncture of an inferior posterior single calyceal access

the insertion of the through-and-through guidewire, the sequential application of fascial, balloon/Alken/silicon dilators and of the Amplatz sheath. Under this retrograde surveillance the percutaneous access could be performed safely and with a reduced radiation exposure, avoiding overadvancement or insufficient insertion of the devices, preventing perforations of the collecting system, fluid extravasation, bleeding and loss of stone fragments in the retroperitoneum.

Unfortunately we soon realized that the Endovision puncture is extremely useful but not always possible, especially in case of impacted or staghorn stones, and also that the retrograde access is not feasible in about 20% of cases for various reasons (non-compliant ureter or ureteral orifice, ureteral spasms and strictures).

At the same time this moment of frustration became a chance of growth exactly when we realized that the conceptual value of ECIRS extends beyond a safe endoscopically guided renal puncture, and that its essence is not retrograde ureteroscopy at any cost with the risk of ureteral damage and related long-term sequelae (in case of non-compliant ureter, the traditional ureteral catheter is retrogradely inserted). On the contrary, the knowledge of the unfavourable features of the low urinary tract and ureter may be of additional help in order to understand the possible causes involved in stone formation and tailor the procedure on the patient's characteristics, planning an effective and safe strategy. Our patients all sign for both RIRS and PNL/ECIRS in the GMSV position and expect us to solve their urolithiasis in one step, choosing intraoperatively whether a retrograde approach is feasible, safe and effective, or whether a percutaneous approach is paradoxically more miniinvasive than a multistep RIRS.

When fully performed, ECIRS is a comprehensive approach to PNL, allowing a versatile and personalized tailoring of all the intraoperative choices in the real-time situation of the patient, the dynamic anatomy of the collecting system and the urolithiasis [2, 5–7, 11].

In ECIRS, retrograde fURS replaces the step of the cystoscopic application of the ureteral catheter for retrograde pyelography, allowing preliminary direct visualization of the urethra, ureteral orifice, ureter, ureteropelvic junction, pelvis and calyces with their infundibula and the instructive evaluation of their dynamic features for an optimal planning of the following strategy.

The diagnostic role of retrograde flexible ureteroscopy goes on intraoperatively, assisting all the steps of the percutaneous renal access (from needle insertion to Amplatz sheath application), stone treatment (lithotripsy and litholapaxy) and exit strategy. We usually say that the use of retrograde fURS puts the eye of the urologist on the tip of the retrograde catheter and the whole procedure in the urologist's hands.

The active role of retrograde flexible ureteroscopy is optional (ECIRS is such also when there is no other retrograde contribution but the diagnostic one) but may be essential for a safe antegrade or retrograde guidewire application to facilitate renal access and to improve stone clearance, managing or treating stones difficult to reach through a single percutaneous tract.

17.6 The Essential Role of Retrograde fURS During PNL and the Step-by-Step Procedure

Retrograde ureteroscopy (first semirigid, then flexible) allows:

- Preliminary lower urinary tract evaluation, timely identifying of urethral strictures, false urethral passages, obstructing or easily bleeding prostatic adenomas, calcified intravesical stents or tight ureteral orifices to deal with
- Passive ureteral dilation thanks to the tapered shape of the semirigid ureteroscope
- Assessment of the dynamic anatomy of the upper urinary tract, integrating the knowledge of the static anatomy deriving from preoperative imaging (evaluation of the elasticity of the collecting system, likelihood of detachment of impacted/staghorn calculi from the mucosa with the creation of a water path around the stone, recognition of suburothelial/parenchy-

mal calcifications looking like stones in non-contrast computed tomography) and driving intraoperative choices concerning size and location of the percutaneous access and type of tract dilation
- Endovision assistance to the percutaneous tract creation
- Generation of a water path around staghorn stones impacted within a calyx by means of retrograde irrigation, facilitating the insertion of the hydrophilic guidewire and supporting the choice of technique of dilation and size of the access tract. In the absence of space between the stone and mucosa, tapered dilators like balloon or silicon dilators (requiring a space of at least 1 cm within the calyx to host their tip) will not be used, but Alken dilators (requiring no other space than that sufficient to host the ball-shaped tip of the first stylet) will be rather employed. If the infundibulum of the access calyx is thin, inelastic instruments and accessories will be adapted to the patient, choosing a miniaturized access to avoid breaking the collecting system causing useless bleeding
- Optional active contribution (about 50% of cases in our experience) in the application of the through and through guidewire (from the percutaneous renal access down the ureter or from below with the antegrade retrieval after the percutaneous access has been gained), the treatment/displacement of stones in calyces difficult to reach antegradely with both rigid and flexible nephroscopes, avoiding the need for multiple percutaneous accesses; and passing the ball through the Amplatz sheath
- Retrograde control of the ongoing antegrade lithotripsy performed by means of both rigid and flexible nephroscope, avoiding descent of fragments below the UPJ
- Final integrated exploration of all calyces allows in search of residual fragments in combination with the flexible nephroscope, aiming at an optimal stone-free status because removable using a basket
- Final evaluation of the collecting system, supporting the decision for a stentless or a stented procedure along with the assessment of the descent of the contrast medium from the pyelocalyceal system below the ureteropelvic junction and within the ureter

In summary, retrograde fURS during PNL has two distinct roles: a fundamental diagnostic one (allowing to adapt the whole surgical strategy to the patient, and sometimes to change the indication from PNL to RIRS in case of friable and retrogradely approachable medium-sized stones), and an optional active one. The diagnostic role being the prominent one, the risk of rupture of the flexible ureteroscope with its high costs is very limited, and, in any case, nowadays there is also the additional option of single-use digital flexible ureteroscopes.

17.7 Conclusions

In the 1970s PNL appeared as a revolutionary procedure for the treatment of large urolithiasis, successfully replacing the traditional invasive open renal surgery required until then. Subsequently PNL reinvented itself instead of simply aging becoming a safer and more effective procedure, thanks to the progresses in patient positioning, the evolution of the techniques of percutaneous renal access, the miniaturization of access tract and of endoscopes/devices/accessories and the improvement in intracorporeal lithotripsy energies [12]. For these reasons, current PNL is for sure much better than that its old version, and ECIRS is part of PNL maturation and improvement, being a comprehensive and versatile approach tailoring all intraoperative choices on the patient.

Conflicts of Interest Dr. C. M. Scoffone is consultant for Boston Scientific, Coloplast Porgés, Cook Medical, DBI, EMS, Olympus, Promed, Storz Medical; Dr. C. M. Cracco is tutor for Boston Scientific.

References

1. Scoffone CM, Cracco CM, Cossu M, et al. Endoscopic combined intrarenal surgery in Galdakao-modified supine Valdivia position: a new standard for percutaneous nephrolithotomy? Eur Urol. 2008;54:1393–403.
2. Scoffone CM, Cracco CM. Invited review: the tale of ECIRS (Endoscopic Combined Intrarenal Surgery)

in the Galdakao-modified supine Valdivia position. Urolithiasis. 2018;46:115–23.
3. https://uroweb.org/wp-content/uploads/EAU-Guidelines-on-Urolithiasis-2018-large-text.pdf. Accessed 15 June 2019.
4. Manzo BO, Lozada E, Vicentini FC, et al. Differences in percutaneous nephrolithotomy practice patterns among Latin American urologists with and without endourology training. Int Braz J Urol. 2018;44:512–23.
5. Scoffone CM, Cracco CM. Chapter 11: Patient positioning, the supine position and the rationale of ECIRS. In: Smith A, Preminger G, Kavoussi L, Badlani G, editors. Smith's textbook of endourology: Wiley-Blackwell; 2019.
6. Scoffone CM, Hoznek A, Cracco CM. Supine percutaneous nephrolithotomy and ECIRS. 1st ed. Paris, France: Springer; 2014.
7. Cracco CM, Knoll T, Liatsikos EN, et al. Rigid-only versus combined rigid and flexible percutaneous nephrolithotomy: a systematic review. Minerva Urol Nefrol. 2017;69(4):330–41.
8. Hamamoto S, Yasui T, Okada A, et al. Efficacy of endoscopic combined intrarenal surgery in the prone split-leg position for staghorn calculi. J Endourol. 2015;29(1):19–24.
9. Cracco CM, Alken P, Scoffone CM. Positioning for percutaneous nephrolithotomy. Curr Opin Urol. 2016;26:81–7.
10. Zhao Z, Fan J, Liu Y, et al. Percutaneous nephrolithotomy: position, position, position! Urolithiasis. 2018;46(1):79–86.
11. Scoffone CM, Cracco CM. The role of retrograde flexible ureteroscopy during percutaneous surgery: trick or treat? In: Autorino R, Liatsikos E, Feds P, editors. New technologies and techniques in minimally invasive urologic surgery. An ESUT collection. Torino: Minerva Medica; 2019. p. 148–54.
12. Ghani KR, Andonian S, Bultitude M, et al. Percutaneous nephrolithotomy: update, trands, and future directions. Eur Urol. 2016;70:382–96.

18 PCNL in Special Situations

Diego M. Carrion, Ramón Cansino, Cristina Ballesteros Ruiz, Juan Gómez Rivas, Juan A. Mainez Rodríguez, Jose R. Pérez-Carral, and Luis Martínez-Piñeiro

18.1 Introduction

There are several kidney anatomical situations in which the management of large urinary calculi presents a unique challenge to urologists.

In this chapter, we will review the management of large lithiasis in the most common kidney anatomical variants we could encounter in clinical practice, which include calyceal diverticula, ectopic (pelvic) kidneys, transplanted kidneys, horseshoe kidneys, spinal deformities, and pregnant patients.

In-depth knowledge of the incidence, pathophysiology, anatomical variations, indications, possible complications and experience in other published series are crucial for pursuing the best results available during percutaneous nephrolithotomy (PCNL). Adequate imaging with contrast-enhanced CT scans is paramount for the surgical planning and prevention of possible complications.

The goals of surgical treatment in these particular situations are similar to those of the normal kidneys. That is the complete clearance of all stone fragments using minimally invasive percutaneous surgery while minimizing secondary procedures and complications.

D. M. Carrion (✉) · R. Cansino · C. Ballesteros Ruiz
J. Gómez Rivas · J. A. Mainez Rodríguez
J. R. Pérez-Carral · L. Martínez-Piñeiro
Department of Urology, La Paz University Hospital, Madrid, Spain

Autonomous University of Madrid, Madrid, Spain
e-mail: joseramon.perez@salud.madrid.org; luis.mpineiro@salud.madrid.org

G. Zeng, K. Sarica (eds.), *Percutaneous Nephrolithotomy*, https://doi.org/10.1007/978-981-15-0575-1_18

18.2 Calyceal Diverticula

18.2.1 Generalities

Calyceal diverticula are defined as congenital, non-secretory cavities within the renal parenchyma, covered by transitional urothelium, which usually maintain a communication with the collecting system through a narrow isthmus [1].

The incidence of calyceal diverticula is thought to be less than 1% of the general population [2]. Theories about their development vary widely, from small divisions of the ureteral bud, which failed to degenerate [1–3], to sequelae of obstruction, infections, or infundibular stenosis [4]. Stone formation inside the diverticula is thought to be caused by urinary stasis inside the cavity, leading to urine crystal precipitation [5, 6]. However, in over 50% of these patients, an underlying metabolic abnormality predisposing to stone formation has been reported [6–9]. Therefore, besides surgical treatment, a complete metabolic evaluation should be done in order to find and treat possible metabolic derangements to prevent future stone recurrence [9].

18.2.2 Diagnosis and Treatment

At present, most patients are asymptomatic [10] and are found to have calyceal diverticula as an incidental finding (around 0.21–0.6% of intravenous pyelographic investigations) [3, 4, 11]. The common presenting symptoms of lithiasis inside calyceal diverticula are lumbar pain, hematuria, and recurrent urinary tract infections. Intradiverticular stones can be found in about 50–96% of patients with calyceal diverticula [3, 4, 10, 12–14].

The most accurate diagnosis for a calyceal diverticulum occupied by lithiasis, which also serves as preoperative planning is made with a contrast-enhanced CT scan. The urinary tract anatomy has to be assessed correctly for considering any other options of treatment and to prevent complications. The widespread use of non-contrast CT scans and intravenous pyelograms (IVP) may delay the accurate diagnosis of calyceal diverticula (Figs. 18.1 and 18.2) [15].

Although the presence of lithiasis does not serve as an indication for the surgical treatment itself, management is recommended for patients who present chronic pain, recurrent infections, hematuria, or progressive damage of the parenchyma.

The best treatment modality for every patient will depend on the size, location, and stone burden of the diverticulum. ESWL is reserved for small diverticula with stones less than 1.5 cm, which have an open neck through which fragments can eventually scape [12, 13].

Flexible ureteroscopy is preferred for diverticula located on the anterior face of the kidney, as well as middle and upper-poles, with small to moderate stone burden [12, 13]. We must have in mind that in most cases, the renal parenchyma surrounding the diverticulum is thin and delicate, and intraluminal pressure during ureteroscopy could result in fistula formation.

Laparoscopic surgery must be reserved for large, anteriorly located diverticula, in which percutaneous access is not safe or feasible.

PCNL is currently the best available treatment for diverticula with a large stone burden, especially on the posterior renal face. Although PCNL is more aggressive than ureteroscopy and ESWL, its stone-free rate is the highest of all the prior described techniques [9, 12, 15–17].

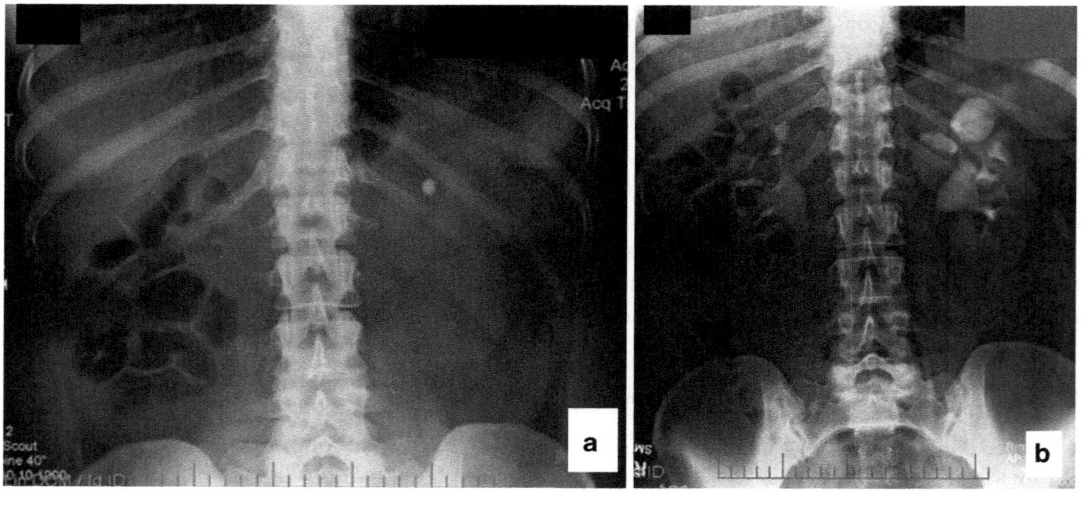

Fig. 18.1 (**a**) Abdominal X-ray demonstrating a calcification in the region of the upper pole of the left kidney. (**b**) IVP of the same patient demonstrating that the calcification is located within an upper pole calyceal diverticulum. (Modified from Mandeville Jessica A, Gnessin Ehud, Lingeman James E. Springer London Heidelberg New York Dorrdech; 2013 ("Percutaneous Management of calyceal diverticula: An American Experience." Difficult cases in endourology), p. 35. Reproduced with permission from Springer)

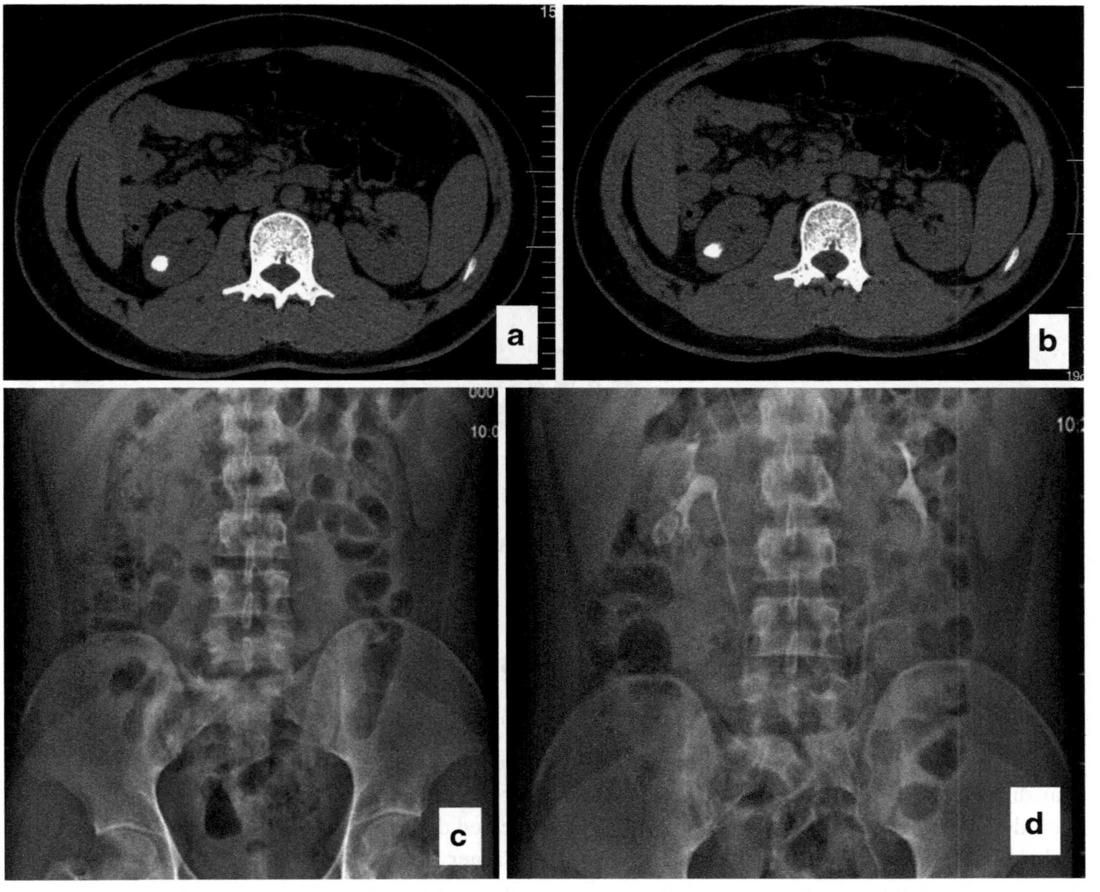

Fig. 18.2 (**a**, **b**) CT scan images from a patient with a right kidney calyceal diverticulum occupied by a stone. (**c**, **d**) Intravenous pyelogram images of a patient with a right lower pole calyceal diverticulum occupied by a lithiasis. (Reproduced with permission from Dr. Wei Zhu)

18.2.3 Considerations and Technique for PCNL

Most commonly, following opacification of the upper urinary tract and the collecting system and the diverticulum through an external ureteral catheter, the puncture can be performed with a large (18-G) needle directly into the diverticular cavity. Some authors have described the puncture directly to radiopaque lithiasis without prior opacification, especially in anterior diverticula [9, 18].

A disadvantage of saline and/or contrast instillation may be the distension of the collecting system, making in some cases a more difficult direct puncture to the diverticulum. Moreover, contrast may also obscure the diverticulum [9]. In such cases, the puncture can be performed under ultrasonographic control.

Tract dilation can be performed through the needle as usual, with metallic Amplatz dilators or with the one-shot dilation method.

An alternative is to perform dilation up to the immediate proximity of the external diverticular wall, with only the tip of the guidewire entering the cavity (Fig. 18.3). After dilation, the nephroscope should be inserted inside the Amplatz sheath, and the puncture orifice of the diverticulum can be widened for its entry with the help of alligator forceps. This method is particularly recommended in the cases of small diverticula [18].

After fragmentation of the lithiasis and the removal of its fragments, different strategies are

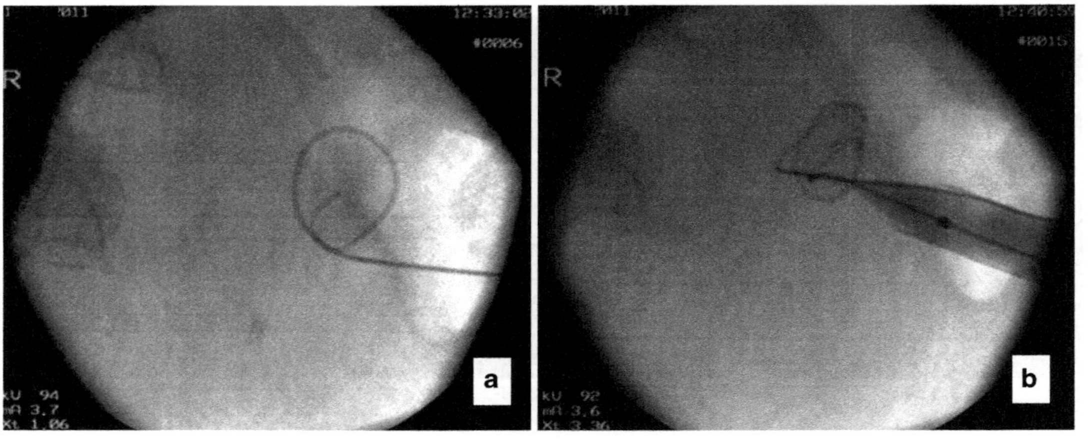

Fig. 18.3 (**a**) J-tipped removable wire coiled within a moderate-sized calyceal diverticulum. (**b**) 30 French Amplatz sheath advanced over the dilating balloon up to the point of the diverticular cavity. (Modified from Mandeville Jessica A, Gnessin Ehud, Lingeman James E. Springer London Heidelberg New York Dorrdech; 2013 ("Percutaneous Management of calyceal diverticula: An American Experience." Difficult cases in endourology, p. 38. Reproduced with permission of Springer)

used for the management of the diverticular cavity and neck.

One approach involves the progressive dilation of the diverticular neck and then placing a transdiverticular nephrostomy catheter, which should continue up to the pelvis [19–21].

In more complicated cases, when the diverticular neck is not easily encountered, methylene blue or indigo carmine can be injected slowly and steadily through the external catheter for easier recognition of the neck.

As a last resource, if the neck cannot be recognized with the prior described method, a possible alternative is to create a neo-neck by placing a nephrostomy catheter through it [22, 23].

The intradiverticular urothelium can be later fulgurated with a Bugbee, bipolar or roller electrode, or even photocoagulated with laser to prevent parenchymal bleeding and to achieve retraction of the cavity to prevent further stone formation [16, 18, 24]. This is debated by some authors who state that the urothelium inside diverticula is non-secretory [25], and others suggest that the mechanical trauma of the percutaneous tract and surgery is sufficient to achieve the disintegration of the cavity [26].

18.2.4 Complications

PCNL offers a more effective treatment than flexible ureteroscopy with a low, but existing concern for major complications, especially in anteriorly located diverticula due to a longer tract involving a larger amount of renal parenchyma. In these cases, another possible complication during surgery is the loss of the percutaneous tract, also because of the reduced space in the diverticular cavity [12, 13, 27, 28].

In the cases where a diverticular neck incision is achieved, there is an increased risk of puncturing an interlobar artery and subsequent bleeding, owing to the proximity of these vessels to the calyceal infundibulum.

18.2.5 Results and Conclusions

The success of PCNL in the cases of intradiverticular stones can be defined in the complete extraction of the stone fragments, the achievement of postoperative absence of symptoms such as pain and recurrent infections, or complete obliteration of the cavity. We could say that the most important achievements of a successful

PCNL are the stone-free status and the absence of symptoms, in which obtaining a wide communication between the pyelocaliceal system and the diverticular cavity is paramount.

The results from PCNL in these cases, with all its variations in techniques, vary between 70 and 100% for the stone-free rate and disappearance of symptoms, and between 66 and 100% for complete obliteration of the diverticular cavity [9, 12, 15–17].

18.3 Pelvic Kidneys

18.3.1 Generalities

Renal ectopia is defined as an atypically located kidney due to the failure of migration from the fetal pelvis during embryologic development. An ectopic kidney can be abdominal, lumbar, or pelvic based on its position in the retroperitoneum.

Incidence of ectopic kidneys in the general population has been reported to be between 1 in 2200 and 1 in 3000 [12, 29], the majority of patients being men and most commonly on the left side [13, 29].

18.3.2 Diagnosis and Treatment

Patients are usually asymptomatic through their lifetime, having no more susceptibility to diseases than patients with normally located kidneys, except for the development of hydronephrosis and lithiasis. The high insertion of the ureter and malrotation predisposes these kidneys to urinary stasis and nephrolithiasis [13, 30]. If presenting symptoms, the most common is usually flank pain, which can be explained due to the same innervation pathway of these kidneys compared to the normally positioned kidneys [13, 30].

Although located in the retroperitoneum, these kidneys are surrounded anteriorly by loops of bowel and posteriorly by the iliac bones, spine, and sacrum. Although a pelvic kidney can be easily recognized in an IVP (Fig. 18.4), imaging with contrast-enhanced CT scan is mandatory to

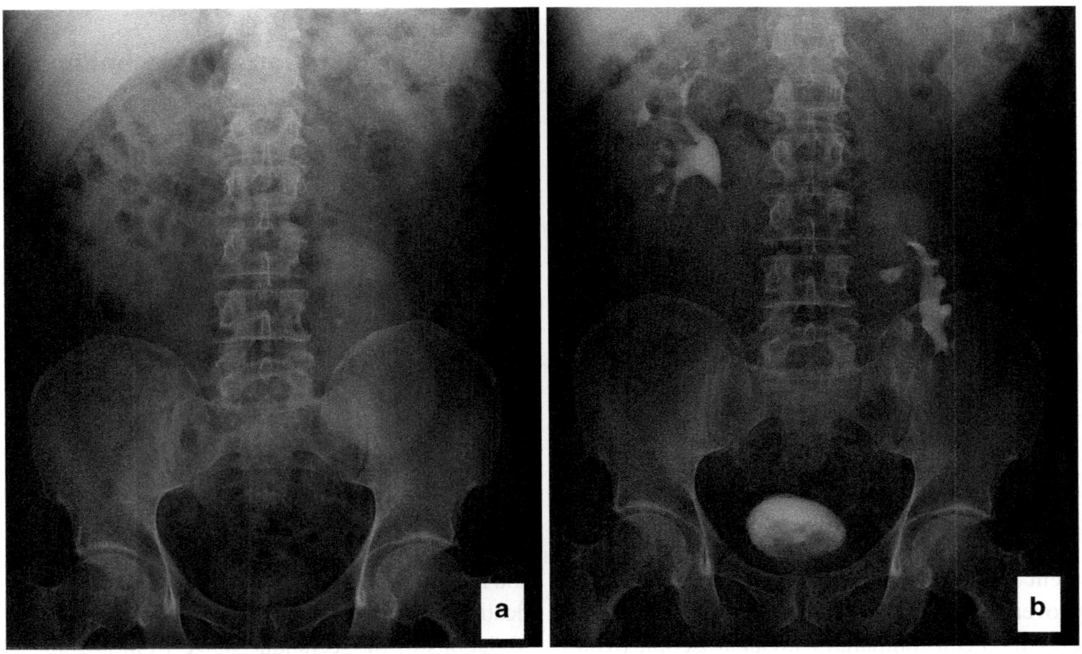

Fig. 18.4 IVP of a 57-year old man presenting a left pelvic kidney

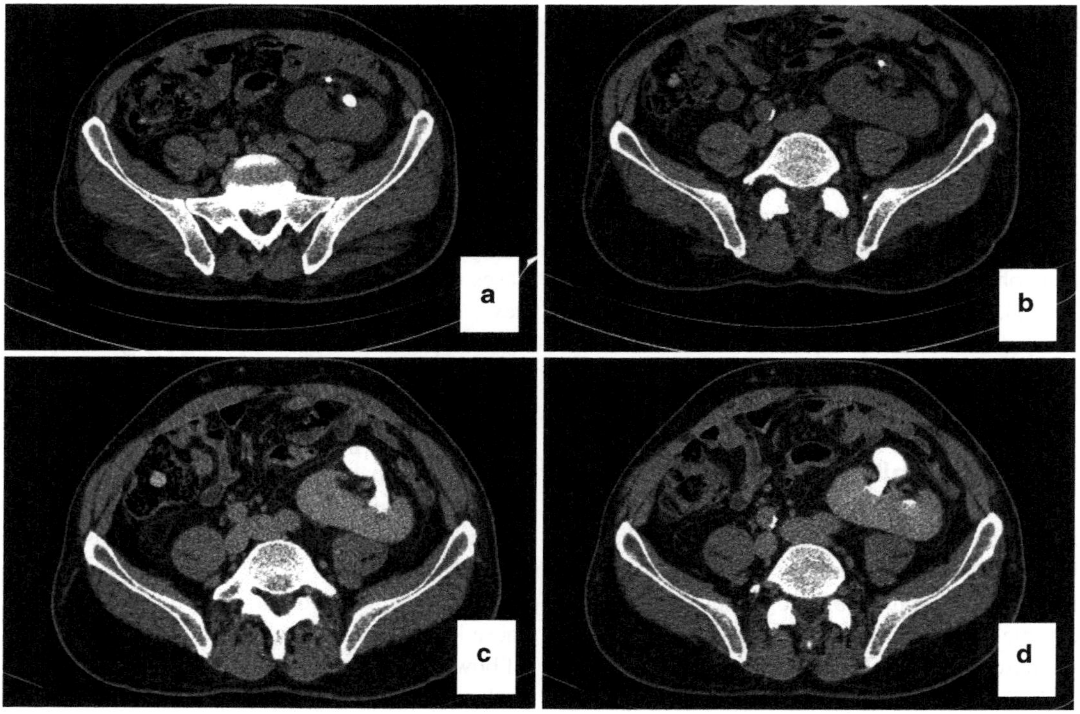

Fig. 18.5 CT scan of a 49-year old man with a left pelvic kidney. (**a**) Lithiasis measuring 14 × 12 mm located in the medial calyx. (**b**) Lithiasis measuring 4 × 3 mm in the renal pelvis. (**c**, **d**) Excretory phases showing the orientation of the upper urinary tract within the abdominal cavity

identify anomalous vasculature and the urinary tract anatomy before surgery (Fig. 18.5).

Pelvic kidneys with lithiasis pose some important challenges for surgical treatments. The efficiency of ESWL is very limited due to the surrounding bowel and bone structures, and a significant proportion of patients will need repeated sessions or further treatments to achieve a stone-free status [31]. Moreover, the clearance of fragments is impaired due to the higher insertion of the ureter, its tortuous anatomy, and abnormal pyeloureteral motility that can be the result of the surrounding fibrous tissue [30]. These latter circumstances make flexible ureteroscopy very challenging [30, 32].

So far, PCNL remains the most effective treatment modality for this particular scenario. It has proven to be as effective as in normal kidneys and even has been compared with laparoscopic pyelolithotomy in terms of achieving stone-free status with a less aggressive intervention [31, 33–36].

18.3.3 Considerations and Technique for PCNL

Two approaches have been well described to obtain an adequate puncture and access into the target calyx in pelvic kidneys, one with the visual guidance of intraperitoneal laparoscopy, and the other with ultrasound-guidance.

Since the first report of a transabdominal laparoscopic-guided PCNL, by Eshghi et al. in 1985 [37], modifications such as using the Trendelenburg position to displace bowel [34] and even intracorporeal suturing of the nephrostomy site after the placement of a ureteral stent have been described [38].

With the intention of reducing the risk of bowel and mesenteric vessel during surgery, several modifications of the tract placement have been described. Variations of the technique range from creating a transabdominal tract which advances transmesenterically between the major mesenteric vessels to allow a better exposure of the kidney, to establishing the access tract totally extraperitoneal [39]. This last approach has the advantage of leaving the peritoneal cavity intact and reducing fluid drainage. Lastly, even posterior access through the greater sciatic foramen has also been described [40].

Percutaneous ultrasound-guided puncture has been reported to be a safe approach in experienced surgeons' hands. Authors stand that abdominal viscera can be easily identified and even manually deflected away with an ultrasound probe. In addition, with the help of color Doppler, significant blood vessels can be identified and avoided [32, 33, 36]. Correct positioning is mandatory if ultrasound is used to direct the puncture. The objective is to separate as much bowel away from the target kidney; a sandbag can be used to bring the pelvic kidney closer to the anterior abdominal wall, and, at the same time, compression with the ultrasound probe can allow safer access into the urinary tract. Drawbacks of this approach are an associated risk of posing injuries to overlying collapsed bowel and the difficulties in the creation of a second tract, if needed. If we plan to do a prone puncture, the sandbag should be positioned between the operating table and the anterior abdominal wall and a superior calyx puncture will be preferred in this scenario. Bowel injuries can be less frequent if the prone position is used, but due to the anatomical variants between cases, not all patients will be suitable for it.

Other benefits of using ultrasound-guided puncture include to discriminate between posterior and anterior calyces easily, to allow 3-dimensional spatial orientation, and identification of the shortest possible puncture to the target calyx with a better perception of deepness [33].

18.3.4 Complications

When the laparoscopic-assisted puncture is being used, we must take into account all the possible complications of abdominal port placement and a longer mean operative time.

The most commonly reported complications of PCNL in these cases include postoperative infection, bleeding from abnormal vasculature, catheter dislodgment, injury to the surrounding bowel, or spillage of fluid into the peritoneum which can cause paralytic ileus [30, 31]. The incidence of nerve and bowel injuries is increased in these cases compared to in the normally located kidneys, with an incidence of 13–27% according to different series [34, 41].

18.3.5 Results and Conclusions

PCNL has proven to be the most effective surgical technique for lithiasis in pelvic kidneys. Several authors report similar effectiveness compared to normally located kidneys, and even compare the stone-clearance rate with laparoscopic pyelolithotomy [31, 33–36]. We believe that with the more extended use of mini-PCNL, the possible complications associated with this surgery will diminish.

At the present time, the ideal method for puncture of ectopic kidneys has not been established but is well known that the most important part of this surgery is to achieve adequate access to the collecting system thought the target calyx.

The decision of laparoscopic or ultrasound-guided access should be carefully and individually decided. Surgeon experience and patient anatomy can favor one approach over the other.

We believe that the endoscopic view and direct mobilization of structures with a laparoscopic approach, associated with the advantage of a possible, safer transmesenteric tract dilation, make this approach more feasible and recommended.

18.4 Transplanted Kidneys

18.4.1 Generalities

The incidence of lithiasis in transplanted kidneys ranges from 0.23 to 6.3% in the most recent series [42, 43]. Rarely, small calculi may have been present beforehand in the donor kidney (graft-gifted lithiasis) [44], but normally they occur de novo due to numerous factors that predispose to stone formation in donated kidneys.

Donors who have a history of stone formation, recurrent lithiasis, or active metabolic diseases are generally excluded from donation. Currently, it is agreed that lithiasis no larger than 4 mm could be left in situ in donor kidneys [45–47].

Kidney recipients with chronic kidney disease often present secondary or tertiary hypothyroidism, which predisposes to them to hypercalcemia and consequent hypercalciuria. Regarding medication, chronic immunosuppression may predispose to recurrent urinary tract infections and other metabolic issues [48]. More specifically, cyclosporine A can predispose to uricosuria, and excessive urate in urine can act as a precursor for calcium oxalate stone formation [13]. The most common composition of lithiasis in transplanted kidneys is calcium oxalate, whereas uric acid stones are relatively uncommon [45, 49].

Other factors predisposing to lithiasis formation are foreign bodies, such as non-absorbable sutures, papillary necrosis, and other less common metabolic abnormalities.

18.4.2 Diagnosis and Treatment

In patients with transplanted kidneys, the typical renal colic is absent due to denervation of the graft. Most commonly, patients will present with signs and symptoms of acute rejection or acute tubular necrosis [50, 51]. The most common presenting signs in a large series include obstructive anuria, acute renal failure, unexplained fever, hematuria, and urinary tract infection [43, 52]. Because transplanted patients depend only on their graft to preserve the renal function, the calculi should be treated quickly and aggressively to avoid graft loss.

The particular location of transplanted kidneys represents a unique situation, which is favorable for a percutaneous approach. The close proximity to the skin makes access easier, although it is recommended to obtain CT images before to exclude overlying abdominal viscera and identify the most appropriate access.

Treatment with ESWL is considered reasonable for calculi smaller than 1.5 cm, although it is very challenging due to the particular location of the kidney inside the bony pelvis [49].

Although previous groups have reported successful treatments with flexible ureteroscopy, these procedures are frequently compromised due to the difficult access to the ureter and the periureteral fibrosis resulting from previous surgery [48].

PCNL for transplanted kidneys is generally recommended for calculi larger than 15–20 mm.

Open surgery in these patients can associate delayed wound healing, sepsis, and fistula formation due to the immunosuppression status. Therefore it should be reserved for those particular patients in whom PCNL has been unsuccessful [51].

18.4.3 Considerations and Technique for PCNL

A favorable detail for PCNL in transplanted kidneys is that part of the management of the acute episode of anuria or oliguria involves the placement of a percutaneous nephrostomy catheter in the acute setting. If by any reason the preexisting nephrostomy has been placed in such a way that is not the ideal for dilation and PCNL access, another more precise puncture should be obtained at the beginning of the surgery [53].

Fluoroscopy and ultrasound can be used together in the operating room to achieve a safer puncture. Percutaneous access can be achieved more easily in the supine position, where access can be best achieved with an ultrasound-guided puncture, or even in the modified lithotomy position if we desire a combined retrograde access through the bladder.

Most commonly, left donor kidneys will be placed into the recipient's right iliac fossa and vice versa. This particular condition rotates the axis of the kidney 180°, thus, making the posterior calyces point anteriorly. This particular condition makes the approach similar to a native kidney.

Although the kidney is relatively close to the abdominal wall, and in the retroperitoneum, the fibrotic capsule in which a transplanted kidney lays makes dilation somewhat more challenging. Thus, balloon fascial dilators can be used as a first step, but if they fail, Amplatz dilators or metal Alken sequential dilators will be helpful to dilate this fibrotic tissue [50, 53, 54]. Another consideration regarding the fibrotic capsule is that excessive torque can lead to massive hemorrhage and parenchymal destruction [13]. To prevent this, a flexible nephroscope and ureteroscope, along with baskets, should be available to use whenever necessary [49].

18.4.4 Complications

Although rare, potential complications include bleeding, sepsis (more risk in immunocompromised patients), delayed wound healing, and urine leaks [13, 53, 55]. A CT scan is always recommended for correct planning and minimizing complications such as bowel or vascular injuries [54, 56].

18.4.5 Results and Conclusions

PCNL is currently considered a feasible and safe approach for the treatment of large calculi in transplanted kidneys. Success rates of up to 100% have been recently reported in case series without major complications [53, 55].

Therefore, PCNL should be considered as the treatment of choice for stones larger than 1.5–2 cm in transplanted kidneys. CT scan should be mandatory in order to plan the best access possible. After surgery, these patients must undergo a complete metabolic evaluation to prevent as much as possible further stone formation.

18.5 Horseshoe Kidneys

18.5.1 Generalities

Among renal fusion anomalies, horseshoe kidneys are the most commonly reported, with a higher incidence in males than females [31].

During embryogenesis (4th to 8th weeks of intrauterine life), the fusion of the lower kidney pole imposes an obstacle to the normal ascent and is responsible for the malrotation and anterior displacement of the collecting system. Furthermore, the insertion of the ureter on the renal pelvis is displaced superiorly and laterally, which is associated with a significantly higher rate of ureteropelvic junction obstruction (15–33%) [57]. Moreover, the aberrant course of the proximal ureter, which courses ventrally over the renal symphysis, may predispose it to be compressed by abnormal vessels that supply the lower renal pole and isthmus.

All the previously mentioned anatomic deviations contribute to impaired drainage and urine stasis, a higher incidence of recurrent urinary tract infections and calculous formation, which has been reported to be approximately 20% [40, 58].

18.5.2 Diagnosis and Treatment

The innervation of horseshoe kidneys does not change in comparison to normal kidneys, so the symptoms of renal colic and ureteral obstruction are the same. Some atypical presentations may be vague abdominal pain or even emesis [12].

Imaging with contrast-enhanced CT is mandatory in order to visualize accordingly aberrant vasculature, anomalies in the collecting system, and interpositions of bowel between the calyces and the skin (Fig. 18.6). Moreover, ureteropelvic junction obstruction should be identified beforehand with an excretory face, as it will pose limitations on the success of certain approaches [13].

ESWL can achieve fragmentation of stones, but fragment passage is often compromised in a substantial number of patients due to the abnormal anatomy [59]. So far, PCNL has become the treatment of choice for stones larger than 2 cm or in the cases that have failed ESWL [60].

18.5.3 Considerations and Technique for PCNL

Despite the abnormal positional anatomy of horseshoe kidneys, PCNL is found to be relatively safe because of favorable calyceal orientation and vascularity.

Most of the vasculature of these kidneys comes from the ventromedial aspect, the opposite side for correct percutaneous access. Furthermore, even dorsal arteries that go directly to the isthmus are protected by the spine and normally situated away from the puncture tract, so the risk of bleeding could be even less than that in normal kidneys [61].

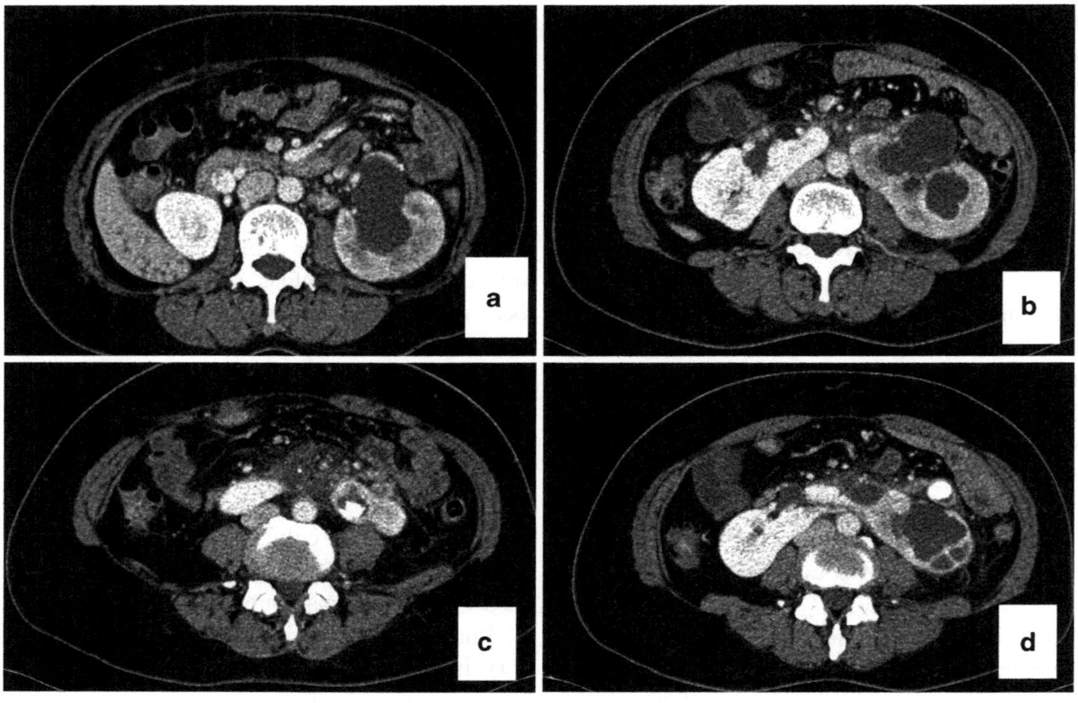

Fig. 18.6 A 36-year old man with a horseshoe kidney. (**a**, **b**) Upper and middle calyces, where puncture and access can be safely done, and adequate parenchymal support is found. (**c**) posteriorly located lithiasis measuring 17 × 16 mm. (**d**) Anteriorly located lithiasis measuring 16 × 14 mm

Regarding calyceal orientation, the lower pole calyces lie within a coronal plane, and they are angled medially, which makes them less suitable for puncture. Meanwhile, the upper pole calyces are located posteriorly and are more lateral (often subcostal); this orientation provides relatively safe access for PCNL puncture. These anatomical changes will result in a lower and medial position of the access tract, whose orientation is dorsoventral [61]. Therefore, the prone position and superior calyx puncture are considered the best approach for these kidneys [62].

Considerations in these patients include a usually lower and more medial tract, even for superior calyx punctures [61]. Medial and lower tracts pose more difficulty in dilation because they traverse through the erector spinae and quadratus lumborum muscles. As tracts can be longer due to the anatomical variants, the usual nephroscope can seem short for this surgery [40]. In order to address the latter problem, some authors have proposed using longer, rigid nephroscopes, mini-PCNL, or even flexible nephroscopes [31, 40]. Upper pole access has become the preferred access in the literature so far, with usage rates of 64–81% [63–66].

Advantages of upper-pole access are access to the renal pelvis, lower pole calyces, pelviureteral junction, and even proximal ureter. In terms of bleeding complications, the long axis of the nephroscope is in alignment with the long axis of the kidney, posing less torque on the renal parenchyma during surgery [40].

18.5.4 Complications

In patients with horseshoe kidneys, upper pole percutaneous access is essential as we have explained before, and it is safer than in normal kidneys owing to their inferior displacement away from the pleura. Accidental entering inside the pleural space is decreased because a supracostal approach is less commonly to be needed. The series from Raj et al. [40] reported pneumothorax in only 6% of cases, while other series have reported none [64–67].

18.5.5 Results and Conclusions

In patients with horseshoe kidneys that present large renal calculi, PCNL seems to be the most efficient treatment. In a few studies in which urinary calculi were managed with either PCNL or ESWL, the first showed a better stone clearance rate, without being perceived as more complex as in normal anatomic kidneys [61, 68].

In a multicenter analysis published by Raj et al. [40], the overall stone-free rate of patients with horseshoe lithiasis treated with PCNL was greater than 90%. The prospective multi-institution study from the Clinical Research Office of the Endourology Society presented results similar to those of normal kidneys regarding the stone-free rate (76.6% vs. 76.2%) with a significantly longer operative time [29]. In order to increase safety and reduce the risk of injuries to the surrounding structures, we believe that a previous CT scan with 3D reconstruction should be mandatory prior to surgery in patients with horseshoe kidneys.

18.6 Spinal Deformities

18.6.1 Generalities

We will focus in this section on various conditions which involve spinal deformities such as scoliosis, spina bifida (SB), and spinal neuropathies. The most important principle is that every patient in this spectrum is different and can pose a wide range of anatomical variations; thus, individualized surgical planning is mandatory.

Patients with skeletal deformities have a significantly increased risk for developing urolithiasis due to abnormal renal anatomy, recurrent urinary tract infection, restricted mobility, a tendency to overweight, urinary stasis and poor urodynamic function [69–71].

Scoliosis is defined as an abnormal deviation of the vertical line of the spinal column. It consists of an exaggerated lateral curvature with a rotation of the vertebrae within their axis. It is not rare that in addition to the lateral curvature, anterior and posterior deformities, such as kyphosis and lordosis, can be present. Although most cases are idiopathic, scoliosis can also be congenital, neuromuscular (acquired), and syndrome-related.

In SB, the neural tube has failed to close; this represents a wide spectrum of diseases which results in variable caudal neurological impairment affecting the function of the lower urinary tract, the bowel, and the lower limb somatosensory function [72].

18.6.2 Diagnosis and Treatment

Surgical planning should include a mandatory CT scan in order to determine the stone size, location, and collecting system anatomy (Fig. 18.7).

Before the introduction of the current techniques such as flexible ureteroscopy, ESWL, and PCNL, surgery was the only method to treat these patients, with the drawbacks of the major complications related to it, including paralytic ileus, delayed wound healing, prolonged postoperative period, wound, and respiratory infections [73].

Currently, ESWL is often considered unsuccessful in patients with severe spinal deformities. Proper positioning is hard to achieve, making wave focus on target a challenge in a substantial number of patients. Moreover, even if ESWL is successful, the next issue encountered is to eliminate the stone fragments spontaneously because its passage can be hindered by aberrant renal locations. This same condition makes flexible ureteroscopy very challenging, presenting considerable difficulty in reaching the lower pole. For these reasons, PCNL remains as the best treatment option for large calculi in these patients at most of the times [62].

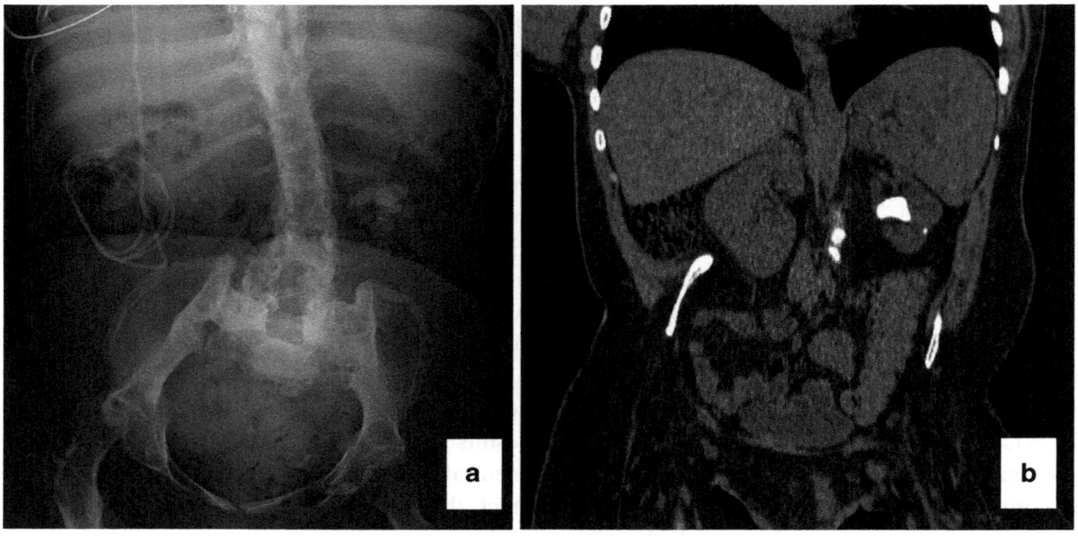

Fig. 18.7 Images from a 41-year old patient with spina bifida presenting with a left incomplete staghorn lithiasis measuring 24 × 13 mm. (**a**) Plain abdominal X-Ray. (**b**) CT scan

18.6.3 Considerations and Technique for PCNL

Interventional treatments in these patients pose a major challenge for urologists as well as for anesthesiologists. As for preoperative considerations, the respiratory and cardiac function should be assessed to determine functional impairments. Physical examination is absolutely important to determine abnormal abdominal and lumbar anatomical landmarks [74].

Spinal deformities impair the respiratory function, commonly causing restrictive pulmonary deficits, which impose reduced the vital and total lung capacity, impaired ventilatory function, and ventilation-perfusion mismatch [74–78]. At some level, cardiac dysfunction can also be present in these patients, resulting in cor pulmonale and pulmonary hypertension [74].

The adequate positioning of the patient within the operating table, and the stabilization of the head and cervical spine can be achieved with the help of head support, and as many pillows and foam pads as necessary to maintain adequate upper body support and to avoid pressure ulcers.

Depending on the spinal deformity and kidney laterality, in most cases only a small window for access can be encountered between the bony structures and bowel; thus, the recommendation of a supine or a prone approach may be individualized. In this situation, being capable of performing either approach will be crucial for obtaining the best possible results [62]. Even in some circumstances, patients will benefit from a combined antegrade and retrograde approach in order to achieve better stone-free results. To create the access tract, we recommend the aid of fluoroscopy, as well as ultrasound in order to minimize complications and provide a safer puncture.

18.6.4 Complications

Difficult surgical access and the possible need of auxiliary second tracts in such a limited space pose a significantly higher risk of complications and high postoperative dependency of inpatient care.

In this particular population, the abnormal relationship with the surrounding intraabdominal and retroperitoneal structures may lead to intraoperative technical problems and increased operative time [79–81].

The use of ultrasound-guided access to ensure a clean puncture, minimizing the surgical time as much as possible, and working with the lowest possible intrarenal pressures may reduce possible complications. An interesting system that could help to achieve the latter point is the minimally invasive PCNL (MIP) system from Karl Storz, which can create a continuous fluid outflow during the procedure [82].

Furthermore, a statistically significant risk of loss of the renal function associated with multiple stone recurrence and repeated surgical interventions can lead these patients to a progressive "end-stage stone disease" within an essentially non-functioning kidney [83].

18.6.5 Results and Conclusions

As for prior sections of this chapter, the lack of prospective trials involving the other alternatives for stone management (flexible ureteroscopy, ESWL), and even within different approaches of PCNL (supine vs. prone), leads conclusions to be based on evidence from case series.

In two series analyzing only patients with SB, stone-free rates after initial PCNL ranged from 46 to 60% [83, 84]. And after a second PCNL and ESWL, stone free-rates reached 100% [84]. Although one series reported no major complications or admissions in the intensive care unit [84], the other compared their patients with a historical cohort, finding an increased risk for a prolonged time spent in the IUC, sepsis, transfusion rate, repeated PCNL, and nephrectomy for the recurrent stone disease [83].

Goumas-Kartalas et al. reported eight patients with spinal deformities, achieving a 55.5% of stone-free rate after initial PCNL, with a 40% overall complication rate (20% blood transfusions and 10% major complications) [85].

Kara et al. reported treatment of five patients with scoliosis with a first PCNL clearance rate of 60% and achieving complete stone-free rate after auxiliary procedures (ureteroscopy in 1 case, and second-look PCNL in 1 case). The complication rate was 60%, none of these being major complications [86].

Symons et al. reported a large series of 39 PCNL procedures in 29 patients with different spinal deformities (spinal cord injury, SB, and other heterogeneous causes for their spinal neuropathy). They achieved a stone-free rate of 62% after initial PCNL, with a 48% complication rate, including two postoperative deaths due to electromechanical dissociation arrest and aspiration pneumonia [69].

Izol V et al. reported 16 patients with multiple spinal deformities (kyphoscoliosis, post-polio syndrome, osteogenesis imperfecta, myotonic dystrophy, and ankylosing spondylitis) that achieved a stone-free rate of 81.2% after prone PCNL in all cases. No anesthetic or cardiopulmonary complications were registered, but one procedure had to be converted to open surgery for uncontrolled hypotension due to severe bleeding [87].

Culkin et al. reported their series of spinal cord injury patients (18 quadriplegic and 5 paraplegic). With an average of 2.04 procedures per patient (47 in total), they achieved a stone-free rate of 90.4%. Major complications were reported in 8.5%, which included respiratory arrest, hydrothorax, and two perirenal abscesses [88].

As a conclusion, in patients with spinal deformities, the choice of treatment should be determined not only by the individual anatomy but also by the stone size and location, the patient's cardiopulmonary impairment and the center and surgeons' experience.

PCNL has been proven to be effective in previous studies, although an increased percentage of surgical related and disease-specific complications and the possibility of needing secondary treatments should be expected and discussed with the patient.

18.7 Pregnancy

Although renal colic is considered the most common non-obstetric complaint responsible for hospital admission during pregnancy, renal calculi are infrequent, and most of the symptomatic lithiasis in these patients pass spontaneously [89, 90]. Intervention is required in about one-third of patients, most usually due to uncontrolled pain, persistent obstruction, or infection. Most commonly, ureteral stent or percutaneous nephrostomy placement are recommended in the cases that require invasive management, being ureteroscopy less frequently required [91–93].

According to the EAU guidelines on interventional treatment for urolithiasis, PCNL is currently contraindicated in cases of pregnancy [92]. Prolonged anesthesia times, the need for fluoroscopy, among others, make this approach unfavorable in pregnant patients.

Little evidence is found in the literature on the use of PCNL in this situation. Hosseini et al. [94] reported a series of seven cases of women in the first trimester of pregnancy that underwent ultrasound-guided PCNL through the lower pole for renal stones (14–40 mm). The procedures were performed under general anesthesia, and pneumatic lithoclast was used in all cases. There were no postoperative complications registered, and all babies were born without complications. Another two case reports have been published of successful PCNLs during the first trimester, without any further complications [95, 96].

References

1. Wulfsohn MA. Pyelocaliceal diverticula. J Urol. 1980;123:1–8.
2. Stunell H, McNeill G, Browne RFJ, Grainger R, Torreggiani WC. The imaging appearances of calyceal diverticula complicated by uroliathasis. Br J Radiol. 2010;83:888–94. https://doi.org/10.1259/bjr/22591022.
3. Middleton AW, Pfister RC. Stone-containing pyelocaliceal diverticulum: embryogenic, anatomic, radiologic and clinical characteristics. J Urol. 1974;111:2–6. https://doi.org/10.1016/S0022-5347(17)59872-9.
4. Timmons JW, Malek RS, Hattery RR, Deweerd JH. Caliceal diverticulum. J Urol. 1975;114:6–9. https://doi.org/10.1016/S0022-5347(17)66930-1.
5. Liatsikos EN, Bernardo NO, Dinlenc CZ, Kapoor R, Smith AD. Caliceal diverticular calculi: is there a role for metabolic evaluation? J Urol. 2000;164:18–20.
6. Matlaga BR, Miller NL, Terry C, Kim SC, Kuo RL, Coe FL, et al. The pathogenesis of calyceal diverticular calculi. Urol Res. 2007;35:35–40. https://doi.org/10.1007/s00240-007-0080-x.
7. Hsu TH, Streem SB. Metabolic abnormalities in patients with caliceal diverticular calculi. J Urol. 1998;160:1640–2.
8. Auge BK, Maloney ME, Mathias BJ, Pietrow PK, Preminger GM. Metabolic abnormalities associated with calyceal diverticular stones. BJU Int. 2006;97:1053–6.https://doi.org/10.1111/j.1464-410X.2006.06134.x.
9. Parkhomenko E, Tran T, Thai J, Blum K, Gupta M. Percutaneous management of stone containing calyceal diverticula: associated factors and outcomes. J Urol. 2017;198:864–8. https://doi.org/10.1016/j.juro.2017.05.007.
10. Rapp DE, Gerber GS. Management of caliceal diverticula. J Endourol. 2004;18:805–10. https://doi.org/10.1089/end.2004.18.805.
11. Michel W, Funke PJ, Tunn UW, Senge T. Pyelocalyceal diverticula. Int Urol Nephrol. 1985;17:225–30.
12. Waingankar N, Hayek S, Smith AD, Okeke Z. Calyceal diverticula: a comprehensive review. Rev Urol. 2014;16:29–43.
13. Tan YK, Cha DY, Gupta M. Management of stones in abnormal situations. Urol Clin North Am. 2013;40:79–97. https://doi.org/10.1016/j.ucl.2012.10.001.
14. Yow RM, Bunts RC. Calyceal diverticulum. J Urol. 1955;73:663–70. https://doi.org/10.1016/S0022-5347(17)67451-2.
15. Ito H, Aboumarzouk OM, Abushamma F, Keeley FX. Systematic review of caliceal diverticulum. J Endourol. 2018;32:961–72. https://doi.org/10.1089/end.2018.0332.
16. Multescu R, Georgescu D, Dragute M, Geavlete PA, Geavlete B. Percutaneous approach of caliceal diverticula. In: Percutaneous surgery of the upper urinary tract. 1st ed: Elsevier; 2016. https://doi.org/10.1016/B978-0-12-802404-1.00004-9.
17. Monga M, Beeman WW. Advanced intrarenal ureteroscopic procedures. Urol Clin North Am. 2004;31:129–35. https://doi.org/10.1016/S0094-0143(03)00086-7.
18. Krambeck AE, Lingeman JE. Percutaneous management of caliceal diverticuli. J Endourol. 2009;23:1723–9. https://doi.org/10.1089/end.2009.1541.
19. Shalhav AL, Soble JJ, Nakada SY, Wolf JS, mcClennan BL, Clayman RV. Long-term outcome of caliceal diverticula following percutaneous endosurgical management. J Urol. 1998;160:1635–9. https://doi.org/10.1016/S0022-5347(01)62366-8.
20. Jones JA, Lingeman JE, Steidle CP. The roles of extracorporeal shock wave lithotripsy and percutaneous nephrostolithotomy in the management of pyelocaliceal diverticula. J Urol. 1991;146:724–7. https://doi.org/10.1016/S0022-5347(17)37906-5.
21. Bellman GC, Silverstein JI, Blickensderfer S, Smith AD. Technique and follow-up of percutaneous management of caliceal diverticula. Urology. 1993;42:21–5. https://doi.org/10.1016/0090-4295(93)90327-7.
22. Auge BK, Munver R, Kourambas J, Newman GE, Preminger GM. Endoscopic management of symptomatic caliceal diverticula: a retrospective comparison of percutaneous nephrolithotripsy and ureteroscopy. J Endourol. 2002;16:557–63. https://doi.org/10.1089/089277902320913233.
23. Al-Basam S, Bennett JD, Layton ZA, Denstedt JD, Razvi H. Treatment of caliceal diverticular stones: transdiverticular percutaneous nephrolithotomy with creation of a neoinfundibulum. J Vasc Interv Radiol. 2000;11:885–9. https://doi.org/10.1016/S1051-0443(07)61806-5.

24. Alwaal A, Azhar RA, Andonian S. Percutaneous holmium laser fulguration of calyceal diverticula. Case Rep Urol. 2012;2012:1–4. https://doi.org/10.1155/2012/716786.
25. Batter SJ, Dretler SP. Ureterorenoscopic approach to the symptomatic caliceal diverticulum. J Urol. 1997;158:709–13. https://doi.org/10.1016/S0022-5347(01)64298-8.
26. Hulbert JC, Reddy PK, Hunter DW, Castaneda-Zuniga W, Amplatz K, Lange PH. Percutaneous techniques for the management of caliceal diverticula containing calculi. J Urol. 1986;135:225–7. https://doi.org/10.1016/S0022-5347(17)45590-X.
27. Turna B, Raza A, Moussa S, Smith G, Tolley DA. Management of calyceal diverticular stones with extracorporeal shock wave lithotripsy and percutaneous nephrolithotomy: long-term outcome. BJU Int. 2007;100:151–6. https://doi.org/10.1111/j.1464-410X.2007.06911.x.
28. Bas O, Ozyuvali E, Aydogmus Y, Sener NC, Dede O, Ozgun S, et al. Management of calyceal diverticular calculi: a comparison of percutaneous nephrolithotomy and flexible ureterorenoscopy. Urolithiasis. 2015;43:155–61. https://doi.org/10.1007/s00240-014-0725-5.
29. Osther PJ, Razvi H, Liatsikos E, Averch T, Crisci A, Garcia JL, et al. Percutaneous nephrolithotomy among patients with renal anomalies: patient characteristics and outcomes; a subgroup analysis of the clinical research office of the endourological society global percutaneous nephrolithotomy study. J Endourol. 2011;25:1627–32. https://doi.org/10.1089/end.2011.0146.
30. Cinman NM, Okeke Z, Smith AD. Pelvic kidney: associated diseases and treatment. J Endourol. 2007;21:836–42. https://doi.org/10.1089/end.2007.9945.
31. Gupta NP, Mishra S, Seth A, Anand A. Percutaneous nephrolithotomy in abnormal kidneys: single-center experience. Urology. 2009;73:710–4. ; discussion 714–5. https://doi.org/10.1016/j.urology.2008.10.070.
32. Ganesamoni R, Sabnis RB, Mishra S, Desai MR. Microperc for the management of renal calculi in pelvic ectopic kidneys. Indian J Urol. 2013;29:257–9. https://doi.org/10.4103/0970-1591.117267.
33. Otaño N, Jairath A, Mishra S, Ganpule A, Sabnis R, Desai M. Percutaneous nephrolithotomy in pelvic kidneys: is the ultrasound-guided puncture safe? Urology. 2015;85:55–8. https://doi.org/10.1016/j.urology.2014.08.015.
34. Holman E, Tóth C. Laparoscopically assisted percutaneous transperitoneal nephrolithotomy in pelvic dystopic kidneys: experience in 15 successful cases. J Laparoendosc Adv Surg Tech A. 1998;8:431–5. https://doi.org/10.1089/lap.1998.8.431.
35. Matlaga BR, Kim SC, Watkins SL, Kuo RL, Munch LC, Lingeman JE. Percutaneous nephrolithotomy for ectopic kidneys: over, around, or through. Urology. 2006;67:513–7. https://doi.org/10.1016/j.urology.2005.09.056.
36. Desai MR, Jasani A. Percutaneous nephrolithotripsy in ectopic kidneys. J Endourol. 2000;14:289–92. https://doi.org/10.1089/end.2000.14.289.
37. Eshghi AM, Roth JS, Smith AD. Percutaneous transperitoneal approach to a pelvic kidney for endourological removal of staghorn calculus. J Urol. 1985;134:525–7.
38. Zafar FS, Lingeman JE. Value of laparoscopy in the management of calculi complicating renal malformations. J Endourol. 1996;10:379–83. https://doi.org/10.1089/end.1996.10.379.
39. Troxel SA, Low RK, Das S. Extraperitoneal laparoscopy-assisted percutaneous nephrolithotomy in a left pelvic kidney. J Endourol. 2002;16:655–7. https://doi.org/10.1089/089277902761402998.
40. Raj GV, Auge BK, Weizer AZ, Denstedt JD, Watterson JD, Beiko DT, et al. Percutaneous management of calculi within horseshoe kidneys. J Urol. 2003;170:48–51. https://doi.org/10.1097/01.ju.0000067620.60404.2d.
41. El-Kappany HA, El-Nahas AR, Shoma AM, El-Tabey NA, Eraky I, El-Kenawy MR. Combination of laparoscopy and nephroscopy for treatment of stones in pelvic ectopic kidneys. J Endourol. 2007;21:1131–6. https://doi.org/10.1089/end.2007.9930.
42. Shoskes DA, Hanbury D, Cranston D, Morris PJ. Urological complications in 1,000 consecutive renal transplant recipients. J Urol. 1995;153:18–21. https://doi.org/10.1097/00005392-199501000-00008.
43. Benoit G, Blanchet P, Eschwege P, Jardin A, Charpentier B. Occurrence and treatment of kidney graft lithiasis in a series of 1500 patients. Clin Transpl. 1996;10:176–80.
44. Pardalidis NP, Waltzer WC, Tellis VA, Jarrett TW, Smith AD. Endourologic management of complications in renal allografts. J Endourol. 1994;8:321–7. https://doi.org/10.1089/end.1994.8.321.
45. Harraz AM, Kamal AI, Shokeir AA. Urolithiasis in renal transplant donors and recipients: an update. Int J Surg. 2016;36:693–7. https://doi.org/10.1016/j.ijsu.2016.11.032.
46. Martin G, Sundaram CP, Sharfuddin A, Govani M. Asymptomatic urolithiasis in living donor transplant kidneys: initial results. Urology. 2007;70:2–5. ; discussion 5–6. https://doi.org/10.1016/j.urology.2007.01.105.
47. Kim IK, Tan JC, Lapasia J, Elihu A, Busque S, Melcher ML. Incidental kidney stones: a single center experience with kidney donor selection. Clin Transpl. 2012;26:558–63. https://doi.org/10.1111/j.1399-0012.2011.01567.x.
48. Del Pizzo JJ, Jacobs SC, Sklar GN. Ureteroscopic evaluation in renal transplant recipients. J Endourol. 1998;12:135–8. https://doi.org/10.1089/end.1998.12.135.
49. Challacombe B, Dasgupta P, Tiptaft R, Glass J, Koffman G, Goldsmith D, et al. Multimodal management of urolithiasis in renal transplantation. BJU Int. 2005;96:385–9. https://doi.org/10.1111/j.1464-410X.2005.05636.x.

50. Harper JM, Samuell CT, Hallson PC, Wood SM, Mansell MA. Risk factors for calculus formation in patients with renal transplants. Br J Urol. 1994;74:147–50.
51. Rhee BK, Bretan PN, Stoller ML. Urolithiasis in renal and combined pancreas/renal transplant recipients. J Urol. 1999;161:1458–62.
52. Krambeck AE, Leroy AJ, Patterson DE, Gettman MT. Percutaneous nephrolithotomy success in the transplant kidney. J Urol. 2008;180:2545–9. https://doi.org/10.1016/j.juro.2008.08.032.
53. Rifaioglu MM, Berger AD, Pengune W, Stoller ML. Percutaneous management of stones in transplanted kidneys. Urology. 2008;72:508–12. https://doi.org/10.1016/j.urology.2008.05.040.
54. Francesca F, Felipetto R, Mosca F, Boggi U, Rizzo G, Puccini R. Percutaneous nephrolithotomy of transplanted kidney. J Endourol. 2002;16:225–7. https://doi.org/10.1089/089277902753752179.
55. He Z, Li X, Chen L, Zeng G, Yuan J. Minimally invasive percutaneous nephrolithotomy for upper urinary tract calculi in transplanted kidneys. BJU Int. 2007;99:1467–71. https://doi.org/10.1111/j.1464-410X.2007.06768.x.
56. Crook TJ, Keoghane SR. Renal transplant lithiasis: rare but time-consuming. BJU Int. 2005;95:931–3. https://doi.org/10.1111/j.1464-410X.2005.05481.x.
57. Jabbour ME, Goldfischer ER, Stravodimos KG, Klima WJ, Smith AD. Endopyelotomy for horseshoe and ectopic kidneys. J Urol. 1998;160:694–7.
58. Evans WP, Resnick MI. Horseshoe kidney and urolithiasis. J Urol. 1981;125:620–1.
59. Kirkali Z, Esen AA, Mungan MU. Effectiveness of extracorporeal shockwave lithotripsy in the management of stone-bearing horseshoe kidneys. J Endourol. 1996;10:13–5. https://doi.org/10.1089/end.1996.10.13.
60. Yohannes P, Smith AD. The endourological management of complications associated with horseshoe kidney. J Urol. 2002;168:5–8.
61. Janetschek G, Kunzel KH. Percutaneous nephrolithotomy in horseshoe kidneys. Applied anatomy and clinical experience. Br J Urol. 1988;62:117–22.
62. Carrion DM, Cansino JR, Quintana LM, Gómez Riva J, Mainez Rodriguez JA, Pérez-Carral JR, et al. Prone percutaneous nephrolithotomy: its advantages and our technique for puncture. Trans Androl Urol. 2018;7:950–9. https://doi.org/10.21037/tau.2018.10.04.
63. Al-Otaibi K, Hosking DH. Percutaneous stone removal in horseshoe kidneys. J Urol. 1999;162:674–7.
64. Satav V, Sabale V, Pramanik P, Kanklia S, Mhaske S. Percutaneous nephrolithotomy of horseshoe kidney: our institutional experience. Urol Ann. 2018;10:258. https://doi.org/10.4103/UA.UA_152_17.
65. Shokeir AA, El-Nahas AR, Shoma AM, Eraky I, El-Kenawy M, Mokhtar A, et al. Percutaneous nephrolithotomy in treatment of large stones within horseshoe kidneys. Urology. 2004;64:426–9. https://doi.org/10.1016/j.urology.2004.04.018.
66. Symons SJ, Ramachandran A, Kurien A, Baiysha R, Desai MR. Urolithiasis in the horseshoe kidney: a single-centre experience. BJU Int. 2008;102:1676–80. https://doi.org/10.1111/j.1464-410X.2008.07987.x.
67. El Ghoneimy MN, Kodera AS, Emran AM, Orban TZ, Shaban AM, El Gammal MM. Percutaneous nephrolithotomy in horseshoe kidneys: is rigid nephroscopy sufficient tool for complete clearance? A case series study. BMC Urol. 2009;9:17. https://doi.org/10.1186/1471-2490-9-17.
68. Jones DJ, Wickham JE, Kellett MJ. Percutaneous nephrolithotomy for calculi in horseshoe kidneys. J Urol. 1991;145:481–3.
69. Symons S, Biyani CS, Bhargava S, Irvine HC, Ellingham J, Cartledge J, et al. Challenge of percutaneous nephrolithotomy in patients with spinal neuropathy. Int J Urol. 2006;13:874–9. https://doi.org/10.1111/j.1442-2042.2006.01431.x.
70. Chen Y, DeVivo MJ, Stover SL, Lloyd LK. Recurrent kidney stone: a 25-year follow-up study in persons with spinal cord injury. Urology. 2002;60:228–32.
71. Levy DA, Resnick MI. Management of urinary stones in the patient with spinal cord injury. Urol Clin North Am. 1993;20:435–42.
72. Nakada SY, Sosa RE, Gill IS, Jarrard DF. Controversial cases in endourology. J Endourol. 1999;13:465–9. https://doi.org/10.1089/end.1999.13.465.
73. Donovan WH, Carter RE, Bedbrook GM, Young JS, Griffiths ER. Incidence of medical complications in spinal cord injury: patients in specialised, compared with non-specialised centres. Paraplegia. 1984;22:282–90. https://doi.org/10.1038/sc.1984.46.
74. Kearon C, Viviani GR, Kirkley A, Killian KJ. Factors determining pulmonary function in adolescent idiopathic thoracic scoliosis. Am Rev Respir Dis. 1993;148:288–94. https://doi.org/10.1164/ajrccm/148.2.288.
75. Buyse B, Meersseman W, Demedts M. Treatment of chronic respiratory failure in kyphoscoliosis: oxygen or ventilation? Eur Respir J. 2003;22:525–8.
76. Campbell RM, Smith MD, Mayes TC, Mangos JA, Willey-Courand DB, Kose N, et al. The characteristics of thoracic insufficiency syndrome associated with fused ribs and congenital scoliosis. J Bone Joint Surg Am. 2003;85-A:399–408.
77. Patel J, Walker JL, Talwalkar VR, Iwinski HJ, Milbrandt TA. Correlation of spine deformity, lung function, and seat pressure in spina bifida. Clin Orthop Relat Res. 2011;469:1302–7. https://doi.org/10.1007/s11999-010-1687-8.
78. Papatsoris A, Masood J, El-Husseiny T, Maan Z, Saunders P, Buchholz N-P. Improving patient positioning to reduce complications in prone percutaneous nephrolithotomy. J Endourol. 2009;23:831–2. https://doi.org/10.1089/end.2008.0611.
79. Al-Kohlany KM, Shokeir AA, Mosbah A, Mohsen T, Shoma AM, Eraky I, et al. Treatment of complete staghorn stones: a prospective randomized comparison of open surgery versus percutaneous nephrolithotomy. J

Urol. 2005;173:469–73. https://doi.org/10.1097/01.ju.0000150519.49495.88.

80. Kukreja R, Desai M, Patel S, Bapat S, Desai M. Factors affecting blood loss during percutaneous nephrolithotomy: prospective study. J Endourol. 2004;18:715–22. https://doi.org/10.1089/end.2004.18.715.
81. Srivastava A, Singh KJ, Suri A, Dubey D, Kumar A, Kapoor R, et al. Vascular complications after percutaneous nephrolithotomy: are there any predictive factors? Urology. 2005;66:38–40. https://doi.org/10.1016/j.urology.2005.02.010.
82. Zanetti SP, Boeri L, Gallioli A, Talso M, Montanari E. Minimally invasive PCNL-MIP. Arch Esp Urol. 2017;70:226–34.
83. Mitchell S, Gurung PMS, Choong S, Morris T, Smith D, Woodhouse C, et al. Percutaneous nephrolithotomy and spina bifida: complex major stone surgery? J Endourol. 2018;32:205–12. https://doi.org/10.1089/end.2017.0775.
84. Alsinnawi M, Torreggiani WC, Flynn R, McDermott TED, Grainger R, Thornhill JA. Percutaneous nephrolithotomy in adult patients with spina bifida, severe spinal deformity and large renal stones. Ir J Med Sci. 2013;182:357–61. https://doi.org/10.1007/s11845-012-0888-4.
85. Goumas-Kartalas I, Montanari E. Percutaneous nephrolithotomy in patients with spinal deformities. J Endourol. 2010;24:1081–9. https://doi.org/10.1089/end.2010.0095.
86. Kara C, Resorlu B, Ozyuvali E, Unsal A. Is percutaneous nephrolithotomy suitable for patients with scoliosis: single-center experience. Urology. 2011;78:37–42. https://doi.org/10.1016/j.urology.2010.11.004.
87. Izol V, Aridogan IA, Borekoglu A, Gokalp F, Hatipoglu Z, Bayazit Y, et al. Percutaneous nephrolithotomy in prone position in patients with spinal deformities. Int J Clin Exp Med. 2015;8:21053–61.
88. Culkin DJ, Wheeler JS, Nemchausky BA, Fruin RC, Canning JR. Percutaneous nephrolithotomy in the spinal cord injury population. J Urol. 1986;136:1181–3.
89. Rodriguez PN, Klein AS. Management of urolithiasis during pregnancy. Surg Gynecol Obstet. 1988;166:103–6.
90. Blanco LT, Socarras MR, Montero RF, Diez EL, Calvo AO, Gregorio SAY, et al. Renal colic during pregnancy: diagnostic and therapeutic aspects. Literature review. Cent Eur J Urol. 2017;70:93–100. https://doi.org/10.5173/ceju.2017.754.
91. Semins MJ, Matlaga BR. Ureteroscopy during pregnancy. Indian J Urol. 2009;25:291–5. https://doi.org/10.4103/0970-1591.56173.
92. Türk C, Petřík A, Sarica K, Seitz C, Skolarikos A, Straub M, et al. EAU guidelines on interventional treatment for urolithiasis. Eur Urol. 2016;69:475–82. https://doi.org/10.1016/j.eururo.2015.07.041.
93. Assimos D, Krambeck A, Miller NL, Monga M, Murad MH, Nelson CP, et al. Surgical management of stones: American Urological Association/Endourological Society guideline, Part I. J Urol. 2016;196:1153–60. https://doi.org/10.1016/j.juro.2016.05.090.
94. Hosseini MM, Hassanpour A, Eslahi A, Malekmakan L. Percutaneous nephrolithotomy during early pregnancy in urgent situations: is it feasible and safe? Urol J. 2017;14:5034–7. https://doi.org/10.22037/uj.v14i6.3617.
95. Shah A, Chandak P, Tiptaft R, Glass J, Dasgupta P. Percutaneous nephrolithotomy in early pregnancy. Int J Clin Pract. 2004;58:809–10.
96. Tóth C, Tóth G, Varga A, Flaskó T, Salah MA. Percutaneous nephrolithotomy in early pregnancy. Int Urol Nephrol. 2005;37:1–3. https://doi.org/10.1007/s11255-004-6087-0.

19 Percutaneous Nephrolithotomy in Children (Pediatric PNL)

Rasim Guzel and Kemal Sarica

Unlike the adult population, due to its relatively uncommon incidence, treatment of the pediatric urinary stones has been challenging to the practicing endourologist. It has been well reported and demonstrated that the risk of stone recurrence is higher in this population, and in light of the small growing kidney, the management needs to aim to render the child completely stone free and maintain the renal function in normal limits. Related to this subject, taking the evident invasive nature of the available stone removal procedures into account, urologists have always been reluctant to perform such procedures to avoid the risk of possible morphological as well as functional adverse effects on the growing pediatric kidney. However, in addition to the experience gained from the manipulations in adults, technological advancements enabling the use of miniaturized, fine instruments in children have significantly altered the surgical management of pediatric calculi where currently the whole spectrum of stone removal procedures could be performed in a safe manner. However, we believe that to select the most appropriate modality, stone-related (location, composition, and size) and patient-related (anatomic characteristics of urinary system, BMI, obstruction) factors should be considered in all cases.

Additionally, as mentioned above, the higher incidence of metabolic and anatomic abnormalities may influence the choice and the ultimate effectiveness of the preferred management option. The preferred modality should render the children stone free with reasonable number of treatment sessions and limited auxiliary procedures. Regarding the minimal invasive stone removal approaches in this specific population, at present all available alternatives, namely SWL, PNL, or ureterorenoscopy (URS), could be performed either alone or in a combined manner, whereas open surgery is needed in a limited percentage of all cases [1–3]. Today, although SWL remains as the treatment of choice with certain indications, and retrograde intrarenal surgery (RIRS) is commonly applied due to the clinical introduction of smaller-diameter flexible ureteroscopes, percutaneous stone removal is also performed on an increasing basis particularly in large and complex stones [4]. However, residual fragments could reside after a successful procedure (particularly in lower pole stones) and may induce distressing symptoms. If untreated, it is clear that such fragments will require additional procedures and promote recurrent stone formation during long-term follow-up of these cases [5].

R. Guzel
Department of Urology, Medistate Hospital, Istanbul, Turkey

K. Sarica (✉)
Department of Urology, Medical School, Biruni University, Istanbul, Turkey

G. Zeng, K. Sarica (eds.), *Percutaneous Nephrolithotomy*,
https://doi.org/10.1007/978-981-15-0575-1_19

As one of the effective management alternative in these cases, following the first report of series in 1985, as a result of increasing experience obtained, PNL has been used either alone or in combination with other approaches in children with relatively larger stones. However, concerns were present for a long period of time regarding the long-term possible renal damage due to the use of relatively large instruments, increased radiation exposure risk and possibility of major complications like bleeding, perforation, and infection. The evident invasive nature of this approach originating from the use of adult-sized large instruments constituted the major concerns, and physicians tended always to be careful for a proper management plan to lower the risk of injury and related complications. In light of all these concerns, physicians tried to limit the risk of injury on the growing child kidney and advancements in instrumentation along with clinical use of more-efficient energy sources for intracorporeal lithotripsy (Ho-YAG laser) have revolutionized the endourological procedures in children. Such efforts resulted in the clinical introduction of smaller nephroscopes, miniaturization has become an important issue, and miniperc procedures became feasible to limit the degree of invasiveness with the same success rates. Additionally, use of ultrasound-guided puncture more commonly than ever in this specific population enabled the physicians to perform stone removal with significantly lower radiation risk. Consequently, mini-PNL procedures began to be used to avoid repeated SWL sessions under anesthesia and lower the risk of residual fragments following the management of large and complex stones in skilled hands. Regarding this issue, endourologists realized well that the use of smaller instruments through miniaturized PNL technique such as "Miniperc" and "Microperc" as well as "ultra-mini PNL (UMP)" could reduce the extent of the damage induced on the renal parenchyma without diminishing its therapeutic efficacy. Acceptable SFRs with lower rates of complications observed in this specific population proved the safety of these techniques [6–12].

19.1 Indications

Like adult cases, PNL application aims the complete removal of stones in cases with high stone volume (>20 mm) in a single session [13–20]. Although adult-sized instruments have been used for a certain period of time in this special population (>5 years), clinical introduction and routine use of smaller nephroscopes have made the procedure more practical and safer than ever [14–18]. The use of small-size nephroscopes (18 Fr, 12 Fr) with holmium:YAG laser with comfortable maneuvers reduced the blood loss significantly, provided shorter hospitalization periods, and replaced open surgery over time in children of all age groups with particularly high stone volumes [19].

The indications are similar to those in adults and PNL is recommended, especially in cases with large stones (>20 mm) in renal pelvis or in the upper pole, >10 mm stones in the lower pole and additionally hard stones such as cystine or sutrivite which cannot be passed spontaneously due to additional anatomic anomalies [21].

19.2 Methods of Percutaneous Stone Removal in Pediatric Cases

19.2.1 Technique

The essential instruments for percutaneous nephrolithotomy technique in children (PNL) are C-arm scopy device, endovision systems, pediatric nephroscopes (18 Fr or 12 Fr), guidewires, Amplatz dilatation set, accessory sheath, intracorporeal lithotripsy systems (laser, pneumatic, or ultrasonographic), baskets, and stone forceps. An adequate experience of the procedure and knowledge in the renal anatomy are certainly needed for a successful and complication-free procedure particularly in this population. The renal artery is divided into the posterior and anterior segmental arteries. The posterior segmental branch is frequently prone to be damaged in endourological interventions. The Brodel line is the avascular area between these vessel branches, and there is no segmental distribution in the veins of kidney. The preferred method is to perform the puncture from the posterior calyx in the Brodel line. Intravenous urography (IVU) and/or non-contrast computed tomography (NCCT) need to be performed to outline the renal anatomy as well as adjacent organs particularly colonic involvement. Many experienced surgeons perform the procedure with retrograde pyelography in the beginning of the procedure after USG evaluation. First, the patient is brought into lithotomy position, then the open end ureteral catheter placed in the ureter is moved up into the ureteropelvic junction. With the help of this catheter, a retrograde contrast agent is given, and the kidney anatomy is visualized. In addition, a Foley catheter should be placed in the bladder to connect the ureteric catheter for free drainage and to keep the bladder empty during the procedure. Then, the patient is placed in the prone position and given the appropriate position for the procedure. Contrast agent is given through the ureteric catheter, and the renal anatomy is once again visualized. Criteria such as infundibulopelvic angle, stone location, and availability of drainage from calyx to pelvis are important factors in the planning of the intervention. The first calyx identified with the USG through the posterior axillary line is the posterior calyx. In order to minimize radiation exposure, it is preferred to make the first access with USG. Intervention is performed towards the target calyx from a small area between the sacrospinous eminentia/line, the posterior axillary line, and 12th rib. For renal pelvic stones, an ox-eye image is created in the lower pole of the posterior calyx, and the percutaneous needle is advanced at an angle of about 45°. After entering into the dependent calyx, the guide wire is advanced through the needle into the kidney, preferably into the bladder and the dilatation of the access tract is started. If mini-PNL with18 Fr pediatric nephroscope is performed, dilatation is done with telescopic metal dilators. But currently, in the clinics dealing with pediatric stone diseases, interventions are usually performed with smaller (12 Fr) nephroscopes. It should be kept in mind that pediatric kidney is positioned more superficially and more mobile than an adult kidney. Control of the location of the sheath with contralateral radiographs and evaluation of the presence of perforation is necessary. Bleeding is very rare in the procedures that are performed appropriately. If the tract is lost or guide wire is dislocated during the procedure, retrograde methylene blue could be given through the ureteric catheter to see the collecting system and re-enter to the kidney. After the procedure, the decision to leave the ureteric catheter and/or placement of a nephrostomy catheter is made depending on the course of the procedure and relevant factors such as whether the disintegrated stone(s) has been completely cleaned and whether the procedure has been performed smoothly. After all procedures, 2 mg/kg lasix IV could be used to remove stone residue with diuresis. PNL is not recommended to the kidneys, whose parenchyma is critically thin, evidently hydronephrotic, and if the kidney function is less than 10%. In cases where the parenchyma is very thin, bleeding during dilatation and long periods of urine leakage has been reported to be high likely.

19.2.2 Standard PNL Application in Children

Since the first report of percutaneous stone surgery for upper-tract stones in adults in 1976, experience has dramatically increased with the common application of PCNL in subsequent years. Nine years later, in 1985, the first pediatric series of PCNL was reported [22, 23]. In contrast to the easy and widespread acceptance of this method among adults, the use and popularization of PCNL were somewhat delayed in children because of some concerns about acute or long-term parenchymal damage, radiation exposure, and risk of major complications such as hemorrhage, colonic injury, and sepsis [24] due to the use of relatively larger instruments in the growing and smaller kidney. As a result, initial publications of pediatric PCNL focused on the complications of PCNL, where the use of "adult-sized" instruments was the main concern as a potential cause of higher complication rates. However, as a result of the accumulated experience obtained from the large number of cases treated, the risk of scarring and loss of renal function after PCNL have not been observed and reported in the literature; the experienced endourologists did continue to perform the procedure as a safe and effective [25]. Related to this issue, in their original study, Dawaba et al. [26] were able to demonstrate no renal scarring in 65 children on a long-term follow-up, indicating the long-term safety of the procedure in children. In another study again Desai et al. [27] found that the size and the number of tracts are main factors for the intraoperative hemorrhage during PCNL in children. Similar observation has been reported by Zeren et al. [28] where a significant association has been identified between the intraoperative bleeding and sheath size, operative time, and stone volume.

As mentioned above, although PCNL was initially not rapidly accepted as a safe and effective management alternative for the removal of large and complex pediatric stones, increasing experience, developments in access techniques, and technological advances use holmium:YAG laser for stone disintegration, PCNL is currently being performed as a safe and efficient method in children as monotherapy in the majority of the cases. Increasing experience coupled with the use of miniaturized systems (mini-ultra mini PNL) particularly in older children has resulted in the use of this approach in a routine manner even in smaller children. In light of all these developments, both EAU and AUA guidelines recommend PNL technique as the treatment of choice in the minimal invasive management of large and complex calculi in pediatric cases [29–31].

Regarding the success rates in terms of stone-free status after the procedure, a wide range of SFR from 58 to 99% have been reported so far in the published data [10, 11, 22, 32, 33]. Patient- and stone-related factors (age or number and size of the stones) have not been found to affect the outcomes. Related to the percutaneous stone management particularly in relatively younger population, Unsal et al. reported a stone-free rate of 94% in kids younger than 7 years of age [34] including even the children with higher stone volumes. Although it is commonly accepted that ESWL is the first treatment option in the management of pediatric stones, some authors aimed to evaluate the efficacy of PCNL in comparison with other available management alternatives. Related to this issue despite the significantly higher success rates obtained with ESWL in medium-sized calculi (10–20 mm), PCNL has been found to be much more effective in the complete removal of larger stones in a single session as reported in adult population [13, 35].

19.2.3 PNL in Children for Staghorn Stones

Concerning the published data, the application of PCNL monotherapy is the initial choice in the management of staghorn stones; a 60–100% overall stone-free rates have been reported for different sized kidney stones in populations of different ages [16]. In their original study for example, Aron et al. [33] found PCNL monotherapy to be highly effective, with stone-free rates approaching 90% in preschool-aged children with staghorn calculi. Additionally, Romanowsky et al. [17] reported complete clearance in eight of nine children (seven of whom had staghorn calculi) after a single stage of PCNL. Lastly, Desai et al. [27] published their results of PCNL for complex calculi (either staghorn or with a large bulk and involving more than one calyx, the upper ureter, or both) in children, and complete clearance of all stones was possible in 90% of the 56 cases undergoing PCNL monotherapy.

Even though it is well confirmed that PCNL is an effective method for removing staghorn stones in children with certain significant advantages (e.g., direct visualization of the fragmentation, clearance of the fragments under vision, minimizing the need for recurrent visits, and multiple/ancillary procedures) [18], some well-known possible severe complications are still a major concern for the practicing endourologists. Regarding this critical issue, in their original publication, Zeren et al. [28] reported a 24% incidence of hemorrhage requiring transfusion after 67 PCNL procedures in 55 children with renal stones. They found a close correlation between transfusion and operative time, stone burden and sheath size. Although much lower transfusion rates (<5%) were reported in subsequent studies, these reports also indicated a close association between both tract number and size and the need for transfusion [16, 23]. Other commonly reported notable complications include transient fever and urinary leakage following the removal of nephrostomy tube [16]. The most serious complication of PCNL in children being treated for staghorn calculi (struvite) is the formation of sepsis, a complication that can result in death [19].

19.2.4 Miniaturized PNL in Children

As a result of the experience obtained in adult population, physicians began to apply percutaneous nephrolithotomy (PNL) also in children with meaningfully higher stone-free rates in one session. However, despite the high efficiency in stone clearance even for larger stones, possible long-term renal damage due to particularly the small size of the child kidney constituted the major concerns raised by the responsible physicians [2, 3]. Majority of the complications have been observed during the puncture of the kidney, and the size of the nephrostomy tract was regarded as the major factor for PCNL-induced morbidity in these specific cases. Regarding this issue, as a result of the technological advancements in recent decades, endourologists looked to search for the use of smaller instruments to limit the presence as well as the degree of invasiveness observed during PNL procedures applied with adult-sized instruments. As a result of these efforts, miniaturized PNL technique has been defined and new techniques using relatively smaller instruments, namely "Miniperc" and "Microperc" as well as "ultra-mini PNL" (UMP) were introduced for clinical practice to reduce the extent of the possible damage on the renal parenchyma without diminishing its therapeutic efficacy [6, 7, 10, 20]. Acceptable SFRs with lower rates of complications observed in this specific population proved the safety of these techniques [9, 27].

Within the frame of this "miniaturization" process, in a recent study, Zeng et al. reported the feasibility of super-mini-PNL (SMP) system in the treatment of urinary stones less than 2.5 cm by describing a new method in the evacuation of stone fragments formed during PNL procedure [21]. Regarding the characteristics of this technique, in addition to the smaller size of the nephrostomy tracts used (ranged from 10F to 14F), active removal of the stone fragments by laser/pneumatic lithotripsy systems through a modified nephrostomy access sheath with continuous negative pressure aspiration was the main advantage of this system. The authors stated well that this approach not only shortens the operating time but also decreases the renal pelvic pressure, a factor that is highly important for the possible infective problems during short-term follow-up. About 85.6% of the children did not require any kind of drainage (totally tubeless) for the collecting system, and complete stone clearance on postoperative CT at 3 months has been reported to be 90.1%.

19.2.5 Advantages of Miniaturized PCNL

Miniaturized PCNL techniques (mini-ultra mini-, super mini-, and micro-PCNL) mainly allow the surgeons to establish relatively smaller sized tracts requiring limited dilatation to get an access to the relevant renal collecting system. As a result of reduced injury to the renal parenchyma by using smaller sheaths, the risk of hemorrhagic complications has decreased to a certain extent as reported in the literature [8, 36–38]. Bleeding risk is particularly of paramount importance in pediatric population because the marked changes in Hb levels originating from excessive bleeding may induce serious problems and even could be fatal. Currently these miniaturized systems could also be used even in infancy period in a safe and successful manner. On the other hand again, puncturing the kidney by performing a single-step dilation procedure with these smaller and fine instruments limits the risk of complications particularly during the first and highly critical phase of the procedure. This approach of course will certainly shorten the total procedural duration from renal access to laser lithotripsy and stone removal phase which can even be performed under spinal anesthesia in selected cases [39]. These advantages will again limit the anesthesia time, the risk of radiation exposure, as well as limited use of irrigation fluid which will lower the risk of hypothermia in children. The safe and effective use of miniaturized techniques has also been demonstrated in children presenting with kidney abnormalities (anomalic, ectopic, solitary, and pelvic kidneys). Last but not least, one of the most important advantages of the miniaturized PNL in children will be the increased chance of performing the procedures in a "tubeless" and even "totally tubeless" manner. This approach will increase the quality of life in the cases by requiring less analgesic need, and also double J stent-related complications will be less likely in these cases.

19.2.6 Disadvantages of Miniaturized PCNL

Despite the evident advantages mentioned above, miniaturized systems may have certain disadvantages which may interfere with a successful and practical procedure. Related to this issue, it is well known that the use smaller caliber instruments may limit the quality of vision where a small amount of bleeding can cause a blurred intraoperative vision. The micro-PNCL technique also does not allow to remove the stone fragments, and such fragments may cause problems during spontaneous passage and also remain in the kidney by increasing the risk of new stone formation particularly in metabolical active children. Again no stone analysis will be available in these cases, and this a major drawback particularly in pediatric cases. Stone removal particularly for larger fragments could be difficult in these systems due to the smaller diameter of the access sheath [40].

Thus accumulated data so far indicated that miniaturized PCNL could be successful enough for relatively smaller kidney stones, and all cases need to be treated with these systems in an individualized manner based on both stone- and patient-related factors. It should be again emphasized that experience (particularly obtained from adult population) is the most crucial factors to perform these techniques in this special population for a successful and complication-free procedure [9, 41].

19.3 Complications

The most important complications of PNL procedure are organ injury (vessel, diaphragm, renal pelvis, and calyx), colonic or duodenal perforation, severe bleeding, hematoma formation, hydrothorax, urine extravasation, UTI, and pyelonephritis. Accumulated experience did clearly show that, as the stone volume increases and the duration of surgery prolongs, the risk for complications increases in a parallel manner [14, 16, 28]. The size and the number of the access tracts are the crucial factors affecting the presence and severity of the complication rates. Kidneys with different anomalies have a higher risk of complications. The use of pediatric instruments instead of adult tools, the dilatation below 20 Fr, operating from a single tract, and lower stone volume reduce the risk of bleeding in a significant manner. Horseshoe kidney, female gender, left kidney, colonic distention, history of surgery, lower pole entry, and lateral access have been reported to be the main risk factors for colonic perforation. PNL in infants did not reveal serious complications and/or blood transfusions after the clinical introduction of smaller (12–14 Fr) tracts [15]. The cut-off value for the tract size was reported to be 24 Fr [15]. The advantages of PNL with larger sheaths in children could be increased efficacy, shorter operational duration, and relatively easier operation, but it is well known that as the sheath diameter increases, the risk of complications such as bleeding and parenchymal damage also increases. Related to this issue, higher complication rates have been reported when PNL is performed with larger instruments especially in children under 7 years of age [1, 28, 31, 38].

References

1. Schultz-Lampel D, Lampel A. The surgical management of stones in children. BJU Int. 2001;87:732–40.
2. Erdenetsesteg G, Manohar T, Singh H, Desai MR. Endourologic management of pediatric uro-

lithiasis: proposed clinical guidelines. J Endourol. 2006;20:737–48.
3. Dogan HS, Tekgul S. Management of pediatric stone disease. Curr Urol Rep. 2007;8:163–73.
4. Tan AH, Al-Omar M, Watterson JD, et al. Results of shockwave lithotripsy for pediatric urolithiasis. J Endourol. 2004;18:527–30.
5. Cass AS. Extracorporeal shockwave lithotripsy or percutaneous nephrolithotomy for lower pole nephrolithiasis? J Endourol. 1996;10:17–20.
6. Datta SN, Solanki R, Desai J. Prospective outcomes of ultra mini percutaneous nephrolithotomy: a consecutive cohort study. J Urol. 2016;195:741–6.
7. Mishra S, Sharma R, Garg C, et al. Prospective comparative study of miniperc and standard PNL for treatment of 1 to 2 cm size renal stone. BJU Int. 2011;108:896–9.
8. Desai MR, Sharma R, Mishra S, et al. Single-step percutaneous nephrolithotomy (microperc): the initial clinical report. J Urol. 2011;186:140–5.
9. Silay MS, Tepeler A, Atis G, et al. Initial report of microperc in the treatment of pediatric nephrolithiasis. J Pediatr Surg. 2013;48:1578–83.
10. Dede O, Sancaktutar AA, Dagguli M, et al. Ultra-mini-percutaneous nephrolithotomy in pediatric nephrolithiasis: both low pressure and high efficiency. J Pediatr Urol. 2015;11:253.e1–6.
11. Samad L, Aquil S, Zaidi Z. Paediatric percutaneous nephrolithotomy: setting new frontiers. BJU Int. 2006;97:359–63.
12. Mor Y, Elmasry YE, Kellet MJ, et al. The role of percutaneous nephrolithotomy in the management of pediatric renal calculi. J Urol. 1997;158:1319–21.
13. Boormans JL, Scheepe JR, Verkoelen CF, Verhagen PCMS. Percutaneous nephrolithotomy for treating renal calculi in children. BJU Int. 2005;95(4):631–4.
14. Walsh DL, Jung C, Pope JC IV et al. An analysis of the efficacy of percutaneous nephrolithotomy versus extracorporeal shock wave lithotripsy for the treatment of large renal calculi in children. Presented at the American Academy of Pediatrics Section on Urology, San Francisco, CA, USA, 2007.
15. Kapoor R, Solanki F, Singhania P, Andankar M, Pathak HR. Safety and efficacy of percutaneous nephrolithotomy in the pediatric population. J Endourol. 2008;22(4):637–40.
16. Gonen M, Turunc T, Ozturk B, Aygun C, Ozkardes H. Outcomes of percutaneous nephrolithotomy in children having complex stones. Urol Int. 2009;83:416–9.
17. Romanowsky I, Lismer L, Asali M, Rosenberg E, Kaneti J. Percutaneous nephrolithotomy for pediatric renal calculus disease. 5 years of local experience. Arch Ital Urol Androl. 2008;80:56–8.
18. Raza A, Turna B, Smith G, Moussa S, Tolley DA. Pediatric urolithiasis: 15 years of local experience with minimally invasive endourological management of pediatric calculi. J Urol. 2005;174:682–5.
19. McAleer IM, Kaplan GW, Bradley JS, Carroll SF. Staghorn calculus endotoxin expression in sepsis. Urology. 2002;59:601.
20. Michel MS, Trojan L, Rassweiler JJ. Complications in percutaneous nephrolithotomy. Eur Urol. 2007;51:899–906.
21. Zeng G, Wan S, Zhao Z, et al. Super-mini percutaneous nephrolithotomy (SMP): a new concept in technique and instrumentation. BJU Int. 2016;117:655–61.
22. Long CJ, Srinivasan AK. Percutaneous nephrolithotomy and ureteroscopy in children: evolutions. Urol Clin North Am. 2015;42(1):1–17.
23. Nouralizadeh A, Basiri A, Javaherforooshzadeh A, Soltani MH, Tajali F. Experience of percutaneous nephrolithotomy using adult-size instruments in children less than 5 years old. J Pediatr Urol. 2009;5(5):351–4.
24. Smaldone MC, Corcoran AT, Docimo SG, Ost MC. Endourological management of pediatric stone disease: present status. J Urol. 2009;181:17–28. https://doi.org/10.1016/j.juro.2008.09.001. [PMID: 19012920].
25. Mayo ME, Krieger JN, Rudd TG. Effect of percutaneous nephrostolithotomy on renal function. J Urol. 1985;133:167–9. [PMID: 3968724].
26. Dawaba MS, Shokeir AA, Hafez AT, et al. Percutaneous nephrolithotomy in children: early and late anatomical and functional results. J Urol. 2004;172(3):1078–81.
27. Desai MR, Kukreja RA, Patel SH, Bapat SD. Percutaneous nephrolithotomy for complex pediatric renal calculus disease. J Endourol. 2004;18:23–7.
28. Zeren S, Satar N, Bayazit Y, Bayazit AK, Payasli K, Ozkeceli R. Percutaneous nephrolithotomy in the management of pediatric renal calculi. J Endourol. 2002;16:75–8.
29. Tekgül S, Riedmiller H, Hoebeke P, Kočvara R, Nijman RJ, Radmayr C, Stein R, Dogan HS. EAU guidelines on vesicoureteral reflux in children. Eur Urol. 2012;62:534–42. https://doi.org/10.1016/j.eururo.2012.05.059. [PMID: 22698573].
30. Davis RB, Farber NJ, Kaplan A, Patel R, Steckler RE, Elsamra SE. Contemporary practice pattern in the treatment of pediatric stone disease. Can J Urol. 2018;25(4):9427–32.
31. Çıtamak B, Altan M, Bozacı AC, Koni A, Doğan HS, Bilen CY, Şahin A, Tekgül S. Percutaneous nephrolithotomy in children: 17-yeras of experience. J Urol. 2016;195(4 Pt 1):1082–7. https://doi.org/10.1016/j.juro.2015.11.070. Epub 2015 Dec 9.
32. Salah MA, oth CT′, Khan AM, Holman E. Percutaneous nephrolithotomy in children: experience with 138 cases in a developing country. World J Urol. 2004;22(4):277–80.
33. Aron M, Yadav R, Goel R, Hemal AK, Gupta NP. Percutaneous nephrolithotomy for complete staghorn calculi in preschool children. J Endourol. 2005;19(8):968–72.
34. Unsal A, Resorlu B, Kara C, Bozkurt OF, Ozyuvali E. Safety and efficacy of percutaneous nephrolithotomy in infants, preschool age, and older children with different sizes of instruments. Urology. 2010;76(1):247–52.

35. Shokeir AA, Sheir KZ, El-Nahas AR, El-Assmy AM, Eassa W, El-Kappany HA. Treatment of renal stones in children: a comparison between percutaneous nephrolithotomy and shock wave lithotripsy. J Urol. 2006;176(2):706–10.
36. Wright A, Rukin N, Smith D, et al. 'Mini, ultra, micro'— nomenclature and cost of these new minimally invasive percutaneous nephrolithotomy (PCNL) techniques. Ther Adv Urol. 2016;8:142–6.
37. Jackman SV, Hedican SP, Peters CA, et al. Percutaneous nephrolithotomy in infants and preschool age children: experience with a new technique. Urology. 1998;52:697–701.
38. Desai J, Zeng G, Zhao Z, et al. A novel technique of ultramini-percutaneous nephrolithotomy: introduction and an initial experience for treatment of upper urinary calculi less than 2 cm. Biomed Res Int. 2013;2013:490793.
39. Karatag T, Tepeler A, Silay MS, et al. A comparison of 2 percutaneous nephrolithotomy techniques for the treatment of pediatric kidney stones of sizes 10–20 mm: Microperc vs miniperc. Urology. 2015;85:1015–8.
40. Liu Y, Wu W, Tuerxun A, Liu Y, Simayi A, Huang J, Batuer A, Zhou Y, Luo J, Zhong W, Zhao Z, Zhu W, Zeng G. Super-mini percutaneous nephrolithotomy in the treatment of pediatric nephrolithiasis: evaluation of initial results. J Endourol. 2017;31:S38–42.
41. Caione P, Collura G, Innocenzi M, et al. Percutaneous endoscopic treatment for urinary stones in pediatric patients: where we are now. Transl Pediatr. 2016;5:266–74.

20 Natural History of Residual Stone Fragments Following PCNL

Mohammad A. Alomar and Alaa A. Mokhtar

Recently, the favored treatment modality for massive and complex renal calculi is percutaneous nephrolithotomy (PCNL) [1, 2]. The outcome in terms of high stone-free rates, which can exceed 90% [3], is the result of continuous improvement of the surgical techniques [4] and innovations of new instruments, endoscopic lithotripters and training models [5–7].

However, residual fragments (RF) of approximately 15–25% post-PCNL were reported at discharge [8, 9]. RF may be asymptomatic, increase in size, or may even lead to recurrence of symptoms, infections along the urinary tract and ureteral obstruction [10, 11].

The term "clinically insignificant residual fragments" (CIRF) refers to asymptomatic remnants that are less than 4 mm and do not cause obstruction or infection [12, 13].

Although the term is widely used, there is no definite maximum size of the stone fragment at which it is considered insignificant. Additionally, it is debatable by the scientific community whether the residual fragment should be labelled as a CIRF or not as the published follow-up results of CIRF are conflicting. Furthermore, there is no agreement regarding the follow-up times needed and the best imaging for CIRF [10, 11, 14–18].

In a study done by Ramana et al., RF following PCNL was 8%. Of them 59.5% were 2 mm or smaller and 78.5% (33 of 42) smaller than 5 mm. Approximately, half of RF was located in the lower calyx. Forty-three percent of these patients had stone-related problems after 32 months. Patients required hospitalization, emergency consultation or subsequent intervention, mostly ureteroscopy (61%). More than half of cases that required active intervention had RFs >2 mm. The authors concluded that fragments with a maximum diameter larger than 2 mm and those positioned in the renal pelvis or ureter independently predicted a future stone-related event and so require immediate intervention [17].

Altunrende et al. identified in their series (22%) of cases to have RF following PCNL by postoperative KUB with more than 60% located in the lower calyx. Thirty-eight patients were followed up for more than 2 years by CT. Of these patients 26.3% became symptomatic and 21% had an increase in RF size. Three of them had magnesium ammonium phosphate stones. Metabolic assessment showed several abnormalities in patients (26.3%). The authors inferred that the progression could be seen in 2-year follow-

M. A. Alomar (✉)
Department of Surgery, Division of Urology, Faculty of Medicine, King Saud University, Riyadh, Saudi Arabia

A. A. Mokhtar
King Faisal Specialist Hospital and Research Center, Riyadh, Saudi Arabia

G. Zeng, K. Sarica (eds.), *Percutaneous Nephrolithotomy*, https://doi.org/10.1007/978-981-15-0575-1_20

up, whereas the presence of risk factors from 24-h urine metabolic analysis could not predict growth of RFs [15].

In another study, Ganpule and Desai examined the follow-up data of 2469 patients who were treated by PCNL. Of them 187 (7.57%) were found to have RF. Follow-up ultrasonography and KUB at 48 h, 1-month and 3-month were done to assess RF. The mean size of RF was 38.6 ± 52 mm^2, and the most common site for residual fragments was the lower calyx (57.7%). Forty-five percent of the patients were stone free without intervention at a mean follow-up of 24 months. Most of the stone fragments (65.47%) spontaneously passed in 3 months. Stone fragments less than 25 mm^2 and in the renal pelvis were the most likely to pass without any complications. The authors concluded that the size and the time of presentation of RF, and the presence of hypercalciuria or hyperuricemia were significant factors that predict the outcome of RF [19].

Osman et al. showed that RF after PCNL increased in size in one-third of patients during a follow-up of 3 years while 29.35% had asymptomatic RFs. Four percent of the patients presented with the RF that migrated into the ureter. The rest of the RF passed spontaneously. Further interventions were performed for 35% of the cases. Only the RF size (>3 mm) correlated significantly with RF growth or ureteral obstruction. The authors concluded that small RF (≤5 mm) after PCNL has to be treated in one-third of cases while single RF (≤3 mm) can be considered clinically insignificant [11].

Olvera et al. showed that after a mean follow-up of 57.9 months, more than half of patients with RF after PCNL (54.5%) developed at least one clinical outcome, and 72.7% patients required surgical intervention. Only four patients had radiological evidence of stone passage. They found that RF >4 mm and struvite or apatite stones were significant predictors for active intervention [20].

Emmott et al. reported true stone-free rates of 55% after performing 658 surgeries as evidenced by CT-KUB on postoperative day 1. Forty-five percent of cases had fragments that were 1 mm or larger. The majorities (70%) of fragments were 4 mm or less. Larger RF size was found to be predictive for higher rates of stone-related events. Re-intervention rates were found to be significantly different based only on RF size. Re-interventions occurred in 28.2% of patients with RFs greater than 4 mm compared to 16.9% of patients with RFs 4 mm or less. Moreover, the rate of spontaneous passage of very small RFs in this study is interestingly low (23.4%). The question is whether these are real RFs or just parenchymal calcifications such as Randall's plaques or even nephrocalcinosis [21].

20.1 Diagnosis of Residual Stone Fragments Post PCNL

The American Urological Association best practice statement and European Association of Urology guidelines recommend that kidneys-ureters-bladder plain radiography (KUB) and ultrasonography (US) should be used for urinary tract stones, even on follow-up, because both imaging modalities eliminate radiation exposure, and the cost compared with unenhanced computerized tomography (CT) is lower [22–24].

Traditionally, KUB or ultrasound was used to determine the stone-free status. However, the sensitivity and specificity of these examinations in detecting small residual fragments are originally low. Additionally, the superimposition of bowel gas, feces and soft tissue calcifications as well as the presence of obesity, faintly radio-opaque stones, nephrostomy tubes and/or pigtails make these diagnostic modalities inaccurate to a certain extent [25–27].

Moreover, plain abdominal film (KUB) may exaggerate the actual stone size by 20% due to magnification error [12]. Also, ultrasonography (US) maybe give an inaccurate stone size compared with unenhanced CT, especially overestimating stones smaller than 5 mm [28].

Many authors reported that linear renal tomography is better than plain radiographs for detecting nephrolithiasis [29–32]. Palmer et al. [33] demonstrated that although US failed to detect stones in 41% of children with stones, unenhanced CT could be relied upon. Thin-slice unenhanced CT, combined with image reconstruction, showed higher sensitivity for the detection of residual stones when it was prospectively compared to other imaging modalities. The sensitivity of the unenhanced CT was almost 100% compared to 47.6% for KUB: 89.2% for linear tomography and 67.8% for US [15, 17, 19, 34–39].

Kanno et al. [40] evaluated the effectiveness of KUB and US for the detection of renal stones, including the combination of both modalities. Of 488 stones detected by plain radiography, 476 stones were also detected by ultrasound with a sensitivity of 89.9% and specificity of 68.1% for the combination of the two modalities. The detection rate for plain radiography for stones less than 5 mm is very low. Stone sizes measured by the two modalities positively correlated with those obtained by computed tomography, and the concordance rate based on size was similar.

Osman et al. [34] evaluated 100 renal units after PCNL by KUB, US and unenhanced CT to detect residual fragments after PCNL. The sensitivity for detecting significant RF was 20% for plain x-ray, 20% for ultrasound, 33.3% for linear tomography and 100% for CT. Sensitivity for detecting significant residual stones was 100% for spiral CT, 85.7% for plain x-ray and 95.2% for linear tomography. The authors recommended the use of unenhanced CT for RF after PCNL except cases with opaque stones where KUB and US could be done because there was no statistically significant increase in the diagnosis of residual stones compared with KUB and US. In spite of this, unenhanced CT has many drawbacks, namely, radiation exposure, cost and overestimation of the stone size in the cranio-caudal dimension [41].

The optimal time for imaging after PCNL is still debatable. Many authors recommended to postpone imaging to allow very small fragments and dust to pass especially if laser lithotripsy was utilised [42, 43]. Immediate imaging has many drawbacks especially if in the presence of ureteral stents or nephrostomy tubes, which might hide residual stones [44]. However, immediate imaging can be done if PCNL was performed with mechanical extraction or if there are no tubes obscuring the assessment. Some authors recommended the use of bone windows during performing unenhanced CT to differentiate tubes from a renal stone [45].

20.2 Management of Post PCNL Residual Fragments

Residual stone fragments have been depicted in recent studies following treatment with SWL, URS or PCNL as being clinically significant and should be treated to render patients stone free, especially if infection stones are suspected. This could be achieved by endoscopic procedures such as second-look nephroscopy and ureterorenoscopy. Non-surgical treatment with antibiotics, urease inhibitors and other supportive measures are not considered a viable alternative except in patients otherwise too ill to tolerate stone removal or when the residual fragments cannot be safely retrieved [46].

20.2.1 Second-Look Flexible Nephroscopy

It is strongly recommended that flexible nephroscopy should be a routine part of standard PCNL [47]. Second-look flexible nephroscopy could be avoided if comprehensive intraoperative evaluation of stone-free status was performed. Portis and his colleagues proved that a combination of high-resolution fluoroscopy and flexible nephroscopy led to sensitive and specific intraoperative detection of RF, allowing immediate extraction [48].

Many studies showed that the use of flexible nephroscopy during PCNL increased stone-free rates. Gücük and colleagues performed a randomized prospective study in which patients underwent rigid nephroscopy during PCNL with or without concomitant flexible nephroscopy, and the stone-free rate was higher with concomitant flexible nephroscopy, 92.5% versus 70%. The stone-free rate was higher in patients with low HU density stones [49].

Furthermore, antegrade flexible nephroscopy can extract stone fragments that might migrate down the ureter.

Based on an evaluated cost comparison of immediate second-look endoscopy against surveillance in post-PCNL RFs, second-look endoscopy was stated by most authors as cost advantageous in patients with RF >4 mm following PCNL that causes stone events [50].

Finally, postoperative imaging may be enough to abort the routine second-look flexible nephroscopy by reliably identifying patients without residual stones. An unnecessary flexible nephroscopy would have been avoided based on unenhanced CT findings in 20% of patients, which reflects significant cost savings [43].

Raman et al. reported that second-look flexible nephroscopy may be used for patients with RFs larger than 2 mm or those with RF located in the renal pelvis or ureter [17]. Preminger et al. concluded that second-look nephroscopy is an efficient method for reducing RF post PCNL [51]. Roth et al. reported that the use of second- and third-look flexible nephroscopies in pediatric patients with urolithiasis treated with PCNL resulted in a 97% stone-free rate [52].

Also, Knudsen rationalized the use for second-look nephroscopy for clinically significant residual renal calculi larger than 2 mm and can be done using flexible nephroscopy as an ambulatory procedure or in the operating room [53].

Borofsky and associates analyzed outcomes of second-look PCNL following initial treatment failure. Stone characteristics significantly differed between those patients undergoing second-look ($n = 31$) and primary PCNL ($n > 1200$). The incidence of staghorn calculi was higher (61.3%) in patients needing second-look PCNL while only 31.4% of the patients had staghorn stones in primary PCNL cohort. Unsuitable access was the most common (80%) reason for prior treatment failure. They also observed that the ultimate stone clearance rate was 97% after second-look PCNL. Secondary SWL was required in 12.8% of these patients [54].

Kumar and his colleagues observed that 86.1% complete clearance rate after second-look PCNL. They concluded that when primary PCNL procedure is discontinued due to bleeding, pelvic perforation or purulent urine coming from access site, second-look PCNL significantly improves stone clearance rates with morbidity comparable to that in primary PCNL. Furthermore, second-look PCNL can be a planned re-intervention for large stone burden, offering better stone clearance. On the other hand, second-look PCNL is associated with prolonged hospital stay, need for anesthesia, antibiotics and increased chances of antibiotic resistance, causing economic burden of patients [55].

20.2.2 Ureterorenoscopy

Few studies scrutinized the use of flexible URS for the management of patients with post-PCNL RFs [56–59].

Xu et al. analyzed the efficacy and safety of flexible ureteroscopy used with holmium laser lithotripsy (F-UL) to treat residual calculi post PCNL in comparison to extracorporeal shockwave lithotripsy (SWL). Residual renal calculi patients (4–20 mm) after PCNL were randomly allocated to be treated by either F-UL or SWL. Follow-up was made 1 month and 3 months after treatment. One month after F-UL the stone-free rate was 84.7%, which rose up to 91.3% in the third month while the stone-free rate in SWL group was 64.6% 1 month after treatment and increased to 72.9% in the third month. For residual stone in the lower calyx, the stone-free rate 3 months after treatment was 90.4% after F-UL compared to 65.2% in SWL group ($P < 0.05$). F-UL provided significantly higher stone-free rate compared with SWL, especially for low-pole calculi [59].

Chen et al. validated the effectiveness and safety of the treatment for residual stones using F-UL and holmium laser lithotripsy. They concluded that combing both PCNL and F-UL could manage complex calculi with a high stone-free rate (SFR) (88.9%), reduce the number of treatment sessions and the number of percutaneous access tracts. Flexible ureteroscopy and holmium laser lithotripsy are other options for residual calculi up to mean stone size of 18 mm [60].

Endoscopic combined intrarenal surgery (ECIRS) is becoming popular for complex renal calculi where primary PCNL can be combined with intraoperative flexible ureteroscopy to reduce the incidence of residual calculi, costs and maximize stone clearance in a single operating session however; proper selection of the patients is of central importance for decreasing complications and avoiding technical errors. Also, randomized control and prospective studies will be needed to further validate this approach [61, 62].

Recent reports showed that SWL is an effective method for treating post PCNL RFs. However, a prospective cohort study is required to compare cost effectiveness, complications and its impact on quality of life [63].

20.3 Medical Therapy

If the patient has a metabolic predisposition to stone formation (hyperuricosuria, hypocitraturia, cystineuria or hypercalciuria), medical therapy is required. Since the underlying medical condition leading to stone formation is still present, stone recurrence and growth may continue and the use of medical therapy based on the stone type and underlying abnormality in 24-h urine metabolic work up will help in decreasing stone growth or recurrence. Thiazide diuretics for hypercalciuric stones, potassium citrate with or without allopurinol for hyperuricosuria and citrate for hypocitraturia [64] are recommended.

Summary Points

- Use of flexible nephroscopy after finishing the PCNL procedure
- If a nephrostomy tube is placed, flexible nephroscopy should be offered to any patient with residual fragments 3 mm or more
- Use of medical therapy for patients with underlying metabolic causes
- Postoperative image at 2–3 months to asses stone-free status
- Offer active removal for residual fragment of infection stones
- To follow up patients with residual stones 2 mm or more and to offer intervention if symptoms or stone growth happens

References

1. Türk C, Knoll T, Petrik A, Sarica K, Straub M, Seitz C. Guidelines on urolithiasis. European Association of Urology, 2016. http://uroweb.org/guideline/urolithiasis/.
2. Preminger GM, Tiselius HG, Assimos DG, et al. 2007 guideline for the management of ureteral calculi. J Urol. 2007;178:2418–34.
3. Kallidonis P, Panagopoulos V, Kyriazis I, et al. Complications of percutaneous nephrolithotomy: classification, management, and prevention. Curr Opin Urol. 2016;26:88.
4. Ghani KR, Sammon JD, Bhojani N, et al. Trends in percutaneous nephrolithotomy use and outcomes in the United States. J Urol. 2013;190:558–64.
5. Borofsky MS, Tayeb MM, El Paonessa JE, et al. Initial experience and comparative intracorporeal ultrasonic lithotriptor. Urology. 2015;85:1279–83.
6. Mishra S, Jagtap J, Sabnis RB, et al. Training in percutaneous nephrolithotomy. Curr Opin Urol. 2013;23:147–51.
7. Ganpule AP, Bhattu AS, Desai M. PCNL in the twenty-first century: role of Microperc, Miniperc, and Ultraminiperc. World J Urol. 2015;33:235–40.
8. Olvera-Posada D, Tailly T, Alenezi H, et al. Risk factors for postoperative complications of percutaneous nephrolithotomy at a tertiary referral center. J Urol. 2015;194:1646–51.
9. de la Rosette J, Assimos D, Desai M, et al. The Clinical Research Office of the Endourological Society Percutaneous Nephrolithotomy Global Study: indications, complications, and outcomes in 5803 patients. J Endourol. 2011;25:11–7.
10. Khaitan A, Gupta NP, Hemal AK, et al. Post-ESWL, clinically insignificant residual stones: reality or myth? Urology. 2002;59:20–4.
11. Osman Y, Harraz AM, El-Nahas AR, et al. Clinically insignificant residual fragments: an acceptable term in the computed tomography era? Urology. 2013;81:723–6.
12. Afshar K, McLorie G, Papanikolaou F, et al. Outcome of small residual stone fragments following shock wave lithotripsy in children. J Urol. 2004;172:1600–3.
13. Dincel N, Resorlu B, Unsal A, Tepeler A, Silay MS, Armağan A, Diri A, Sancaktutar AA, Ziypak T, Mir S. Are small residual stone fragments really insignificant in children? J Pediatr Surg. 2013;48(4):840–4.
14. Streem SB, Yost A, Mascha E. Clinical implications of clinically insignificant store fragments after extracorporeal shock wave lithotripsy. J Urol. 1996;155:1186–90.
15. Altunrende F, Tefekli A, Stein RJ, et al. Clinically insignificant residual fragments after percutaneous nephrolithotomy: medium term follow-up. J Endourol. 2011;25:941–5.
16. Chew BH, Brotherhood HL, Sur RL, et al. Natural history, complications and re-intervention rates of asymptomatic residual stone fragments after ureteroscopy: a report from the EDGE research consortium. J Urol. 2016;95(4 Pt 1):982–6.

17. Raman JD, Bagrodia A, Gupta A, et al. Natural history of residual fragments following percutaneous nephrostolithotomy. J Urol. 2009;181:1163–8.
18. Assimos DG. Re: clinically insignificant residual fragments: is it an appropriate term in children? J Urol. 2016;195:170.
19. Ganpule A, Desai M. Fate of residual stones after percutaneous nephrolithotomy: a critical analysis. J Endourol. 2009;23(3):399–403.
20. Olvera-Posada D, Ali S, Marie Dion M, Alenezi H, Denstedt J, Razv H. Natural history of residual fragments after percutaneous nephrolithotomy: evaluation of factors related to clinical events and intervention. J Urol. 2016;97:46–50.
21. Anthony S, Emmott A, Brotherhood H, Paterson R, Lange D, Ben H. Chew complications, re-intervention rates, and natural history of residual stone fragments after percutaneous nephrolithotomy. J Endourol. 2018;32(1):33.
22. Turk C, Knoll T, Petrik A, Sarica K, Straub M, Seitz C. Guidelines on urolithiasis. Eur Urol. 2014;14:1102–6.
23. Fulgham PF, Assimos DG, Pearle MS, Preminger GM. Clinical effectiveness protocols for imaging in the management of ureteral calculous disease: AUA technology assessment. J Urol. 2013;189:1203–13.
24. Pearle MS, Goldfarb DS, Assimos DG, et al. Medical management of kidney stones: AUA guideline. J Urol. 2014;192:316–24.
25. Delvecchio FC, Preminger GM. Management of residual stones. Urol Clin North Am. 2000;27:347–54.
26. Denstedt JD, Clayman RV, Picus DD. Comparison of endoscopic and radiological residual fragment rate following percutaneous nephrolithotripsy. J Urol. 1991;145:703–5.
27. Lehtoranta K, Mankinen P, Taari K, Rannikko S, Lehtonen T, Salo J. Residual stones after percutaneous nephrolithotomy; sensitivities of different imaging methods in renal stone detection. Ann Chir Gynaecol. 1995;84:43–9.
28. Ray AA, Ghiculete PKT, Honey RJ. Limitations to ultrasound in the detection and measurement of urinary tract calculi. Urology. 2010;76:295–300.
29. Dundee P, Bouchier-Hayes D, Haxhimolla H, Dowling R, Costello A. Renal tract calculi: comparison of stone size on plain radiography and noncontrast spiral CT scan. J Endourol. 2006;20:1005–9.
30. Van Appledorn S, Ball AJ, Patel VR, Kim S, Leveillee RJ. Limitations of noncontrast CT for measuring ureteral stones. J Endourol. 2003;17:851–4.
31. Sacks E, Fajardo L, Hillman B, Drach G, Gaines J, Claypool H, et al. Prospective comparison of plain abdominal radiography with conventional and digital renal tomography in assessing renal extracorporeal shock wave lithotripsy patients. J Urol. 1990;144:1341–6.
32. Jewett M, Bombardier C, Caron D, Ryan M, Gray R, St. Louis E, et al. Potential for inter-observer and intra-observer variability in x-ray review to establish stone-free rates after lithotripsy. J Urol. 1992;147:559–62.
33. Palmer J, Donaher E, O'Riordan M, Dell K. Diagnosis of pediatric urolithiasis: role of ultrasound and computerized tomography. J Urol. 2005;174:1413–6.
34. Osman Y, El-Tabey N, Refai H, Elnahas A, Shoma A, Eraky I, et al. Detection of residual stones after percutaneous nephrolithotomy: role of non-enhanced spiral computerized tomography. J Urol. 2008;179:198–200.
35. Rassweiler JJ, Renner C, Chaussy C, Thuroff S. Treatment of renal stones by extracorporeal shockwave lithotripsy: an update. EurUrol. 2001;39:187–99.
36. Carr LK, D'A Honey J, Jewett MA, Ibanez D, Ryan M, Bombardier C. New stone formation: a comparison of extracorporeal shock wave lithotripsy and percutaneous nephrolithotomy. J Urol. 1996;155:1565–7.
37. Candau C, Saussine C, Lang H, Roy C, Faure F, Jacqmin D. Natural history of residual renal stone fragments after ESWL. Eur Urol. 2000;37:18–22.
38. Olcott EW, Sommer FG, Napel S. Accuracy of detection and measurement of renal calculi: in vitro comparison of three-dimensional spiral CT, radiography and nephrotomography. Radiology. 1997;204:19–25.
39. Park J, Hong B, Park T, Park HK. Effectiveness of non- contrast computed tomography in evaluation of residual stones after percutaneous nephrolithotomy. J Endourol. 2007;21:684–7.
40. Kanno T, Kubota M, Funada S, Okada T, Higashi Y, Yamada H. The utility of the kidneys-ureters-bladder radiograph as the sole imaging modality and its combination with ultrasonography for the detection of renal stones. Urology. 2017;104:40–4.
41. Jackman SV, Potter SR, Regan F, Jarrett TW. Plain abdominal x ray versus computerized tomography screening: sensitivity for stone localization after nonenhanced spiral computerized tomography. J Urol. 2000;164:308–10.
42. Eisner BH, McQuaid JW, Hyams E, Matlaga BR. Nephrolithiasis: what surgeons need to know. AJR. 2011;196:1274–8.
43. Pearle MS, Watamull LM, Mullican MA. Sensitivity of noncontrast helical computerized tomography and plain film radiography compared to flexible nephroscopy for detecting residual fragments after percutaneous nephrostolithotomy. J Urol. 1999;162:23–6.
44. Portis AJ, Laliberte MA, Holtz C, Ma W, Rosenberg MS, Bretzke CA. Confident intra- operative decision making during percutaneous nephrolithotomy: does this patient need a second look? Urology. 2008;71:218–22.
45. Tanrikut C, Sahani D, Dretler SP. Distinguishing stent from stone: use of bone windows. Urology. 2004;63:823–7.
46. Assimos D, Krambeck A, Miller N, Monga M, Murad H, Nelson C, Pace KT, Pais VM Jr, Pearle M, Preminger G, Razvi H, Shah O, Matlaga B. Surgical Management of Stones: American Urological Association/Endourological Society Guideline, PART II. J Urol. 2016;196(4):1161–9.

47. Assimos D, Krambeck A, Miller N, Monga M, Murad H, Nelson C, Pace KT, Pais VM Jr, Pearle M, Preminger G, Razvi H, Shah O, Matlaga B. Surgical Management of Stones: American Urological Association/Endourological Society Guideline, PART I. J Urol. 2016;196(4):1153–60. https://doi.org/10.1016/j.juro.2016.05.090. Published online 2016 May 27.
48. Portis AJ, Laliberte MA, Drake S, Holtz C, Rosenberg MS, Bretzke CA. Intraoperative fragment detection during percutaneous nephrolithotomy: evaluation of high magnification rotational fluoroscopy combined with aggressive nephroscopy. J Urol. 2006;175:162–6.
49. Gücük A, Kemahli E, Uyeturk U, et al. Routine flexible nephroscopy for percutaneous nephrolithotomy for renal stones with low density: a prospective randomized study. J Urol. 2013;190:144.
50. Raman JDA, Bagrodia A, Bensalah K, Pearle MS, Lotan Y. Residual fragments after percutaneous nephrolithotomy: cost comparison of immediate second look flexible nephroscopy versus expectant management. J Urol. 2010;183(1):188–93.
51. Preminger GM, Assimos DG, Lingeman JE, Nakada SY, Pearle MS, Wolf JS Jr, AUA Nephrolithiasis Guideline Panel. Chapter 1: AUA guideline on management of staghorn calculi: diagnosis and treatment recommendations. J Urol. 2005;173:1991–2000.
52. Roth CC, Donovan BO, Adams JM, Kibar Y, Frimberger D, Kropp BP. Use of second look nephroscopy in children undergoing percutaneous nephrolithotomy. J Urol. 2009;181:796–800.
53. Knudsen BE. Second-look nephroscopy after percutaneous nephrolithotomy. Ther Adv Urol. 2009;1:27–31.
54. Borofsky MS, Wollin DA, Reddy T, Shah O, Assimos DG, Lingeman JE. Salvage percutaneous nephrolithotomy: analysis of outcomes following initial treatment failure. J Urol. 2016;195:977–81.
55. Kumar S, Karthikeyan V, Mallya A, Keshavamurthy R. Outcomes of second-look percutaneous nephrolithotomy in renal calculi-a single Centre experience. Turk J Urol. 2018;44(5):406–10.
56. Andonian S, Okeke Z, Smith AD. Digital ureteroscopy: the next step. J Endourol. 2008;22:603–6.
57. Mitchell S, Havranek E, Patel A. First digital flexible ureterorenoscope: initial experience. J Endourol. 2008;22:47–50.
58. Menezes P, Dickinson A, Timoney AG. Flexible ureterorenoscopy for the treatment of refractory upper urinary tract stones. BJU Int. 1999;84:257–60.
59. Xu G, Wen J, Li Z, et al. A comparative study to analyze the efficacy and safety of flexible ureteroscopy combined with holmium laser lithotripsy for residual calculi after percutaneous nephrolithotripsy. Int J Clin Exp Med. 2015;8(3):4501–7.
60. Chen L, Sha ML, Li D, Zhuo J, Jiang CY, Zhu YP, et al. Treatment for residual stones using flexible ureteroscopy and holmium laser lithotripsy after the management of complex calculi with single-tract percutaneous nephrolithotomy. Lasers Med Sci. 2017;32:649–54.
61. Hamamoto S, Yasui T, Okada A, Taguchi K, Kawai N, Ando R, et al. Endoscopic combined intrarenal surgery for large calculi: simultaneous use of flexible ureteroscopy and mini-percutaneous nephrolithotomy overcomes the disadvantageous of percutaneous nephrolithotomy monotherapy. J Endourol. 2014;28:28–33.
62. Scarpa RM, Scoffone CM, Cracco CM. Letter about: treatment for residual stones using flexible ureteroscopy and holmium laser lithotripsy after the management of complex calculi with single-tract percutaneous nephrolithotomy. Lasers Med Sci. 2018;33:451.
63. Aminsharifi A, Irani D, Amirzargar H. Shock wave lithotripsy is more effective for residual fragments after percutaneous nephrolithotomy than for primary stones of the same size: a matched pair cohort study. Curr Urol. 2018;12(1):27–32.
64. Kang DE, Maloney MM, Haleblian GE. Effect of medical management on recurrent stone formation following percutaneous nephrolithotomy. J Urol. 2007;177:1785–9.

21 Training in Percutaneous Nephrolithotomy

Abdullatif Aydın, Ahmed Al-Jabir, Brandon Smith, and Kamran Ahmed

Over the last few decades, there has been a momentous rise in the number of minimally invasive procedures and technologies to supplant open procedures within urology. These procedures are often associated with a greater number of training hours to develop the skillsets required for competency and proficiency [1]. Percutaneous nephrolithotomy (PCNL) is known to be particularly challenging, with much difficulty attributed to renal access [2].

Furthermore, transformations in contemporary employment legislation such as the European Working Time Directive, financial constraints in healthcare organisations and subsequently increasing demands in service provision have significantly reduced training hours [3], not taking into account the educational requirements of the resident surgeon [4].

A. Aydın
MRC Centre for Transplantation, King's College London, London, UK

The London Clinic Centre for Robotics, London, UK

A. Al-Jabir · B. Smith
MRC Centre for Transplantation, King's College London, London, UK

K. Ahmed (✉)
MRC Centre for Transplantation, King's College London, London, UK

Department of Urology, King's College Hospital NHS Foundation Trust, London, UK
e-mail: kamran.ahmed@kcl.ac.uk

For a profession like surgery, which is subservient on the development, acquisition and application of psychomotor skills such as fine manual dexterity and visuospatial awareness [5, 6], this reduction in working hours, and ultimately opportunities to train in the operating room (OR), may have negative consequences on a trainee's surgical education [7].

The rising complexity of surgical cases and the changing attitudes of the medico-legal aspects in a surgeon's training (in that it is ethically unacceptable to train on patients, regardless of supervision) have led to radical changes in surgical training. The traditional Halstedian apprenticeship model of "see one, do one, teach one" is no longer feasible [8]. Surgical simulation has, therefore, emerged to occupy a central position within surgical training as a useful adjunct to the traditional learning methods such as observership and mentorship [9], providing safe and controlled environments for trainees to acquire, augment and maintain their surgical skillset through structured and repetitive self-practice, without endangering patients [10]. However, before utilising models and simulators in training and assessment, they must undergo a scientific evaluation across a variety of suggested scientific parameters (Fig. 21.1) [11, 12].

To date, the majority of simulators and training models pertaining to percutaneous nephrolithotomy produced exist as bench models. Despite this, there remains a paucity in the scientific eval-

G. Zeng, K. Sarica (eds.), *Percutaneous Nephrolithotomy*,
https://doi.org/10.1007/978-981-15-0575-1_21

Face Validity – Opinions, including of non-experts, regarding the realism of the simulator
Content Validity – Opinions of experts about the simulator and its appropriateness for training
Construct Validity

- Within one group – Ability of the simulator to assess and differentiate between the level of experience of an individual or group measured over time
- Between groups – Ability of the simulator to distinguish between different levels of experience

Concurrent Validity – Comparison of the new model against the older and gold standard, usually by OSATS
Predictive Validity – Correlation of performance with operating room performance, usually measured by OSATS

Fig. 21.1 Definitions of validity, based on definitions by McDougall et al. [11] and van Nortwick et al. [12]. *OSATS* Objective Structured Assessment of Technical Skills

uation and validation of the majority of these simulators.

21.1 Virtual Reality Simulators

Virtual reality (VR) simulators have the added benefit of reusability and providing statistical feedback through objective performance evaluation reports. PERC Mentor™ (Simbionix, South Carolina, USA) is the only reported VR simulator for PCNL, to date, and comprises of a mannequin and computer-based components with modules to simulate percutaneous access in normal and obese patients under fluoroscopic guidance.

It has been thoroughly assessed for validity (Fig. 21.1), demonstrating face, construct, content and predictive validities [13–17]. Knudsen et al. [15] concluded that the group in their study utilising the PERC Mentor significantly improved performance compared to the control arm that received no training and therefore upheld this model's ability to adhere to theoretical relationships. Khan et al. [13] described the use of the PERC Mentor amongst other simulators within a urology simulation programme, demonstrating the model's ability at depicting a realistic environment (with 90% of participants rating it as realistic). Senior trainees significantly outperformed junior trainees in all simulation sessions.

Although expensive, this simulator provides the opportunity to practice radiation-free percutaneous access using a biplanar virtual reality C-arm, whereby a number of clinical scenarios can be simulated, including vascular injury, aspiration and respiration-induced renal movement. In addition, performance parameters such as procedural time, puncture attempts, and number of unintended injuries are automatically measured allowing for immediate feedback and assessment.

21.2 Organic and Synthetic Models

Surgical simulation utilising non-biological bench models refers to the use of a range of physical models made from synthetic or organic materials to represent pathological states. These can be utilised for specific procedures with the benefit of recreating the tactile sensations of the surgical environment. Such models may also be useful for improving motor skills and hand-eye co-ordination. However, replacement of the models may be required following each use [18].

Fruit and vegetable models such as aubergines and water melons are widely used to simulate the task of renal access but are not described in the literature. Sinha et al. [19] (NU Hospitals, Bangalore, India) reported the use of a courgette model with a bottle gourd to simulate both the time taken and accuracy of fluoroscopically-guided needle punctures in the posterior abdominal wall in a cost-effective and simple way. Such affordable and potentially widely available models should be methodologically evaluated.

The Perc Trainer (Mediskills Ltd., Edinburgh, UK) is a commercially available synthetic bench model with the ability to reproduce ultrasound and fluoroscopic features of the human kidney using standard equipment, allowing for stone identification practice. Despite this, re-use is limited depending on the stage of PCNL simulated; although its "resealing" material allows for repeated needle punctures in the collecting system; once the tract has been dilated the simulator becomes limited to nephroscopic manoeuvres [20]. Similarly, the PCNL Trainer (Limbs and Things Ltd., Bristol, UK) is another non-biological model, comprising a slab with multiple calices where stones may be placed, allowing for simulated needle and guidewire insertion. Utilising a unique combination of a translucent nephrolithotomy slab and lightbox, X-ray imaging can be simulated for renal calyx identification, allowing for the subsequent placement of instruments [1]. Both models lack scientific validation studies evaluating their effectiveness.

The Fluoro-less SimPORTAL C-arm Trainer (CAT; SimPORTAL, University of Minnesota, Minneapolis, USA) offers a unique approach to imaging guidance in percutaneous nephrolithotomy simulation. Utilising dual webcams in opposition to each other, the C-arm is capable of producing a simulated X-ray image despite the external surface of the model being covered by an opaque synthetic skin. The model was preliminarily validated by its developers, demonstrating face and content validity in a sample of 14 urologists in their first post-residency year [21]. A second study was conducted during an American Urological Association post-graduate PCNL course to ascertain the construct validity of the CAT [22]. The results from this cohort established the model's ability to correlate with independent variables such as experience/training. There was a significant improvement in performance after undertaking training in upper pole renal access ($p = 0.0015$); however, no improvement was displayed in lower pole access.

Finally, the "PCNL Boz Kidney Trainer" or "PCNL BOZX" (Encoris Corporation, Michigan, USA) appears to offer much more realistic simulation through application of reusable kidney cartridges, containing simulated stones, within an enclosure formed of synthetic skin, subcutaneous tissue and bony landmarks including the iliac crest, ribs and spine. The model allows for ultrasound or fluoroscopy, with the potential to simulate different stone morphologies and orientations through its interchangeable kidney cartridges. Bozzini et al. [23] trained 25 residents in needle access and tract dilatation and compared to two other simulators. The authors found that it was effective and well-rated with the added benefit of being reusable.

These commercially available models may be utilised alongside the VR simulator, and efforts must be made for further scientific evaluation of their effectiveness.

21.3 Wet-Lab and Cadaveric Simulation

Animal models offer many benefits over bench models, such as respiratory movement and haptic feedback [24]. However, their availability is often limited and thus senior-level fellows and surgeons, requiring advanced training in a high-fidelity environment, are given priority. Despite being more cost effective in comparison to cadavers, further issues exist due to licensing and ethics [25]. Travelling to international wet-lab courses is becoming very common to overcome such hurdles. Both ex-vivo and in-vivo animal models have been used for PCNL and a handful of studies have highlighted the use of porcine and bovine kidneys in PCNL simulation [9, 26]. Various styles of implementation have been demonstrated, including kidneys simulated in-vivo [14], wrapped in foam [27], silicone [28, 29] or within a chicken carcass to simulate the posterior tissue layers [30, 31]; the latter implementation of these porcine-based simulators has demonstrated face validity [31]. Other studies also reported several training procedures using live porcine [14, 32, 33].

Zhang et al. [34] described a porcine kidney wrapped in thick porcine skin containing subcutaneous fascia and muscle. Forty-two urologists performed percutaneous procedures on the model and rated it either "helpful" or "very helpful."

Live anaesthetised pigs were utilised by Mishra et al. [14] in a study including 24 experts performing percutaneous renal access in a live porcine model and the PERC Mentor VR simulator. Using a five-point Likert scale, the study concluded that the overall usefulness of both models was equivalent, with the live porcine model providing a more realistic assessment tool for access ($p < 0.001$), whilst the PERC Mentor was superior at repetitive tasking and feasibility ($p < 0.001$).

Fresh frozen cadavers are known to provide excellent tissue handling, human anatomical structures, preserved tissue planes and realistic haptic feedback [35]. However, validated cadaveric training programmes are limited and none have been published in the literature regarding the use of cadaveric simulation for PCNL training despite student feedback on cadaveric masterclasses for other procedures proving its superiority over animal tissue and bench models. Due to the expense and lack of cadavers for surgical education, it is recommended that training is done as part of modular masterclasses in conjunction with training for other urological procedures for maximum efficiency and benefit for the trainee.

21.4 Non-Technical Skills Training

The importance of non-technical skills (NTS) training for surgeons is becoming increasingly recognised with evidence supporting its utilisation in the clinical setting. An audit evaluating surgical mortality found that only 4.3% of operative errors constitute technical errors, with far more operative errors stemming from poor decision making [36]. Ounounou et al. [37] divided simulation-based NTS training into three main categories: full immersion/distributed simulation (FIDS), high fidelity OR simulation (HFORS) and crisis resource management (CRM). Although the literature does not describe PCNL-specific NTS training, each of these suggested modalities have been successfully utilised in urologically-themed NTS training and may be done so with appropriate scenarios for PCNL.

The highest reported modality of training is FIDS, a 360° inflatable and mobile "Igloo" (Imperial College, London, UK) that can be set up with real OR equipment to create a realistic environment [38–41]. Brewin et al. [39] investigated the combined teaching of technical skills (TURP) and NTS within this environment and demonstrated face, content and construct validity. The course received positive qualitative feedback and the NTS of the experienced urologists was significantly better than those of trainees. The results of this study were further supported by Brunckhorst et al. [38], where novices ($n = 31$) were recruited by Brunckhorst et al. [38] in a randomised controlled trial. Participants who received simulation training for ureteroscopy (including NTS), as opposed to simple didactic teaching, performed significantly better in both technical and NTS, demonstrating its consistency with theoretical relations and independent variables. The authors also found a significant correlation between technical and non-technical skills [42]. Similarly, the ureteroscopy procedure-specific NTS curriculum reported by Aydin et al. [40], for junior urology residents, also demonstrated an educational impact and a significant improvement in NTS with consecutive scenarios ($p = 0.0037$) in groups of up to four residents ($n = 42$). Development and execution of similar scenarios for percutaneous access may be worthwhile to better prepare urolithiasis fellows in NTS for a highly technically demanding procedure.

HFORS uses a dedicated OR simulated for training and assessment of non-technical surgical skills. In a prospective cohort study by Abdelshehid et al. [43], urology residents performed laparoscopic partial nephrectomy, using a validated training model within a simulated environment as part of a team-training scenario. The level of urology resident training significantly affected the NTS performance, thereby demonstrating construct validity. A similar study [44] conducted alongside anaesthetic residents highlighted that 94% rated the session useful and stated that it should be included in residency training, demonstrating face validity. Similar training may be conducted for PCNL-based scenarios.

Training must also address the surgeon's wider role, including outside the OR, in clinics and wards, since different skills may be required for different settings [45]. CRM training, which addresses NTS in emergency scenarios, has been used successfully in aviation and acute care and is associated with a reduction in errors [46, 47]. Many studies exclusively use the OR setting for simulation but there are some examples of simulated ward rounds, such as the UK urology boot camp initiative [48], an intense 1-week training curriculum and course for newly-starting trainees. Simulated wards and clinics have also been employed as part of a larger programme in a urology-focused course by Khan et al. [13], using the "SimMan" model, and for general NTS training with multiprofessional groups. The authors suggest that repeated training is important for trainees to develop NTS and improve their stress management earlier on in their careers [13].

21.5 Assessment

Surgical competence comprises technical skills, theoretical knowledge, decision making and communication skills [49] and develops from novice to proficiency to mastery of a procedure. Traditionally, this has been done in a subjective manner with logbooks, non-criteria based direct observation of procedures as well as a purely numerical "time taken for a procedure." However, this is often reliant on the observer and lacks validity and reliability. Objective methods of assessment have been validated for use, including checklists and global rating scales. These have been combined to form an objective structured assessment of technical skills (OSATS) [50], long-considered the gold-standard in surgical assessment.

Procedure specific checklists have been implemented in other urological procedures such as ureteroscopy [51] and in robot–assisted radical prostatectomy, where scores obtained using the tool have been used to establish learning curves in this procedure [52]. Quirke et al. [53] reported the development of an assessment tool for PCNL technical skills (Percutaneous Nephrolithotomy Assessment Score) using a healthcare failure mode and an effect analysis method where the most hazardous steps of the procedure were identified. The assessment score contains 10 phases, from pre-operative preparation to tract dilatation and patient transfer at the end of the procedure, 21 processes and 47 sub-processes as part of a comprehensive analysis of a trainee's performance in the procedure. Both OSATS and this newly-developed tool may be utilised in simulation and OR settings, as part of continuous assessment and structured feedback.

21.6 Learning Curves and OR Training

Training must inevitably continue on the OR to reach a level of competency in the learning curve. The learning curve of a procedure is the period in which the operator finds the technique more difficult and subsequently the operation may be associated with lower efficacy, higher complication rates and longer operative times [54]. A systematic review by Quirke et al. [2] reported on the learning curves of urolithiasis procedures. Although the lack of comparable outcome measures between studies means that a definitive learning curve for PCNL has not yet been established, the majority discuss learning curves in relation to operative time and demonstrate that a surgeon is required to complete between 30 and 60 cases to reach a plateau [55–65]. The authors identified a wider range of cases required to reach a plateau for other parameters such as the fluoroscopic screening time (20–115 cases) and the stone-free rate (30–105 cases) [2].

The number of cases required to attain competence in PCNL is also dependent on the type of PCNL conducted and the outcome measure utilised to measure competence [2]. With regards to prone PCNL, the learning curve varies significantly depending on the outcome measure and was demonstrated to be completed between 30 and 60 cases when observing the operative time, 105 cases for an acceptable stone-free rate and 30–115 cases for a plateau regarding the fluoroscopic screening time. As for supine PCNL, the operative time reaches an acceptable length after 36 cases. For gaining access to the kidney in PCNL, studies found that the learning curve for the operative time was completed after 60 cases and that the fluoroscopic screening time reached an acceptable level between 20 and 40 cases. As such, residents and surgical mentors are advised to perform a minimum of 30 cases before being deemed competent in the procedure.

21.7 Conclusion

Based on the available literature and training tools, a variety of physical models and the PERC Mentor VR simulator can be utilised at the initial phase of the PCNL training, with particular emphasis on percutaneous renal access. This may be useful for junior trainees in grasping new concepts and familiarizing themselves with surgical instruments. The next phase of the training should incorporate porcine kidney/reno-ureteral tissue due to its accuracy in reflecting human tissue followed by wet lab training with fresh or live porcine tissue and/or cadaveric simulation masterclasses in multiple procedures, as they replicate the OR to the highest degree and are expensive to maintain [35]. NTS should be incorporated alongside the selected models using the validated full immersion simulation environment or within a designated OR. Trainees should be assessed using generic assessment tools such as OSATS and the newly-available Percutaneous Nephrolithotomy Assessment Score, as part of a continual assessment. A minimum of 30 cases must be performed in the OR to be deemed competent in the PCNL (subjective to the method and personal progress).

References

1. Wignall GR, Denstedt JD, Preminger GM, Cadeddu JA, Pearle MS, Sweet RM, et al. Surgical simulation: a urological perspective. J Urol. 2008;179(5):1690–9. https://doi.org/10.1016/j.juro.2008.01.014.
2. Quirke K, Aydin A, Brunckhorst O, Bultitude M, Khan MS, Dasgupta P, et al. Learning curves in urolithiasis surgery: a systematic review. J Endourol. 2018;32(11):1008–20. https://doi.org/10.1089/end.2018.0425.
3. Chikwe J, de Souza AC, Pepper JR. No time to train the surgeons. BMJ. 2004;328(7437):418–9. https://doi.org/10.1136/bmj.328.7437.418.
4. Wade RG, Henderson J. Perceived impact of EWTD on UK doctors. Bulletin R Coll Surg Engl. 2009;91(4):132–4. https://doi.org/10.1308/147363509x424264.
5. Schueneman AL, Pickleman J, Hesslein R, Freeark RJ. Neuropsychologic predictors of operative skill among general surgery residents. Surgery. 1984;96(2):288–95.
6. Gibbons RD, Baker RJ, Skinner DB. Field articulation testing: a predictor of technical skills in surgical residents. J Surg Res. 1986;41(1):53–7. https://doi.org/10.1016/0022-4804(86)90008-9.
7. RCoS. The implementation of the working time directive, and its impact on the NHS and health professionals—report of the independent working time regulations taskforce to the Department of Health: Royal College of surgeons. 2004.
8. Brewin J, Ahmed K, Challacombe B. An update and review of simulation in urological training. Int J Surg. 2014;12(2):103–8. https://doi.org/10.1016/j.ijsu.2013.11.012.
9. Aydin A, Raison N, Khan MS, Dasgupta P, Ahmed K. Simulation-based training and assessment in urological surgery. Nat Rev Urol. 2016;13(9):503–19. https://doi.org/10.1038/nrurol.2016.147.
10. Kneebone RL, Scott W, Darzi A, Horrocks M. Simulation and clinical practice: strengthening the relationship. Med Educ. 2004;38(10):1095–102. https://doi.org/10.1111/j.1365-2929.2004.01959.x.
11. McDougall EM. Validation of surgical simulators. J Endourol. 2007;21(3):244–7. https://doi.org/10.1089/end.2007.9985.
12. Van Nortwick SS, Lendvay TS, Jensen AR, Wright AS, Horvath KD, Kim S. Methodologies for establishing validity in surgical simulation studies. Surgery. 2010;147(5):622–30. https://doi.org/10.1016/j.surg.2009.10.068.
13. Shamim Khan M, Ahmed K, Gavazzi A, Gohil R, Thomas L, Poulsen J, et al. Development and implementation of centralized simulation training: evaluation of feasibility, acceptability and construct validity. BJU Int. 2013;111(3):518–23. https://doi.org/10.1111/j.1464-410X.2012.11204.x.
14. Mishra S, Kurien A, Ganpule A, Muthu V, Sabnis R, Desai M. Percutaneous renal access training: content validation comparison between a live porcine and a virtual reality (VR) simulation model. BJU Int. 2010;106(11):1753–6. https://doi.org/10.1111/j.1464-410X.2010.09753.x.
15. Knudsen BE, Matsumoto ED, Chew BH, Johnson B, Margulis V, Cadeddu JA, et al. A randomized, controlled, prospective study validating the acquisition of percutaneous renal collecting system access skills using a computer based hybrid virtual reality surgical simulator: phase I. J Urol. 2006;176(5):2173–8. https://doi.org/10.1016/j.juro.2006.07.011.
16. Patel D, El-Husseiny T, Moraitis K, Shaikh T, Buchholz N, Masood J, et al. 1332 assessing and developing percutaneous renal access skills of trainees using the state of the art PERC Mentor™ simu-

lation trainer. J Urol. 2010;183(4S):e514. https://doi.org/10.1016/j.juro.2010.02.938.
17. Ganpule AP, Mishra S, Sabnis RB, Muthu V, Desai MR. Evaluation and validation of virtual reality (VR) based simulation to develop endourological percutaneous renal access technique for urological trainees. J Urol. 2009;181(4S):491–2. https://doi.org/10.1016/s0022-5347(09)61389-6.
18. Khan R, Aydin A, Khan MS, Dasgupta P, Ahmed K. Simulation-based training for prostate surgery. BJU Int. 2015;116(4):665–74. https://doi.org/10.1111/bju.12721.
19. Sinha M, Krishnamoorthy V. Use of a vegetable model as a training tool for PCNL puncture. Indian J Urol. 2015;31(2):156–9. https://doi.org/10.4103/0970-1591.152922.
20. Hoznek A, Salomon L, de la Taille A, Yiou R, Vordos D, Larre S, et al. Simulation training in video-assisted urologic surgery. Curr Urol Rep. 2006;7(2):107–13. https://doi.org/10.1007/s11934-006-0068-z.
21. Veneziano D, Smith A, Reihsen T, Speich J, Sweet RM. The SimPORTAL fluoro-less C-arm trainer: an innovative device for percutaneous kidney access. J Endourol. 2015;29(2):240–5. https://doi.org/10.1089/end.2014.0401.
22. Chrouser K, Marsh B, Sweet R. MP20-03 percutaneous access skill improvement after the AUA PCNL training course using the simportal fluoro-less C-arm trainer. J Urol. 2016;195(4S):e213. https://doi.org/10.1016/j.juro.2016.02.2772.
23. Bozzini G, Provenzano M, Seveso M, Mandressi A, Buffi N, Guazzoni G, et al. MP20-01 realising a new model to train residents in nephrostomy tube placement and PCNL. J Urol. 2016;195(4):e212. https://doi.org/10.1016/j.juro.2016.02.2770.
24. Ahmed K, Jawad M, Dasgupta P, Darzi A, Athanasiou T, Khan MS. Assessment and maintenance of competence in urology. Nat Rev Urol. 2010;7(7):403–13. https://doi.org/10.1038/nrurol.2010.81.
25. Hart R, Karthigasu K. The benefits of virtual reality simulator training for laparoscopic surgery. Curr Opin Obstet Gynecol. 2007;19(4):297–302. https://doi.org/10.1097/GCO.0b013e328216f5b7.
26. Noureldin YA, Andonian S. Simulation for percutaneous renal access: where are we? J Endourol. 2017;31(S1):S10–S9. https://doi.org/10.1089/end.2016.0587.
27. de Sá Earp PP. Percutaneous renal surgery – new model for learning and training. Int Braz J Urol. 2003;29(2):151. https://doi.org/10.1590/S1677-55382003000200011.
28. Strohmaier WL, Giese A. Ex vivo training model for percutaneous renal surgery. Urol Res. 2005;33(3):191–3. https://doi.org/10.1007/s00240-005-0478-2.
29. Strohmaier WL, Giese A. Improved ex vivo training model for percutaneous renal surgery. Urol Res. 2009;37(2):107–10. https://doi.org/10.1007/s00240-009-0180-x.
30. Hacker A, Wendt-Nordahl G, Honeck P, Michel MS, Alken P, Knoll T. A biological model to teach percutaneous nephrolithotomy technique with ultrasound- and fluoroscopy-guided access. J Endourol. 2007;21(5):545–50. https://doi.org/10.1089/end.2006.0327.
31. Hammond L, Ketchum J, Schwartz BF. A new approach to urology training: a laboratory model for percutaneous nephrolithotomy. J Urol. 2004;172(5 Pt 1):1950–2.
32. Jagtap J. 1333 surgical skills lab for percutaneous renal access training: content validation comparison between live porcine and VR simulation model. J Urol. 2010;183(4S):e515. https://doi.org/10.1016/j.juro.2010.02.939.
33. Mishra S, Kurien A, Patel R, Patil P, Ganpule A, Muthu V, et al. Validation of virtual reality simulation for percutaneous renal access training. J Endourol. 2010;24(4):635–40. https://doi.org/10.1089/end.2009.0166.
34. Zhang Y, Ou TW, Jia HG, Gao W, Cui X, Wu JT, et al. Novel biologic model for percutaneous renal surgery learning and training in the laboratory. Urology. 2008;72(3):513–6. https://doi.org/10.1016/j.urology.2008.05.016.
35. Ahmed K, Aydin A, Dasgupta P, Khan MS, McCabe JE. A novel cadaveric simulation program in urology. J Surg Educ. 2015;72(4):556–65. https://doi.org/10.1016/j.jsurg.2015.01.005.
36. Mortality SAoS. The Scottish audit of surgical mortality. Annual Report 2010. 2010.
37. Ounounou E, Aydin A, Brunckhorst O, Khan MS, Dasgupta P, Ahmed K. Nontechnical skills in surgery: a systematic review of current training modalities. J Surg Educ. 2018;76:14. https://doi.org/10.1016/j.jsurg.2018.05.017.
38. Brunckhorst O, Shahid S, Aydin A, McIlhenny C, Khan S, Raza SJ, et al. Simulation-based ureteroscopy skills training curriculum with integration of technical and non-technical skills: a randomised controlled trial. Surg Endosc. 2015;29(9):2728–35. https://doi.org/10.1007/s00464-014-3996-6.
39. Brewin J, Tang J, Dasgupta P, Khan MS, Ahmed K, Bello F, et al. Full immersion simulation: validation of a distributed simulation environment for technical and non-technical skills training in urology. BJU Int. 2015;116(1):156–62. https://doi.org/10.1111/bju.12875.
40. Aydin A, Brunckhorst O, Aya H, Eldred-Evans D, Al-Jabir A, Brewin J, et al. MP20-04 development and validation of a Ureterorenoscopy non-technical skills curriculum. J Urol. 2016;195(4S):e213–4. https://doi.org/10.1016/j.juro.2016.02.2773.
41. Kassab E, Tun JK, Arora S, King D, Ahmed K, Miskovic D, et al. "Blowing up the barriers" in surgical training: exploring and validating the concept of distributed simulation. Ann Surg. 2011;254(6):1059–65. https://doi.org/10.1097/SLA.0b013e318228944a.
42. Brunckhorst O, Shahid S, Aydin A, Khan S, McIlhenny C, Brewin J, et al. The relationship between technical and nontechnical skills within a simulation-based ureteroscopy training environment. J Surg

Educ. 2015;72(5):1039–44. https://doi.org/10.1016/j.jsurg.2015.04.002.
43. Abdelshehid CS, Quach S, Nelson C, Graversen J, Lusch A, Zarraga J, et al. High-fidelity simulation-based team training in urology: evaluation of technical and nontechnical skills of urology residents during laparoscopic partial nephrectomy. J Surg Educ. 2013;70(5):588–95. https://doi.org/10.1016/j.jsurg.2013.04.009.
44. Lee JY, Mucksavage P, Canales C, McDougall EM, Lin S. High fidelity simulation based team training in urology: a preliminary interdisciplinary study of technical and nontechnical skills in laparoscopic complications management. J Urol. 2012;187(4):1385–91. https://doi.org/10.1016/j.juro.2011.11.106.
45. Rashid P, Gianduzzo TR. Urology technical and non-technical skills development: the emerging role of simulation. BJU Int. 2016;117(Suppl 4):9–16. https://doi.org/10.1111/bju.13259.
46. Truta TS, Boeriu CM, Copotoiu SM, Petrisor M, Turucz E, Vatau D, et al. Improving nontechnical skills of an interprofessional emergency medical team through a one day crisis resource management training. Medicine (Baltimore). 2018;97(32):e11828. https://doi.org/10.1097/md.0000000000011828.
47. Yee B, Naik VN, Joo HS, Savoldelli GL, Chung DY, Houston PL, et al. Nontechnical skills in anesthesia crisis management with repeated exposure to simulation-based education. Anesthesiology. 2005;103(2):241–8.
48. Somasundram K, Spence H, Colquhoun AJ, McIlhenny C, Biyani CS, Jain S. Simulation in urology to train non-technical skills in ward rounds. BJU Int. 2018;122(4):705–12. https://doi.org/10.1111/bju.14402.
49. Cuschieri A, Francis N, Crosby J, Hanna GB. What do master surgeons think of surgical competence and revalidation? Am J Surg. 2001;182(2):110–6.
50. Martin JA, Regehr G, Reznick R, MacRae H, Murnaghan J, Hutchison C, et al. Objective structured assessment of technical skill (OSATS) for surgical residents. Br J Surg. 1997;84(2):273–8.
51. Sarica K, Ahmed K, Abdullatif A, Veneziano D, Van Cleynenbreugel B, Serdar A et al. Education; Training|Uroweb. 2017. http://uroweb.org/section/eulis/education-training/.
52. Lovegrove C, Novara G, Mottrie A, Guru KA, Brown M, Challacombe B, et al. Structured and modular training pathway for robot-assisted radical prostatectomy (RARP): validation of the RARP assessment score and learning curve assessment. Eur Urol. 2016;69(3):526–35. https://doi.org/10.1016/j.eururo.2015.10.048.
53. Quirke K, Aydin A, Lovegrove C, Bultitude M, Denstedt J, Dragos LB, et al. MP19–15 development and validation of a modular training and assessment score for percutaneous nephrolithotomy. J Endourol. 2018;32:A187. https://doi.org/10.1089/end.2018.29043.abstracts.
54. Artibani W, Novara G. Cancer-related outcome and learning curve in retropubic radical prostatectomy: "if you need an operation, the most important step is to choose the right surgeon". Eur Urol. 2008;53(5):874–6. https://doi.org/10.1016/j.eururo.2008.01.087.
55. Allen D, O'Brien T, Tiptaft R, Glass J. Defining the learning curve for percutaneous nephrolithotomy. J Endourol. 2005;19(3):279–82. https://doi.org/10.1089/end.2005.19.279.
56. Bergmann T, Herrmann TRW, Schiller T, Zimmermann U, Burchardt M. Implementation of minimally invasive percutaneous nephrolithotomy (MIP): comparison of the initial learning curve with the later on clinical routine in a tertiary centre. World J Urol. 2017;35(12):1933–8. https://doi.org/10.1007/s00345-017-2069-6.
57. Bucuras V, Bardan R, Muresan A, Cumpanas A, Balarie C, Secasan C, et al. VP04–09 The role of the learning curve in supine percutaneous nephrolithotomy. J Endourol. 2011;25(S1):A292. https://doi.org/10.1089/end.2011.2001.supp.
58. Garg A, Yadav SS, Tomar V, Priyadarshi S, Giri V, Vyas N, et al. Prospective evaluation of learning curve of urology residents for percutaneous nephrolithotomy. Urol Pract. 2016;3(3):230–5. https://doi.org/10.1016/j.urpr.2015.06.009.
59. Jang WS, Choi KH, Yang SC, Han WK. The learning curve for flank percutaneous nephrolithotomy for kidney calculi: a single surgeon's experience. Korean J Urol. 2011;52(4):284–8. https://doi.org/10.4111/kju.2011.52.4.284.
60. Jessen JP, Honeck P, Knoll T, Wendt-Nordahl G. Percutaneous nephrolithotomy under combined sonographic/radiologic guided puncture: results of a learning curve using the modified Clavien grading system. World J Urol. 2013;31(6):1599–603. https://doi.org/10.1007/s00345-012-1016-9.
61. Kallidonis P, Kyriazis I, Vasilas M, Panagopoulos V, Georgiopoulos I, Ozsoy M, et al. Modular training for percutaneous nephrolithotripsy: the safe way to go. Arab J Urol. 2015;13(4):270–6. https://doi.org/10.1016/j.aju.2015.07.005.
62. Schilling D, Gakis G, Walcher U, Stenzl A, Nagele U. The learning curve in minimally invasive percutaneous nephrolitholapaxy: a 1-year retrospective evaluation of a novice and an expert. World J Urol. 2011;29(6):749–53. https://doi.org/10.1007/s00345-010-0553-3.
63. Song Y, Ma Y, Song Y, Fei X. Evaluating the learning curve for percutaneous nephrolithotomy under total ultrasound guidance. PLoS One. 2015;10(8):e0132986. https://doi.org/10.1371/journal.pone.0132986.
64. Tanriverdi O, Boylu U, Kendirci M, Kadihasanoglu M, Horasanli K, Miroglu C. The learning curve in the training of percutaneous nephrolithotomy. Eur Urol. 2007;52(1):206–11. https://doi.org/10.1016/j.eururo.2007.01.001.
65. Ziaee SA, Sichani MM, Kashi AH, Samzadeh M. Evaluation of the learning curve for percutaneous nephrolithotomy. Urol J. 2010;7(4):226–31.

9789811505744